# Drugs
## for the
# Heart

## FOURTH EDITION

# Drugs for the Heart

## FOURTH EDITION

### Lionel H. Opie, M.D., D.Phil., F.R.C.P.
Professor of Medicine, University of Cape Town,
Cape Town, South Africa;
Visiting Professor, Division of Cardiology,
Stanford University Medical Center
Stanford, California

WITH THE COLLABORATION OF

- Kanu Chatterjee, M.D., F.R.C.P.
- William H. Frishman, M.D.
- Bernard J. Gersh, M.B.Ch.B., D.Phil., F.R.C.P.
- Norman Kaplan, M.D.
- Frank I. Marcus, M.D.
- Philip A. Poole-Wilson, M.D., F.R.C.P.
- Edmund H. Sonnenblick, M.D.
- Udho Thadani, M.B.B.S., M.R.C.P., F.R.C.P.(C.)

FOREWORD BY

Eugene Braunwald, M.D.

## W. B. SAUNDERS COMPANY
A Division of Harcourt Brace & Company
PHILADELPHIA, LONDON, TORONTO, MONTREAL, SYDNEY, TOKYO

**W. B. SAUNDERS COMPANY**

*A Division of Harcourt Brace & Company*

The Curtis Center
Independence Square West
Philadelphia, PA 19106

**Library of Congress Cataloging-in-Publication Data**

Drugs for the heart / Lionel H. Opie : with the collaboration of Kanu
 Chatterjee . . . [et al.] : foreword by Eugene Braunwald.—4th ed.
  p.  cm
  Includes bibliographical references and index.
  ISBN 0-7216-5943-8
   1. Cardiovascular agents.  I. Opie, Lionel H.  II. Chatterjee, Kanu.
  [DNLM: 1. Cardiovascular Agents—adverse effects.
  2. Cardiovascular Agents—therapeutic use.  3. Heart—drug effects.
  QV  150  D7938  1995]
  RM345.D784    1995
 615′.71—dc20
 DNLM/DLC
 for Library of Congress                                        94-36995
                                                                     CIP

International Edition                          ISBN  0-7216-6281-1

DRUGS FOR THE HEART                            ISBN  0-7216-5943-8

Last digit is the print number:    9   8   7   6   5   4   3   2   1

*DISCLAIMER*

Every effort has been made to check generic and trade names, and to verify drug doses as correct according to the standards accepted at the time of publication. The ultimate responsibility lies with prescribing physicians based on their professional experience and knowledge of the patient, to determine dosages and the best course of treatment for the patient. The reader is advised to check the product information currently provided by the manufacturer of each drug to be administered to ascertain any change in drug dosage, method of administration or contraindications. In no case can the institutions with which the authors are affiliated or the publisher be held responsible for the views expressed in this book, which reflects the combined opinions of several authors. Please call any errors to the attention of the authors.

"When an approved treatment is considered for an unapproved indication, the physician must evaluate the safety of the medication, its value in related conditions, and the individual patient. What is asked is that he make a prudent decision based upon full knowledge of the available evidence."

*Judge's instruction to jury*

# Foreword

During the past decade, an extraordinary array of new cardiovascular drugs has become available, and both students and practitioners of medicine have difficulty deciding how to choose the proper drugs for their patients. Professor Opie's book provides a rational approach to help with this important decision. This marvelous book is a concise yet complete presentation of cardiac pharmacology and therapeutics. It presents, in a very readable and eminently understandable fashion, an extraordinary amount of important information on the effects of drugs on the heart and circulation. Professor Opie and his colleagues have the unique ability to explain in a straightforward manner the mechanism of action of drugs without oversimplifying these complex matters. Simultaneously, this book provides important practical information to the clinician.

The fourth edition of this now well-established book builds on the strengths of its predecessors. The excellent explanatory diagrams (an Opie trademark) are even better than in previous editions, and the text and references in this rapidly moving field are as fresh as this morning's newspaper. This concise volume should be of value and interest to all—specialists, generalists, clinicians, students, teachers and scientists—who wish to gain a clear understanding of cardiovascular therapeutics.

*Eugene Braunwald, M.D.*
*Boston, Massachusetts*

# List of Contributors

**Eugene Braunwald MD (Foreword)**
Hersey Professor of Medicine
Harvard Medical School
Chairman, Department of Medicine
Brigham and Women's Hospital
75 Francis Street
Boston, MA 02115

**Kanu Chatterjee MD FRCP**
Professor of Medicine
Lucie Stern Professor of Cardiology
University of California, San Francisco
Associate Chief, Cardiovascular Division
Moffitt Hospital—Room 1186
505 Parnassus Avenue
San Francisco, CA 94143

**William Frishman MD**
Professor and Associate Chairman
Department of Medicine
Albert Einstein College of Medicine
1825 Eastchester Road
Bronx, NY 10461

**Bernard J Gersh MD DPhil FRCP**
W Proctor Harvey Teaching Professor of Cardiology
Chief, Division of Cardiology
Georgetown University Medical Center
3800 Reservoir Road NW
Washington DC 20007

**Norman Kaplan MD**
Professor of Internal Medicine
University of Texas Health Sciences Center
5323 Harry Hines Boulevard
Dallas, TX 75235-8852

**Frank I Marcus MD**
Distinguished Professor of Medicine
Cardiology Section
Health Sciences Center
University of Arizona
Tucson, AZ 85724

**Lionel H Opie MD DPhil FRCP**
Professor of Medicine
University of Cape Town
Cape Town, South Africa;
Visiting Professor
Division of Cardiology
Stanford University Medical Center
Stanford, CA 94305

**Philip A Poole-Wilson MD FRCP**
Professor of Cardiology
National Heart and Lung Institute
Dovehouse Street
London SW3 6LY
United Kingdom

**Edmund H Sonnenblick MD**
Chief, Division of Cardiology
Olson Professor of Medicine
Albert Einstein College of Medicine
1300 Morris Park Avenue
Bronx, NY 10461
USA

**Udho Thadani MBBS MRCP FRCP(C)**
Professor of Medicine
University of Oklahoma Health Sciences Center
Director of Clinical Research
Vice Chief, Cardiology Section
Oklahoma Memorial Hospital and Veterans Administration Center
P O Box 26901
Oklahoma City, OK 73190

# *The Lancet* Editorial, 1980

(An Editorial from *The Lancet*, March 29, 1980, to introduce a series of articles on Drugs and the Heart)

Cardiovascular times are achanging. After a mere ten years' repose the medical Rip van Winkle would be thoroughly bewildered. For instance, there has been a big switch in attitudes to the failing heart. What would he make of those soft voices which now preach unloading or "afterload reduction"? Experience with beta-blockers has shown the fundamental importance of sympathetic activity in regulating cardiac contraction, and this activity can now be adjusted readily in either direction. Likewise, from calcium antagonists much has been discovered about the function of this ion at cellular level and its importance in the generation of necrosis and cardiac arrhythmia. New radionuclide and angiographic techniques have redirected attention to spasm in coronary arteries and fresh means to forestall it. Continuous ambulatory electrocardiography and special electrophysiological techniques have eased the assessment of arrhythmias, and, again, of drugs to stop or prevent them. Many new drugs have come on the scene, and increasingly they have been devised to act at specific points on pathways to cellular metabolism.

Dr. van Winkle apart, there may be one or two other physicians who regard with alarm the new flood of cardioactive drugs. For such as these, Professor Lionel Opie has written the series of articles which begin on the next page. As Professor Opie remarks, drugs should be given not because they *ought* to work but because they *do* work. We hope that this series will help stimulate the critical approach to cardiovascular pharmacology that will be much needed in the coming decade.

# Acknowledgements

The rapid appearance of this newly revised fourth edition has once again been made possible by the willing and unstinting cooperation of many people. I again thank my co-authors for generously sharing their expertise and clinical skills on which this book is based, and for undertaking their meticulous updating of the third edition. I extend a special welcome to Dr William Frishman, Professor and Associate Chairman, Department of Medicine, Albert Einstein College of Medicine, New York, who has now joined us for the first time. Sadly we must bid farewell to an old friend, Dr. Bramah Singh, who has been with us from 1984, and is an acknowledged international expert in arrhythmia management. He is now in the throes of establishing an important new journal. I again thank Richard Zorab and the staff of WB Saunders for so efficiently dealing with the deadline and preparing such a well-produced book. The figures (my copyright unless otherwise stated) are hand-drawn by myself and recreated by Jeanne Walker, an illustrator without peer. I thank Professor Patrick Commerford and his colleagues of the Department of Cardiology at Groote Schuur Hospital, Cape Town, for generous help with proofreading. Victor Claasen provided an infallible reference-retrieval service. Last, but certainly not least, my secretary June Chambers is thanked for prodigious patience and unfailing skills. She has also helped rewrite many parts of the book which needed verbal polishing and any excellence of style (which from time to time has been mentioned to me) is at least in part thanks to her constant vigilance.

L H Opie
Cape Town
South Africa

# Preface

*"On presenting this book once more to the profession in what I conceive to be a very improved form, it is quite unnecessary to trouble the reader with a long and tedious Preface."*
The Practice of Surgery, designed as an introduction for students, S Cooper, London, Longman, 1819.

*"Encouraged by the public reception of the former editions, the author has spared neither labour nor expense, to render this as perfect as his opportunities and abilities would permit. The progress of knowledge is so rapid, and the discoveries so numerous, both at home and abroad, that this may rather be regarded as a new work than as a re-publication of an old one. On this account, a short enumeration of the more important changes may possibly be expected by the reader."*
William Withering, from Botany, 3rd Edition, 1801

I think the advice of these two early authors is profound. Withering suggests that the changes should be enumerated, and Cooper that the Preface should not be long and tedious. The changes for this new edition are:

1. **Co-authors**
   Dr William Frishman has come in to fortify the sections on lipids (an area of growing concern for cardiologists) and antianginal agents.
2. **Illustrations**
   The creative and hopefully didactic illustrations stem from conjoint work with Jeanne Walker, my illustrator. In every chapter almost all illustrations are either new or newly recreated with the aim of conveying maximum clarity. The introduction of two colors and several tones in the illustrations is also aimed at enhancing the final quality of the book and the appeal to readers. These trends are in keeping with the increasingly visual times in which we live.
3. **References**
   A concerted effort has been made to provide the reader with all the major new references from 1991 for each chapter. A few statistics follow. The chapters with the largest number of new references are Chapter 11 (Which Drug for Which Disease?) and Chapter 5 (ACE Inhibitors), each with 107 new references. Then follows Chapter 9 (Antithrombotic Agents) with 95 new references. Which area is growing fastest? When the rate of addition of new references in this edition is compared with that in the previous edition, then the ACE inhibitors again come first with a 3.3-fold growth. Next, perhaps surprisingly, come Diuretics with a 2-fold growth.
4. **Clarity of text**
   Each sentence of each chapter has been toothcombed to simplify and clarify the meaning whilst maintaining the scientific message.
5. **Update sections**
   The major text was completed in mid-1994, updated to include new information provided at the European and World Congress of Cardiology in September 1994 in Berlin and at the American Heart Association Meeting in November 1994. Update sections at the end of each chapter will be revised with each new printing of the book and the Fifth Edition is planned to appear in the year 2000 or earlier.

A final comment. Our aim is not to produce a textbook of Cardiology nor of Cardiovascular Pharmacology, but to continue to provide a pocket-size guide to cardiovascular drugs, in a style and format that is unique. This compact book, in the widely acclaimed Michelin size, gives crucial information in a readily accessible format for Residents, Cardiology Fellows, and senior students. We believe that the new Fourth Edition will be as much in demand as were the previous editions.

# Contents

Foreword
  *Eugene Braunwald*

Preface

*The Lancet* Editorial, 1980

Acknowledgements

Contributors

Commonly Used Abbreviations

## Antianginal Agents

## Antifailure Agents

## Other Cardiac Drugs

# Commonly Used Abbreviations

| | | |
|---|---|---|
| ACE inhibitor | = | angiotensin-converting enzyme inhibitor |
| AF | = | atrial fibrillation |
| AMI | = | acute myocardial infarction |
| AV | = | atrioventricular |
| BP | = | blood pressure |
| CHF | = | congestive heart failure |
| CNS | = | central nervous system |
| DBP | = | diastolic blood pressure |
| E | = | epinephrine |
| FDA | = | Food and Drug Administration (USA) |
| GI | = | gastrointestinal |
| GU | = | genito-urinary |
| GFR | = | glomerular filtration rate |
| IV | = | intravenous |
| IM | = | intramuscular |
| ISA | = | intrinsic sympathomimetic activity (partial agonist activity of some beta-blockers) |
| $K^+$ | = | blood potassium |
| NE | = | norepinephrine |
| NIH | = | National Institute of Health (USA) |
| NYHA | = | New York Heart Association (grading of CHF) |
| NYHA Grade I | = | no symptoms with ordinary physical activity |
| NYHA Grade II | = | symptoms with ordinary activity |
| NYHA Grade III | = | symptoms with less than ordinary activity |
| NYHA Grade IV | = | symptoms with any physical activity or at rest |
| LVF | = | left ventricular failure |
| LVH | = | left ventricular hypertrophy |
| PVC | = | premature ventricular contractions |
| SA | = | sinoatrial |
| SBP | = | systolic blood pressure |
| VF | = | ventricular fibrillation |
| VT | = | ventricular tachycardia |
| WHO | = | World Health Organization |
| WPW | = | Wolff-Parkinson-White syndrome |

# 1    Beta-Blocking Agents

L.H. Opie  ♦  E.H. Sonnenblick  ♦  W. Frishman
U. Thadani

Beta-adrenergic receptor antagonist agents remain a cornerstone in the therapy of all stages of ischemic heart disease, with the exception of Prinzmetal's vasospastic variant angina. Beta-blockade is standard therapy for effort angina, mixed effort and rest angina, and unstable angina. Beta-blockers decrease mortality in acute phase myocardial infarction and in the postinfarct period. Beta-blockers retain their position among basic therapies for numerous other conditions including hypertension arrhythmias and cardiomyopathy (Table 1–1). Beta-blockers are now recognized by the new American guidelines as one of the two preferred first-line therapies for hypertension, the other being diuretics (Chapter 7). These agents may also play an important role in altering the progression of idiopathic dilated cardiomyopathy.

## The Beta-Adrenoceptor and Signal Transduction

The beta-receptors classically are divided into the $beta_1$-receptors found in heart muscle and the $beta_2$-receptors of bronchial and vascular smooth muscle. There also are sizeable populations—about 20% to 25%—of $beta_2$-receptors in the myocardium. Some metabolic $beta_2$-receptors cannot easily be classified. Situated on the cell membrane, the beta-receptor is part of the adenylate cyclase system (Fig. 1–1). The G-protein system links the receptor to adenylate cyclase (AC), when the G-protein is in the stimulatory configuration ($G_s$). The link is interrupted by the inhibitory form ($G_i$), the formation of which results from muscarinic stimulation following vagal activation. When activated, adenylate cyclase produces cyclic AMP from ATP. Cyclic AMP is the intracellular messenger of beta-stimulation; among its actions is the "opening" of calcium channels to promote a positive inotropic effect and increased re-uptake of cytosolic calcium into the sarcoplasmic reticulum (relaxing or lusitropic effect). In the sinus node the pacemaker current is increased (positive chronotropic effect), while the rate of conduction is accelerated (positive dromotropic effect). The effect of a given beta-blocking agent depends not only on the way it is absorbed, bound to plasma proteins, and on its metabolites, but also on the extent to which it inhibits the beta-receptor (lock and key fit). Some beta-blockers also have the capacity to activate the receptor, hence the term partial agonist activity (PAA), also called intrinsic sympathomimetic activity (ISA), as epitomized in pindolol. ISA tends to avoid resting bradycardia and confers some vasodilatory capacity on the beta-blocker.

RECEPTOR DOWNREGULATION. Experimentally, Hausdorff and coworkers[48] have exposed intact beta-receptors on isolated membranes to prolonged beta-adrenergic stimulation. The beta-receptors responded by internalization so that the beta-adrenergic response was diminished (Fig. 1–2). Such downregulation could be viewed as a self-protective mechanism in view of the known adverse effects of excess levels of the second messenger, cyclic AMP, and the third

TABLE **1–1**

| INDICATIONS FOR BETA-BLOCKADE | FDA-APPROVED DRUGS |
|---|---|
| **1.** Ischemic heart disease | |
| Angina pectoris | propranolol, nadolol, atenolol, metoprolol |
| Silent ischemia | none |
| AMI, early phase | atenolol, metoprolol |
| AMI, follow-up | propranolol, timolol, atenolol, metoprolol |
| **2.** Hypertension | |
| Hypertension, systemic | acebutolol, atenolol, betoxalol, bisoprolol, carteolol, labetalol, metoprolol, nadolol, penbutolol, pindolol, propranolol, timolol |
| Hypertension, severe, urgent | labetalol |
| Hypertension with LVH | (? all) |
| Hypertension, systolic | (? all) |
| Pheochromocytoma (already receiving alpha-blockade) | propranolol |
| Hypertension, severe peri-operative | esmolol |
| **3.** Arrhythmias | |
| Tachycardias (SVT and VT) | propranolol |
| Supraventricular, peri-operative | esmolol |
| Digitalis-induced tachyarrhythmias | propranolol |
| Anesthetic arrhythmias | propranolol |
| PVC control | acebutolol |
| Serious ventricular tachycardia | sotalol |
| **4.** Cardiomyopathy | |
| Dilated cardiomyopathy | (metoprolol, carvedilol) |
| Hypertrophic obstructive cardiomyopathy (subaortic stenosis) | propranolol |
| **5.** Other cardiovascular indications | |
| Vasovagal syncope, aortic dissection, Marfan's syndrome, mitral valve prolapse, congenital QT prolongation, Tetralogy of Fallot, fetal tachycardia | (propranolol; ? all) |
| **6.** Central indications | |
| Anxiety | (propranolol) |
| Essential tremor | propranolol |
| Migraine prophylaxis | propranolol, nadolol |
| Alcohol withdrawal | (propranolol, atenolol) |
| **7.** Endocrine | |
| Thyrotoxicosis (arrhythmias) | propranolol |
| **8.** Gastrointestinal | |
| Esophageal varices | (propranolol) |
| **9.** Glaucoma (local use) | timolol, betoxalol, carteolol, levobunolol, metipranolol |

( ) = well tested but not FDA approved; SVT = supraventricular tachycardia; VT = ventricular tachycardia; PVC = premature ventricular contractions.

## CARDIAC BETA-ADRENERGIC SIGNAL SYSTEM

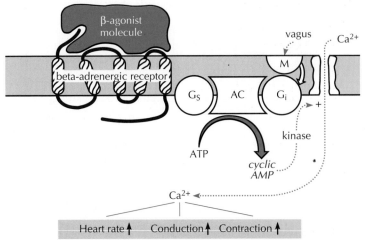

**FIGURE 1–1.** The cardiac beta-adrenoceptor and signaling system. The beta-antagonist molecule interacts with the beta-receptor, whose molecular structure has recently been revealed and the amino acid sequence characterized. In the presence of the stimulatory form of the G-protein ($G_s$), adenylate cyclase (AC) converts ATP to cyclic AMP which acting via a protein kinase enhances phosphorylation of the calcium channel and permits more calcium to enter through the calcium channel during voltage-induced depolarization. Such calcium releases much more from the sarcoplasmic reticulum (calcium-induced calcium release) to increase cytosolic calcium, heart rate, conduction and contraction as well as the rate of relaxation (the latter via phosphorylation of the protein phospholamban in the sarcoplasmic reticulum). $G_i$ = inhibitory G-protein, part of signaling system for vagal muscarinic stimulation. Fig. copyright L.H. Opie and modified from Reference 1.

messenger, calcium ions. If the beta-stimulation is sustained, then the internalized receptors may undergo lysosomal destruction with a true loss of receptor density. Otherwise the internalized receptors may regain their surface location once more to be active. This whole process is sometimes called the receptor round-trip cycle.

In clinical practice, beta-receptor downregulation occurs during prolonged beta-agonist therapy or in severe congestive heart failure (CHF). During continued infusion of dobutamine, a beta-agonist, there may be a progressive loss or decrease of therapeutic efficacy, which is termed tachyphylaxis. The time taken and the extent of receptor downgrading depend on multiple factors including the dose and rate of infusion, the age of the patient, and the degree of pre-existing downgrading of receptors as a result of CHF. For example, one-third of the hemodynamic response to dobutamine may be lost after 72 hours (p 161). Second, in CHF, beta-receptors are downgraded, especially the beta$_1$ variety, so that the response to beta$_1$-stimulation is diminished.[40] Cardiac beta$_2$-receptors are not downregulated but "uncoupled," therefore also responding less well to stimulation.[37] Recent research in the therapy of CHF shows that low doses of beta-blockers may restore beta-adrenergic receptor sensitivity with therapeutic benefits.[47]

RECEPTOR UPREGULATION. Conversely, when beta-receptors are chronically blocked, as during sustained beta-blocker therapy, the number of beta-receptors increases. There is nonetheless a decreased overall response to beta-adrenergic stimulation because the receptors are occupied by the beta-blocker. If the beta-blocker were abruptly stopped, the increased receptor density may precipitate a hyperreaction to physiologic adrenergic stimulation, so that ischemic events can be precipitated (withdrawal syndrome).

## β-RECEPTOR DOWNREGULATION

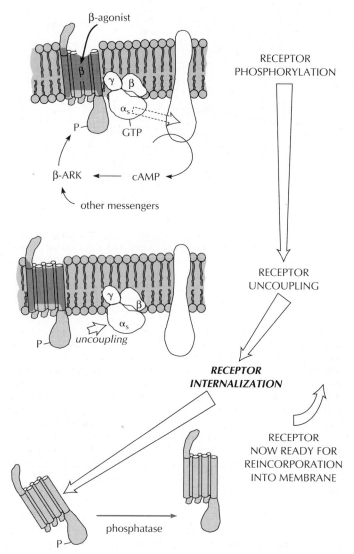

**FIGURE 1–2.** Proposed mechanism for beta-receptor downregulation by means of internalization. Fig. copyright L.H. Opie.

## Cardiovascular Effects of Beta-blockade

Beta-blockers were originally designed by Sir James Black, working at Imperial Chemical Industries in the United Kingdom, to counteract the cardiac effects of adrenergic stimulation. The latter, he reasoned, increased myocardial oxygen demand and worsened angina. His work led to the design of the prototype beta-blocker, propranolol. By blocking the cardiac beta-receptors, these agents induce the well-known inhibitory effects on the sinus node, atrioventricular node, and on myocardial contraction. These are respectively the negative chronotropic, dromotropic, and inotropic effects (Fig. 1–3). Of these, it is especially the bradycardic and negative inotropic effects that are relevant to the therapeutic effect in angina pectoris, because these changes decrease the myocardial oxygen demand. The inhibitory effect on the AV node is of special relevance in the therapy of supraventricular tachycardia (Table 11–4), or when beta-blockade is used to control the ventricular response rate in atrial fibrillation.

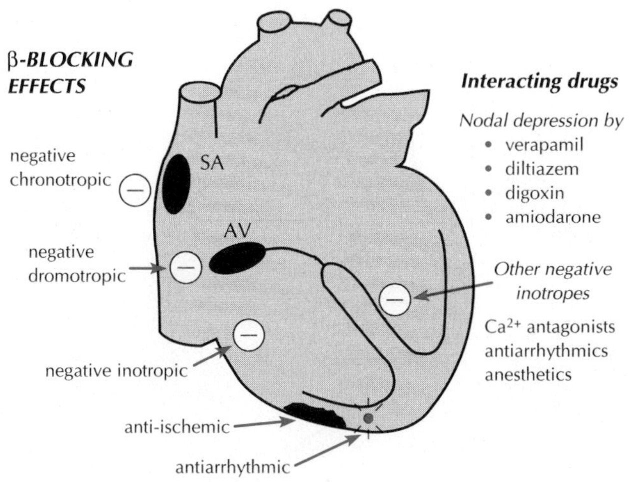

β-BLOCKING
EFFECTS

negative
chronotropic

negative
dromotropic

negative inotropic

anti-ischemic

antiarrhythmic

SA

AV

**Interacting drugs**

*Nodal depression by*
- verapamil
- diltiazem
- digoxin
- amiodarone

*Other negative
inotropes*

$Ca^{2+}$ antagonists
antiarrhythmics
anesthetics

FIGURE 1–3. Cardiac effects of beta-adrenergic blocking drugs at the levels of the SA node, AV node, conduction system, and myocardium. Some drug interactions are shown on the right. SA = sinoatrial; AV = atrioventricular. Fig. copyright L.H. Opie.

### Effects on Coronary Flow and Myocardial Perfusion

Enhanced beta-adrenergic stimulation, as in exercise, leads to beta-mediated coronary vasodilation. The signaling system in vascular smooth muscle again involves the formation of cyclic AMP, but whereas the latter agent increases cytosolic calcium in the heart, it paradoxically decreases calcium levels in vascular muscle cells (Fig. 3–2). Thus, during exercise, the heart pumps faster and more forcefully, while the coronary flow is increased—a logical combination. Conversely, it might be expected that beta-blockade would of necessity have a coronary vasoconstrictive effect with a rise in coronary vascular resistance.[75] However, the longer diastolic filling time, resulting from the decreased heart rate in exercise, leads to better diastolic myocardial perfusion, which is an important therapeutic benefit.

### Effects on Systemic Circulation

The above effects explain why beta-blockers are antianginal as predicted by their developers. Antihypertensive effects are less well understood. In the absence of the peripheral dilatory actions of some beta-blockers (see Vasodilatory Beta-blockers), beta-blockers initially decrease the resting cardiac output by about 20% with a compensatory reflex rise in the peripheral vascular resistance. Thus, within the first 24 hours of therapy, the arterial pressure is unchanged. The peripheral resistance then starts to fall after 1 to 2 days and the arterial pressure declines. The mechanism of this hypotensive process is unclear, but may involve (1) inhibition of those beta-receptors on the terminal neurons that facilitate the release of norepinephrine (prejunctional beta-receptors), (2) central nervous effects with reduction of adrenergic outflow, and (3) lessening of the activity of the renin-angiotensin system, because beta-receptors mediate renin release. All beta-blockers reduce circulating renin levels, yet the antihypertensive effect is not directly related to the reduction of circulating levels. An effect on the local renin-angiotensin system in vascular tissue cannot, however, be excluded.

## Angina Pectoris

Beta-blockade reduces the oxygen demand of the heart (Fig. 1–4) by reducing the double product (heart rate × blood pressure) and

## BETA-BLOCKADE EFFECTS ON ISCHEMIC HEART

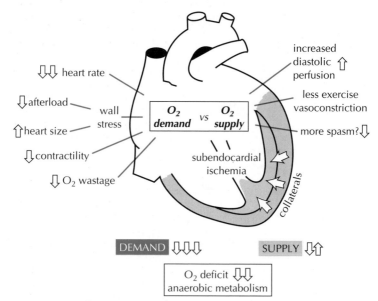

FIGURE 1–4. Effects of beta-blockade on ischemic heart. Beta-blockade has a beneficial effect on the ischemic myocardium, unless (1) the preload rises substantially as in left heart failure or (2) there is vasospastic angina when spasm may be promoted in some patients. Note recent proposal that beta-blockade diminishes exercise-induced vasoconstriction. Fig. copyright L.H. Opie and modified from Reference 1.

by limiting exercise-induced increases in contractility. Of these, the most important and easiest to measure is the reduction in heart rate. In addition, an aspect frequently neglected is the increased oxygen demand resulting from left ventricular (LV) dilation, so that any accompanying ventricular failure needs active therapy.

*All beta-blockers are potentially equally effective in angina pectoris (Table 1–1) and the choice of drug matters little in those who do not have concomitant diseases.* But about 20% of patients do not respond to any beta-blocker,[1] because of (1) underlying severe obstructive coronary artery disease, responsible for angina at a low level of exertion and at heart rates of 100 beats/min or lower, or (2) an abnormal increase in LV end-diastolic pressure resulting from an excess negative inotropic effect and a resultant decrease in subendocardial blood flow. Although it is conventional to adjust the dose of a beta-blocker to secure a resting heart rate of 55 to 60 beats/min, rates below 50 beats/min may be acceptable provided that heart block is avoided and there are no symptoms. The reduced heart rate at rest reflects the persistent vagal tone that accompanies the decrease in adrenergic effects. A major benefit is the limitation of the increase in the heart rate during exercise, which ideally should not exceed 100 beats/min in patients with angina. In the case of beta-blockers with added vasodilatory properties (p 16), it may not be possible nor desirable to achieve low resting heart rates because reduction of the afterload plays an increasingly larger role in reducing the myocardial oxygen demand. Nonetheless, in general, vasodilatory beta-blockers have not been well tested against angina.

COMBINATION THERAPY OF ANGINA PECTORIS. Beta-blockers are often combined with nitrate vasodilators and calcium antagonists in the therapy of angina. It is conventional to start with two agents, nitrates plus beta-blockers or calcium antagonists, and then to go onto combined triple therapy (Table 2–4) while watching for adverse side-effects, such as hypotension. The mechanism of action of the three types of agents is different and may be additive. Thus beta-blockers act chiefly by decreasing the myocardial oxygen demand, whereas nitrates dilate coronary collaterals and reduce the preload (Fig. 2–1), while calcium antagonists prevent exercise-induced coronary constriction and reduce the afterload. Beta-blockers may also improve myocardial blood flow by increased time for diastolic coronary blood flow.

Of the possible *combinations of beta-blockers with calcium antagonists*, that with nifedipine is hemodynamically the soundest, as the tendency to tachycardia with nifedipine and related compounds is antagonized by the beta-blocker, whereas the nifedipine-like compounds contribute vasodilation to the mechanism of antianginal effect. Beta-blockers should only be combined with verapamil and diltiazem with caution, as extreme bradycardia or atrioventricular (AV) block may occasionally occur and, in the case of verapamil, a marked negative inotropic effect is possible.[30] In any case, the benefits of adding beta-blockade to high doses of diltiazem are questionable and fatigue often results.[12] Therefore the decision to add a calcium antagonist to beta-blocker plus nitrate therapy requires, first of all, a knowledge of the hemodynamics of the combination of beta-blocker plus calcium antagonist (Fig. 3–8), a careful examination of the cardiovascular system, and a certain amount of judicious guesswork. Of the combinations, beta-blocker plus a DHP is likely to be simplest, beta-blocker plus diltiazem is almost as simple but without much increased benefit, and that with verapamil is most likely to cause problems.[30] Beta-blocker plus diltiazem is more likely to cause excess sinus bradycardia, and beta-blocker plus verapamil results in excess AV nodal inhibition.

Hemodynamically, the combination of beta-blockade plus any of the second generation calcium antagonists, such as amlodipine, felodipine, isradipine, and others, is similar to that of the beta-blocker plus nifedipine combination. Of interest would be to test the effects of the combination of ultralong-acting compounds of each category, for example amlodipine and nadolol.

The combination beta-blockade and calcium antagonism (atenolol plus nifedipine) improves hard end-points in patients with effort angina (see Outcome Studies).

IMPAIRED LV FUNCTION. In angina pectoris with abnormal LV function, beta-blockade may decrease angina at the cost of lessening exercise tolerance because of the increased LV size and wall tension; diuretics and digitalis can prevent clinical deterioration and reverse the cardiac enlargement.[1] The current trend is to replace digitalis by ACE inhibitors. Theoretically, vasodilatory beta-blockers should depress myocardial function less.

UNSTABLE ANGINA WITH THREAT OF MYOCARDIAL INFARCTION. Unstable angina is an all-purpose term including a large number of clinical entities. In view of the complex etiology, different therapies may be appropriate (Fig. 1–5). Short-lived attacks of chest pain at rest, although correctly described as angina at rest, may have a very different connotation from increasingly severe and prolonged pain with threat of myocardial infarction, the sense in which the term "unstable angina" is now increasingly used. At present, plaque fissuring with partial coronary thrombosis or platelet aggregation is seen as the basic pathology in threatened infarction, so that urgent antithrombotic therapy by heparin followed by aspirin is basic. Added beta-blockade is usual, especially in patients with elevated blood pressure and heart rate. *Logically the lower the heart rate, the less the risk of recurrent ischemia.* Hence standard blockers are preferred to the vasodilatory agents. The actual objective evidence favoring the use of beta-blockers in unstable angina is limited to one placebo-controlled trial.[19] Patients who were not on prior beta-blockade were randomized either to metoprolol or nifedipine, or to the combination. Patients on prior beta-blockade were randomized to placebo or nifedipine. "Of all the treatments studied, only the addition of nifedipine

## UNSTABLE ANGINA AT REST

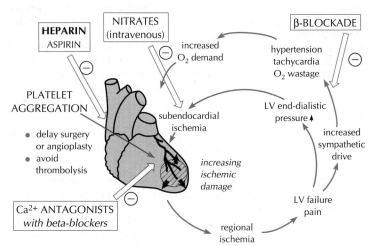

**FIGURE 1–5.** Hypothetical mechanisms for unstable angina at rest and proposed therapy. Increasing emphasis is being placed on the role of antithrombotics and antiplatelet agents. Beta-blockade may be particularly effective in the presence of sympathetic activation with increased heart rate and blood pressure. Calcium antagonists, especially nifedipine, should be used with care and nifedipine only in combination with beta-blockade. Fig. copyright L.H. Opie and modified from Reference 1.

to previous maintenance with a beta-blocker was clearly beneficial," as judged by recurrent ischemia or myocardial infarction at 48 hours. In the case of beta-blockade alone, statistical proof of a reduction in recurrent ischemia was not achieved. An important conclusion of this study was a trend to increased complications with nifedipine alone, which is therefore relatively contraindicated in unstable angina in the absence of beta-blockade.[13,19]

In patients with crescendo angina or prolonged ischemic chest pain poorly relieved by intravenous nitroglycerin and without evidence of Prinzmetal's angina, propranolol (initial dose 40 mg, increased to 80 mg 3 times daily) was as effective as the calcium antagonist diltiazem (initial dose 60 mg, followed by 120 mg also 3 times daily).[1]

In patients with unstable angina, once the acute phase is over, coronary angiography is likely to lead to coronary artery bypass grafting or to angioplasty in selected patients. Occasionally acute intervention is attempted when pain does not respond to standard therapy.

PRINZMETAL'S VARIANT ANGINA. Beta-blockade is commonly held to be ineffective and even harmful, supposedly because of enhanced coronary spasm from unopposed alpha-receptor activity.[27] On the other hand, there is excellent evidence for the benefit of calcium antagonist therapy, which is standard. Although some reports[15] have reported relief of variant angina with propranolol (mean dose 391 mg daily), such therapy is not standard. In the case of exercise-induced anginal attacks in patients with variant angina, there is good evidence, obtained from a prospective randomized study in 20 patients, that nifedipine is considerably more effective than propranolol.[24]

COLD INTOLERANCE AND ANGINA. During exposure to severe cold, effort angina may occur more easily.[25] Conventional beta-blockade by propranolol is not as good as vasodilatory therapy by nifedipine. Speculatively, vasodilatory beta-blockers may also be better than propranolol.

MIXED OR DOUBLE-COMPONENT ANGINA. In the past, much was made of the possibility that coronary spasm contributes to the symptomatology of mixed or double-component angina where, in addition to ordinary effort angina, there is angina at rest. However, in a double-blind comparison of atenolol 100 mg daily, nifedipine 60 mg daily, and isosorbide mononitrate 80 mg daily, atenolol was the best overall agent and was as effective as nifedipine is abolishing nocturnal ST-segment changes.[26] Likewise, propranolol (80 mg 4 times daily) was more effective than nifedipine (20 mg 4 times daily) in double-component angina as assessed by the incidence of silent and symptomatic ischemic episodes.[10]

VARIABLE THRESHOLD ANGINA. This condition, once regarded as an indication for calcium antagonists rather than beta-blockers, responds equally well to atenolol or diltiazem.[56]

SILENT MYOCARDIAL ISCHEMIA. Increasing emphasis is now placed on the importance of silent myocardial ischemia in patients with angina. Attacks, monitored by continuous ECG recordings, may be precipitated by minor elevations of heart rate, probably explaining why beta-blockers are very effective in reducing the frequency and number of episodes of silent ischemic attacks[35] and are probably superior to nitrates and calcium antagonists.[29,34] In patients with silent ischemia and mild or no angina, atenolol given for 1 year lessened new events (angina aggravation, revascularization) and reduced combined end-points.[35]

BETA-BLOCKADE WITHDRAWAL. When beta-blockers are suddenly withdrawn, angina may be exacerbated, sometimes resulting in myocardial infarction. In the case of poorly compliant patients, the use of a beta-blocker with added ISA such as pindolol appears to lessen the role of withdrawal effects. Treatment of the withdrawal syndrome is by reintroduction of beta-blockade.

## Acute Myocardial Infarction (AMI)

### Very Early AMI

In AMI without obvious clinical contraindications, very early intravenous beta-blockade in patients is now increasingly used despite occasional unpredictable hemodynamic effects. The risk of ventricular fibrillation (VF) and chest pain may be lessened.[1] Whether "infarct size" is reduced remains controversial. Theoretically, intravenous beta-blockade is of most use in about the first 4 hours after the onset when the adrenergic reflex response is most evident and when VF might be most prevalent. For this use against VF, a nonselective agent like propranolol is probably best (**Inderal,** 0.5 mg increments intravenous up to a total of 0.1 mg/kg[1]), although no formal comparisons exist between selective and nonselective agents. Early intravenous metoprolol (**Lopressor,** 5 mg every 5 minutes to a total of 15 mg) followed by 100 mg twice daily for 3 months lessens VF[1] and decreases mortality.[18] The first ISIS trial[20] showed that about 150 patients needed to be treated by early intravenous atenolol (**Tenormin** 5 to 10 mg) followed by oral therapy for one week to save one life; the mechanism was probably by prevention of cardiac rupture. Most of the benefit was achieved on the first day, at least in the case of atenolol. In the USA, metoprolol and atenolol are the only beta-blockers licensed for intravenous use in AMI. If there are doubts about the effects of beta-blockade on the hemodynamic status, then ultrashort-acting esmolol is the drug of choice.[62]

The current widespread use of thrombolytic agents within the first 6 hours of AMI has overshadowed the possible benefits of early intravenous beta-blockade (p 275). In the TIMI-II study,[72] the addition of intravenous metoprolol to thrombolytic therapy improved the early outcome although there was no real long-term advantage. Further prospective studies regarding this combination are required.

## Postinfarct Follow-up

In the postinfarct phase, beta-blockade reduces the risk of sudden death and reinfarction by about one-quarter.[68] Timolol, propranolol, metoprolol, and atenolol are all effective and licensed for this purpose.[1] Beta-blockers such as oxprenolol with ISA are supposedly ineffective[1] because of the higher heart rates caused by the ISA. Nonetheless, acebutolol, a cardioselective agent also with ISA, reduced total and vascular mortality in higher-risk postinfarct patients.[3] On the assumption that beta-blockade prevents reinfarction and sudden death at least in part by preventing the effects of catecholamine surges, it should not matter which type of beta-blocker is used.

The only outstanding questions are (1) whether low-risk patients should also be given beta-blockade; (2) which beta-blocker should be used—here it is safest to stick to those with documented efficacy and follow-up; (3) when to start—taking together the data on metoprolol and timolol, it seems reasonable to start either by early intravenous beta-blockade or as soon as the patient's condition allows, but optimally once the patient has stabilized at about 1 to 2 weeks; and (4) how long beta-blockade should be continued. In the absence of data to prove this point and bearing in mind the risk of beta-blockade withdrawal in patients with angina, many clinicians continue beta-blockade administration forever once a seemingly successful result has been obtained. Yet unless adequate stratification of risk is undertaken postinfarct, many patients have to be treated for a long time before there is any benefit (an estimated 30 patient years of treatment for one extra year of life).[1] The high-risk patients who should benefit most also have most contraindications to beta-blockade.[1] Although *congestive heart failure* is classically regarded as a contraindication to beta-blockade, postinfarct patients with heart failure appear to benefit more than others from beta-blockade.[51A,53] Today this category of patient would also be treated by ACE inhibitors and often diuretics.

The recent SAVE trial[60] has shown that reduced mortality achieved by ACE inhibitors and beta-blockade following myocardial infarction are additive, at least in patients with reduced ejection fractions. This benefit should be most important in patients with larger infarcts. The benefits of beta-blockers are greatest in the first year postinfarct, while the benefits of ACE inhibitors are most evident by the second or third year, perhaps due to improved ventricular remodeling with less dilation and reduced reinfarction.[76]

# Outcome Studies in Angina and Myocardial Ischemia

Solid evidence for a decrease in mortality in acute AMI and in postinfarct follow-up achieved by beta-blockade has led to the assumption that this type of treatment must also improve the outcome in effort angina and unstable angina. Unfortunately, there are no good outcome studies to support this proposal. In unstable angina, the short-term benefits of metoprolol were borderline.[19] In mixed effort and silent ischemia, an important European study, thus far not published in full, shows that after about 1,200 patient years of treatment, the beta-blocker atenolol and the calcium antagonist nifedipine were equally effective as judged by the incidence of hard end-points (cardiac death, myocardial infarction or unstable angina), whereas the combination reduced these end-points by about 30%.[71] A possible mechanism could have been a greater reduction of blood pressure. Unfortunately, there was no placebo group. The possible benefit of beta-blockade itself on clinical events in silent ischemia with mild or no angina seems settled by the ASIST study[35] in which atenolol increased event-free survival at one year, but major events, such as death, AMI, or unstable angina, were not reduced. Adding

BP AND β-BLOCKERS

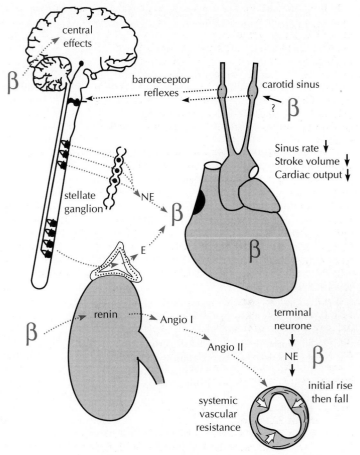

**FIGURE 1–6.** Possible sites of action of beta-blockers (B) relevant to hypertension. NE = norepinephrine; E = epinephrine; Angio = angiotensin. Fig. copyright L.H. Opie.

aspirin to beta-blockade in patients with overt angina reduces hard end-points including all cause mortality.[51]

## Beta-blockers for Hypertension

Beta-blockers are, with diuretics, currently recommended by the Joint National Council of the USA as first-line treatment for hypertension, probably because of the importance attached to the favorable effects of beta-blockade in a number of prospective outcome studies. It is especially the reduction of stroke that is well documented.

Despite the widespread use of beta-blockers for hypertension, the exact mechanism whereby beta-blockade lowers blood pressure remains an open question (Fig. 1–6). A sustained fall of cardiac output and a late decrease in peripheral vascular resistance (after an initial rise) appear to be important.

Of the large number of beta-blockers now available, all have been shown to be antihypertensive. There are currently eleven beta-blockers registered for hypertension in the USA. Of those available, particularly propranolol, atenolol and metoprolol have been well studied in long-term outcome trials. Logically, propranolol is not the ideal agent because of the high incidence of central side-effects,[9] whereas atenolol, acebutolol, metoprolol, and many other beta-blockers give a good quality of life.

CORONARY MORTALITY. Can beta-blockade reduce coronary mortality in hypertensives? In middle-aged patients, the answer has been elusive, with positive data only available for propranolol in non-smoking males.[55] A large meta-analysis suggests that blood pressure reduction is not as effective as it should be in reducing coronary heart disease,[39] when a combined attack on all the risk factors seems more logical.

ELDERLY PATIENTS. Contrary to a common opinion, beta-blockade is at least as effective in elderly as in younger patients, at least as far as whites are concerned.[54] That these advantages of beta-blockade do not appear to be commonly known is suggested by the observation that American physicians are increasingly using ACE inhibitors and calcium antagonists for the treatment of elderly hypertensives.[61]

Recently the Swedish STOP study[67] in elderly hypertensives found a reduction in mortality by beta-blockade (often combined with diuretic) in mortality with, however, the dominant effect being on stroke and the effect on myocardial infarction being only marginal. In the SHEP study[64] on systolic hypertension in the elderly, atenolol 25 to 50 mg daily was the second agent used after a diuretic. After nearly 5 years of follow-up, coronary heart disease was reduced by about one-quarter. Again, there was a major effect on stroke reduction. These favorable results of beta-blockade might not apply to black patients.

BLACK PATIENTS. In elderly blacks, Materson et al.[54] showed that atenolol was only marginally more effective than placebo. The ACE inhibitor, captopril, was less effective than placebo, while the calcium antagonist, diltiazem, was most effective. Unexpectedly, in younger blacks (age less than 60 years), atenolol was the second most effective agent, following diltiazem, and more effective than the diuretic hydrochlorothiazide.[54] Thus, although beta-blockade is generally held to be ineffective as monotherapy in black patients, this reservation may be largely restricted to those over 60 years.

BETA-BLOCKERS AND LEFT VENTRICULAR HYPERTROPHY (LVH). Although retrospective analyses have suggested that beta-blockade might be less effective in achieving regression of LVH than ACE inhibitors,[41] prospective studies are sparse. In a preliminary communication, Senior et al.[63] compared the effects of beta-blockade by atenolol, with nifedipine, the diuretic indapamide, and the diuretic hydrochlorothiazide in a parallel double-blind series on 149 hypertensive patients. All these agents caused a significant reduction in diastolic blood pressure, but of the four agents only hydrochlorothiazide did not decrease left ventricular mass.

COMBINATION ANTIHYPERTENSIVE THERAPY. Beta-blockers may be combined with diuretics, calcium antagonists, alpha-blockers, and centrally active agents in the therapy of hypertension. Because beta-blockers reduce renin levels, combination with ACE inhibitors is less logical. Ziac is bisoprolol (2.5 to 10 mg) with a very low dose of hydrochlorothiazide (6.25 mg). This drug combination has been approved as first-line therapy (starting with bisoprolol 2.5 mg plus thiazide 6.25 mg) for systemic hypertension by the FDA, an approval never before given to a combination product. To get this approval, there had to be a demonstration that both low-dose components (the diuretic and the beta-blocker) were themselves only marginally effective with a response rate at 12 weeks of below 30%, and that when added together the agents were more efficacious with a response rate of 60% or more, and with a demonstration that each component contributed to the blood-pressure-lowering effect of the combination.[44,45] The side-effects of each type of drug, beta-blocker and diuretic, are dose-dependent and different in nature. It makes sense that the combined low doses of each type gave fewer side-effects than the higher doses of each agent alone that would be required to drop the blood pressure by the same amount. Thus, the

## ANTIARRHYTHMIC EFFECTS OF β-BLOCKERS

*All β-blockers have anti-ischemic effects*

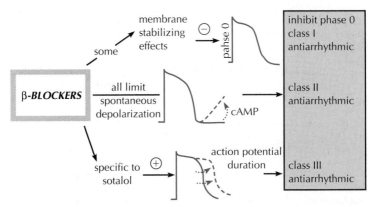

**FIGURE 1–7.** Antiarrhythmic properties of beta-blockers. Note that only sotalol has a Class-III antiarrhythmic effect. It is questionable whether the membrane stabilizing effects of propranolol and related agents confer additional antiarrhythmic properties. Fig. copyright L.H. Opie and modified from Reference 1.

metabolic side-effects of higher thiazide doses were minimized and the side-effect profile of the combination differed little from placebo with only a small increase in fatigue and dizziness. In Europe, several combinations of beta-blocker plus low-dose diuretic are available (Tenoret 50, Secadrex, Lopresoretic), yet none with the diuretic dose so low. In the USA, **Tenoretic** and **Lopressor HCT** are combinations widely used, yet they contain too high doses of diuretics (chlorthalidone 25 mg, see Chapter 7).

## Beta-blockers for Arrhythmias

Although beta-blockers have long been regarded as effective agents for supraventricular tachycardias, it was only recently that their remarkable efficacy and safety as ventricular antiarrhythmics has come to be appreciated. First, an important European trial showed that empirical use of metoprolol was as effective as electrophysiologically guided antiarrhythmic therapy.[66] Second, the ESVEM study[43] showed that sotalol, a beta-blocker with added Class III activity (Fig. 1–7), was more effective than a variety of Class I antiarrhythmics when used against ventricular tachyarrhythmias. These studies are supported by the earlier finding that in patients with severe ventricular tachycardia or fibrillation, long-term beta-blockade was successful in most, especially those with a LV ejection fraction exceeding 45% and, surprisingly, even in the absence of coronary disease.[5]

In **postinfarct patients** with depressed LV function and ventricular arrhythmias, a retrospective analysis of data from the CAST study (p 225) shows that beta-blockade reduced all cause mortality and arrhythmia deaths.[51A]

Beta-blockers have multiple antiarrhythmic mechanisms (Fig. 1–7). Among the beta-blockers used for ventricular arrhythmias, sotalol with added Class III activity may be best, but there is the risk of occasional torsades de pointes especially during diuretic cotherapy (Chapter 8). In the USA, sotalol is licensed only for sustained **life-threatening ventricular tachycardia.** Logically, beta-blockers should be particularly effective in arrhythmias caused by **increased circulating catecholamines** (early phase AMI, pheochromocytoma, anxiety, anesthesia, postoperative states, and some exercise-related arrhythmias, as well as mitral valve prolapse) or by increased cardiac sensitivity to catecholamines (thyrotoxicosis).

In **acute supraventricular tachycardias,** intravenous esmolol is challenging the otherwise standard use of verapamil or diltiazem in the perioperative period, although otherwise adenosine is preferred (Chapter 8). Beta-blockade may be effective in the prophylaxis of SVT by inhibiting the initiating atrial ectopics and effective in the treatment of SVT by slowing the AV node and lessening the ventricular response rate.

Intravenous esmolol may be used in **atrial fibrillation/flutter** to acutely reduce the rapid ventricular response rate.

## Cardiomyopathy and CHF

In **hypertrophic obstructive cardiomyopathy,** propranolol is standard therapy although verapamil and disopyramide are effective alternatives. High-dose propranolol (average 462 mg/day)[1] is thought to reduce ventricular arrhythmias. Lower-dose beta-blockade (mean 280 mg propranolol or equivalent per day)[1] has been ineffective against the arrhythmias; amiodarone therapy may be required in patients at risk of sudden death.[1]

In **congestive cardiomyopathy,** metoprolol is best tested. Low-dose beta-blockade may be added cautiously to conventional therapy especially when there is resting tachycardia. This indication, initially highly controversial, is increasingly supported. In a prospective study on 383 patients, there was improvement of symptoms and prevention of clinical deterioration.[73] Furthermore, long-term metoprolol (mean dose 100 to 150 mg daily) causes a moderate upregulation of ventricular beta$_1$-receptors.[47] The *initial dose* of metoprolol may have to be *extremely low,* as little as 5 mg daily, and there may be an initial period when the patient feels worse than before.[36]

Other beta-blockers that may also be effective include the vasodilatory agents bucindolol, labetalol, and carvedilol. Carvedilol, a beta-blocker with added alpha-blocking capacity, improves LV function without upgrading myocardial beta-receptors.[47]

In **ischemic cardiomyopathy,** it has not been so clear that beta-blockade improves the situation, yet a recent study with bucindolol in 30 patients suggests benefit, at least as much as in dilated cardiomyopathy.[38]

Propranolol has not been well studied in heart failure. In postinfarct patients, a retrospective analysis suggests that it is most effective in patients with pre-existing CHF.[53]

## Other Cardiac Indications

In **mitral stenosis** with sinus rhythm, beta-blockade benefits by decreasing resting and exercise heart rates, thereby allowing longer diastolic filling and improved exercise tolerance.[1] In mitral stenosis with chronic atrial fibrillation, beta-blockade may have to be added to digoxin to obtain sufficient ventricular slowing during exercise. Occasionally beta-blockers, verapamil and digoxin are all combined.

In **mitral valve prolapse,** beta-blockade is the standard procedure for control of associated arrhythmias.

In **dissecting aneurysms,** in the hyperacute phase, intravenous propranolol has been standard, although it could be replaced by esmolol. Thereafter oral beta-blockade is continued.

In **Marfan's syndrome** with aortic root involvement, propranolol is likewise used against aortic dilation and possible dissection.

In **vasovagal syncope,** beta-blockade helps to control the episodic adrenergic reflex discharge believed to contribute to symptoms.[70]

In **Fallot's tetralogy,** propranolol 2 mg/kg twice daily is usually effective against the cyanotic spells, probably acting by inhibition of right ventricular contractility.

In **congenital QT-prolongation,** propranolol is standard therapy, perhaps acting to restore an imbalance between left and right stellate ganglia.

# Noncardiac Indications for Beta-blockade

## Thyrotoxicosis

Together with antithyroid drugs or radioiodine, or as the sole agent before surgery,[1] beta-blockade is commonly used in thyrotoxicosis to control symptoms, although the hypermetabolic state is not decreased. Beta-blockade controls tachycardia, palpitations, tremor, and nervousness and reduces the vascularity of the thyroid gland, thereby facilitating operation.[1] In **thyroid storm,** intravenous propranolol can be useful at a rate of 1 mg/min (to a total of 5 mg at a time); circulatory collapse is a risk, so that beta-blockade should only be used in thyroid storm if LV function is normal as shown by conventional noninvasive tests. Because control of tachycardia is important, the choice of agent usually falls on those without ISA. A cardioselective agent is advisable when there is bronchospasm.

## Anxiety States

Although propranolol is most widely used in anxiety (and is licensed for this purpose in several countries, including the USA), probably all beta-blockers are effective, acting not centrally but by a reduction of peripheral manifestations of anxiety such as tremor and tachycardia.[1] In a double-blind study of anxiety in hypertensive patients (not the same as nonhypertensive patients presenting with anxiety), atenolol was considerably better than propranolol.[8]

## Other Central Nervous Indications

Atenolol and propranolol are very effective in **postalcoholic withdrawal syndrome.**[23]

In **subarachnoid hemorrhage,** early treatment by propranolol with long-term follow-up appeared to be beneficial,[33] although the study design was imperfect.

In **acute stroke,** on the contrary, atenolol or propranolol not only failed to benefit the patient but increased mortality. In contrast, patients taking beta-blockers at the start of the stroke appeared to have some protection.[4]

## Glaucoma

The use of local beta-blocker eye solutions is now established for open-angle glaucoma; care needs to be exerted with occasional systemic side-effects such as sexual dysfunction,[1] bronchospasm, and cardiac depression. Among the agents approved for treatment of glaucoma in the USA are the nonselective agents timolol (**Timoptic**), carteolol, levobunolol, and metipranolol. The cardioselective **betaxolol** may be an advantage in avoiding side-effects in patients with bronchospasm.

## Migraine

Propranolol (80 to 240 mg daily, licensed for this purpose in the USA) acts prophylactically to reduce the incidence of migraine attacks in 60% of patients. The mechanism is presumably by beneficial vasoconstriction. The antimigraine effect is prophylactic and not for attacks once they have occurred. If there is no benefit within 4 to 6 weeks of top doses, the drug should be discontinued.

# Pharmacologic Properties of Various Beta-blockers

## Beta-blocker Generations

First-generation agents such as propranolol nonselectively block all the beta-receptors (both $beta_1$ and $beta_2$). Second-generation agents such as atenolol, metoprolol, acebutolol, bisoprolol, and others have relative selectivity when given in low doses for the $beta_1$ (largely cardiac) receptors. Third-generation agents have added vasodilatory properties, acting chiefly through two mechanisms: (1) $beta_2$ intrinsic sympathomimetic activity (ISA) which stimulates blood vessels to relax; and (2) added alpha-adrenergic blockade as in labetalol and carvedilol.

Other marked differences between beta-blockers lie in the pharmacokinetic properties, with half-lives varying from about 10 minutes to over 30 hours, and in differing lipid or water solubility. Hence the side-effects may vary from agent to agent. Nonetheless, there is no evidence that any of these ancillary properties has any compelling therapeutic advantage, *although for the individual patient the art of minimizing beta-blocker side-effects may be of great importance.* For example, a patient with chronic obstructive airways disease needs a cardioselective agent, whereas a patient with early morning angina may need an ultralong-acting beta-blocker. Likewise, a patient with cold extremities or a resting bradycardia might benefit from a vasodilatory agent.

## Nonselective Agents (Beta₁ plus Beta₂-blockers)

The prototype beta-blocker is propranolol which is still used more than any other agent and is a WHO essential drug. By blocking $beta_1$-receptors it affects heart rate, conduction, and contractility, yet by blocking $beta_2$-receptors it tends to cause smooth muscle contraction with risk of bronchospasm in predisposed individuals. This same quality might, however, explain the benefit in migraine when vasoconstriction could inhibit the attack. Among the nonselective blockers, nadolol and sotalol are much longer-acting and lipid-insoluble.

## Cardioselective Agents (Beta₁-selectivity)

Cardioselective agents (acebutolol, atenolol, betoxalol, bisoprolol, celiprolol, and metoprolol) are preferable in patients with chronic lung disease, asthma or chronic smoking, and insulin-requiring diabetes mellitus (Fig. 1–8). Cardioselectivity varies between agents. As judged by bronchospasm in asthmatics (fall in forced expiratory volume), atenolol is somewhat more cardiospecific than metoprolol and both are more so than acebutolol.[1] Cardioselectivity declines or is lost at high doses. *No beta-blocker is completely safe in the presence of asthma; low-dose cardioselective agents can be used with care in patients with bronchospasm or chronic lung disease or chronic smoking.* In angina and hypertension, cardioselective agents are just as effective as noncardioselective agents. In acute myocardial infarction (AMI) complicated by stress-induced hypokalemia, nonselective blockers theoretically should be better antiarrhythmics than $beta_1$-selective blockers.[1]

## Vasodilatory Beta-blockers

The two chief mechanisms of vasodilation are, first, intrinsic sympathomimetic activity and, second, added alpha-adrenergic blockade (Fig. 1–9).

INTRINSIC SYMPATHOMIMETIC ACTIVITY (ISA OR PARTIAL AGONIST ACTIVITY). Beta-blockers with ISA lower resting heart rate and cardiac output to a lesser extent than those without ISA.[32] **Pindolol** is the beta-blocker with most ISA and nonselective beta-blocking qualities. **Acebutolol** has less ISA which in clinical practice is not enough to

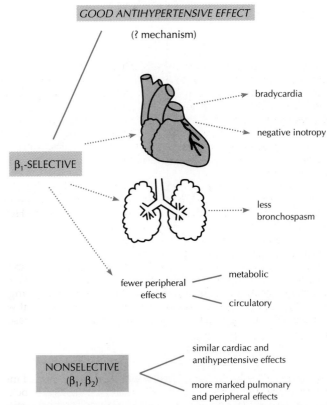

FIGURE 1–8.   Beta-antagonist agents may be either beta$_1$-cardioselective or non-cardioselective (beta$_1$-beta$_2$ antagonism). In general, note several advantages of cardioselective beta-blockers. There may be occasional disadvantages as in hypokalemia associated with acute myocardial infarction. Fig. copyright L.H. Opie.

distinguish it from metoprolol.[6] The effect of a beta-blocker with ISA on resting heart rate depends on the degree of sympathetic stimulation at rest and the relative ratios of beta$_1$ or beta$_2$ agonism. Beta$_1$-stimulation acts chiefly on the heart, beta$_2$ on the peripheral arterioles and the bronchi. **Pindolol** has both beta$_1$ and beta$_2$ agonist activity with beta$_2$ greater than beta$_1$. If the resting sympathetic tone is high, a beta-blocker with beta$_1$ ISA reduces the resting heart rate. As with beta-blockade, ISA may be selective for beta$_1$- or beta$_2$-receptors or may be nonselective. ISA introduces a quality of potential beta-receptor stimulation that is probably useful in patients with hypertension because of peripheral vasodilation; in elderly patients in whom fatigue might be caused by limitation of cardiac output; or in black patients in whom vasodilation appears to improve the antihypertensive effect. In patients with ischemic heart disease, however, a slower heart rate might be better, and ISA is a potential disadvantage.

Another potential disadvantage of ISA is the stimulation of the central nervous system at night, when sympathetic tone is low, causing sleep impairment.[22]

ADDED ALPHA-BLOCKING ACTIVITY.   **Labetalol** is a combined alpha- and beta-blocking agent that causes less bronchospasm and vasoconstriction than propranolol, lowers the blood pressure acutely unlike standard beta-blockers, and works better than propranolol in black hypertensives.[1] These advantages are bought at the cost of two potential side-effects: postural hypotension with high doses and occasional retrograde ejaculation (alpha-blockade relaxes the bladder neck sphincter and is used in the therapy of prostatism). Besides alpha-

## VASODILATORY β-BLOCKERS

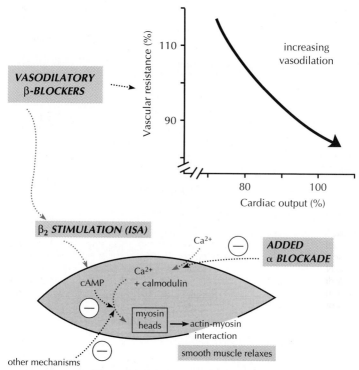

**FIGURE 1–9.**  Vasodilatory mechanisms and effects. Vasodilatory beta-blockers tend to decrease the cardiac output less as the systemic vascular resistance falls. Vasodilatory mechanisms include alpha-blockade, nonspecific mechanisms, and intrinsic sympathomimetic activity (ISA). ISA has a specific effect in increasing sympathetic tone when it is low, as at night, and increasing nocturnal heart rate which might be disadvantageous in nocturnal angina or unstable angina. Fig. copyright L.H. Opie and modified from Reference 1.

blockade, labetalol may possess significant ISA.[1] Labetalol is a more powerful beta-blocker than alpha-blocker (beta:alpha ratio 3:1 after oral and 7:1 after intravenous dosage), so that a high dose may be required for adequate alpha-blockade. A standard dose of labetalol (200 mg twice daily) was as effective as atenolol (100 mg daily) in controlling angina in patients with coexisting hypertension.[1] For angina without hypertension, the efficacy of labetalol is not well documented. Intravenous labetalol has a rapid onset of action in severe hypertension and is well tested in **pregnancy hypertension** (intravenous or oral). Even oral labetalol leads to a rapid fall of blood pressure, in contrast to propranolol or other conventional beta-blockers.

OTHER VASODILATORY BETA-BLOCKING MOLECULES.  **Carvedilol,** under investigation, has added alpha-blockade. **Bucindolol,** another drug in clinical trials, has a hydralazine-like moiety built into the molecule. **Celiprolol** (in Europe) is a highly cardioselective agent with $beta_2$ agonism and another nonspecific vasodilatory quality.

ANTIARRHYTHMIC BETA-BLOCKERS.  All beta-blockers are potentially antiarrhythmic (Class II activity). Propranolol and some others have, in addition, a quinidine-like quality called membrane stabilizing activity (MSA), that is to say Class I activity. Such experimental activity is not clinically relevant except in cases of overdose when MSA contributes to fatality.[49] **Sotalol** is a unique beta-blocker with prominent added Class III antiarrhythmic activity (Chapter 8).

ROUTE OF ELIMINATION

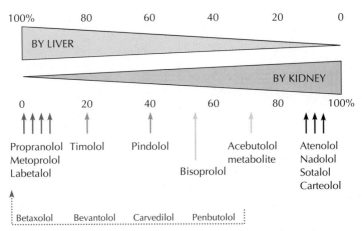

FIGURE 1–10. Comparative routes of elimination of beta-blockers. Those most hydrophilic and least lipid-soluble are excreted unchanged by the kidneys. Those most lipophilic and least water-soluble are largely metabolized by the liver. Note that the metabolite of acebutolol, diacetolol, is largely excreted by the kidney, in contrast to the parent compound. (For derivation of figure, see previous edition. Estimated data points for acebutolol, and newer agents added). Fig. copyright L.H. Opie and modified from Reference 1.

## Pharmacokinetic Properties of Beta-blockers

PLASMA HALF-LIVES. That of propranolol (Table 1–2) is only 3 hours, but continued administration saturates the hepatic process that removes propranolol from the circulation; the active metabolite 4-hydroxypropranolol is formed, and the effective half-life then becomes longer. The biological half-life of propranolol and metoprolol (and all other beta-blockers) exceeds the plasma half-life considerably, so that twice-daily dosage of standard propranolol is effective even in angina pectoris. Clearly, the higher the dose of any beta-blocker, the longer the biologic effects. Longer-acting compounds such as nadolol, sotalol, atenolol, and slow-release propranolol (**Inderal-LA**) or extended-release metoprolol (**Toprol-XL**) should be better for hypertension and ordinary angina, whereas ultrashort-acting intravenous esmolol is preferable in unstable angina and threatened infarction when hemodynamic changes may call for withdrawal of beta-blockade. In the case of early morning angina when protection is given by the beta-blocker taken the previous day, the ultralong-acting compound nadolol is better than atenolol.[21]

PROTEIN BINDING. Propranolol is highly bound, as are pindolol, labetalol and bisoprolol. Hypoproteinemia calls for lower doses of such compounds.

FIRST-PASS LIVER METABOLISM. This is found especially with the highly lipid-soluble compounds, such as propranolol, labetalol, and oxprenolol; acebutolol, metoprolol, and timolol have only modest lipid solubility, yet with hepatic clearance; first-pass metabolism varies greatly among patients and alters the dose required. In liver disease or low-output states the dose should be decreased. First-pass metabolism produces active metabolites with, in the case of propranolol, properties different from those of the parent compound. Acebutolol produces large amounts of diacetolol, also cardioselective with ISA, but with a longer half-life and chiefly excreted by the kidneys (Fig. 1–10).[2]

IDEAL KINETICS. Lipid-insoluble hydrophilic compounds (**atenolol, sotalol, nadolol**) are excreted only by the kidneys (Fig. 1–10) and have low brain penetration. In patients with renal or liver disease, the simpler pharmacokinetic patterns of lipid-insoluble agents make dosage easier. As a group, these agents have low protein binding (Table 1–2).

**TABLE 1–2    PROPERTIES OF VARIOUS BETA-ADRENOCEPTOR ANTAGONIST AGENTS, NONSELECTIVE VERSUS CARDIOSELECTIVE AND VASODILATORY AGENTS**

| GENERIC NAME (TRADE NAME) | ISA | PLASMA HALF-LIFE (h) | LIPID++ SOLUBILITY | FIRST-PASS EFFECT | LOSS BY LIVER OR KIDNEY | PLASMA PROTEIN BINDING (%) | USUAL DOSE FOR ANGINA (OTHER INDICATIONS IN BRACKETS) | USUAL DOSES AS SOLE THERAPY FOR MILD/MODERATE HYPERTENSION | INTRAVENOUS DOSE (AS LICENSED IN USA) |
|---|---|---|---|---|---|---|---|---|---|
| **Noncardioselective** | | | | | | | | | |
| Propranolol*† (Inderal) | − | 1–6 | +++ | ++ | Liver | 90 | 80 mg 2× daily usually adequate (may give 160 mg 2×) | Start with 10–40 mg 2× daily. Mean 160–320 mg/day, 1–2 doses. | 1–6 mg |
| (Inderal-LA) | − | 8–11 | +++ | ++ | Liver | 90 | 80–320 mg 1× daily | 80–320 mg 1× daily | — |
| Carteolol* (Cartrol) | + | 5–6 | 0/+ | 0 | Kidney | 20–30 | (Not evaluated) | 2.5–10 mg single dose | — |
| Nadolol*† (Corgard) | − | 20–24 | 0 | 0 | Kidney | 30 | 40–80 mg 1× daily; up to 240 mg. | 40–80 mg/day 1× daily; up to 320 mg. | — |
| Penbutolol* (Levatol) | + | 20–25 | +++ | ++ | Liver | 98 | (Not studied) | 10–20 mg daily | — |
| Sotalol** (Betapace) | − | 7–18 (mean 12) | 0 | 0 | Kidney | 5 | (240–480 mg/day in two doses for arrhythmias) | 80–320 mg/day; mean 190 mg. | — |
| Timolol* (Blocadren) | − | 4–5 | + | + | L, K | 60 | (post-AMI—10 mg 2× daily) | 10–30 mg 2× daily | — |
| **Cardioselective** | | | | | | | | | |
| Acebutolol* (Sectral) | ++ | 8–13 (diacetolol) | 0 (diacetolol) | ++ | L, K | 15 | (400–1200)/day in 2 doses for PVC) | 400–1200 mg/day; can be given as a single dose. | — |
| Atenolol*† (Tenormin) | − | 6–7 | 0 | 0 | Kidney | 10 | 50–200 mg 1× daily | 50–100 mg/day 1× daily | 5 mg over 5 min; repeat 5 min later |

| | | | | | Elimination | Bioavailability (%) | Oral dose (hypertension) | Oral dose | Intravenous dose |
|---|---|---|---|---|---|---|---|---|---|
| Betaxolol* (Kerlone) | 14–22 | — | + + | + + | L, then K | 50 | 10–20 mg 1× daily (use pending approval) | 10–20 mg 1× daily | — |
| Bisoprolol* (Zebeta) | 9–12 | — | + | 0 | L, K | 30 | 10 mg 1× daily (not in USA) | 2.5–40 mg 1× daily (see also Ziac) | — |
| Metoprolol*† (Lopressor) | 3–7 | — | + | + + | Liver | 12 | 50–200 mg 2× daily | 50–400 mg/day in 1 or 2 doses | 5 mg 3× at 2 min intervals |
| **Vasodilatory beta-blockers, nonselective** | | | | | | | | | |
| Labetalol* (Trandate) (Normodyne) | 6–8 | — | + + + | + + | L, some K | 90 | As for hypertension. | 300–600 mg/day in 3 doses; top dose 2400 mg/day. | Up to 2 mg/min, up to 300 mg for severe HT |
| Pindolol* (Visken) | 4 | + + + | $\beta_1\beta_2$ | + | L, K | 55 | 2.5–7.5 mg 3× daily (In UK, not USA) | 5–30 mg/day 2× daily | — |
| Carvedilol (investigational) | 6 | — | + | + + | Liver | 95 | 25–50 mg 2× daily | 25–50 mg 1× daily | — |
| **Vasodilatory beta-blockers, selective** | | | | | | | | | |
| Celiprolol (Celectol in UK; not in USA) | 6–8 | + $\beta_2$ | 0/+ | 0 | Chiefly kidneys also L | | 400 mg once daily | 400 mg once daily | — |

†† Octanol-water distribution coefficient (pH 7.4, 37° C) where 0 = < 0.5; + = 0.5–2.0; + + = 2–10; + + + = > 10; L = liver; K = kidney; HT = hypertension; PVC = premature ventricular contractions

* Approved by FDA for hypertension

† Approved by FDA for angina pectoris

** Approved for life-threatening ventricular tachyarrhythmias.

### Drug Interactions with Beta-blockers

These are relatively few.[58] Pharmacodynamic interactions can be predicted and are with other drugs depressing the SA or AV nodes, or with other negative inotropic agents (Fig. 1–3). Pharmacokinetic interactions are chiefly at the level of the liver. Cimetidine reduces hepatic blood flow and increases blood levels of beta-blockers highly metabolized by the liver, especially propranolol. Verapamil inhibits the hepatic breakdown of metoprolol and possibly other beta-blockers metabolized by the liver. To avoid such hepatic interactions, it is simpler to use those beta-blockers not metabolized by the liver (Fig. 1–10). Beta-blockers, in turn, depress hepatic blood flow so that the blood levels of lidocaine increase with greater risk of lidocaine toxicity.

## Concomitant Diseases and Choice of Beta-blocker

RESPIRATORY DISEASE. Cardioselective beta$_1$-blockers in low doses are best for patients with reversible bronchospasm. ISA or added alpha-blockade may confer a lesser degree of protection. In patients with a history of asthma, no beta-blocker can be considered safe.

ASSOCIATED CARDIOVASCULAR DISEASE. In patients with **sick sinus syndrome,** beta-blockade can be dangerous. Added ISA may be best. In patients with **Raynaud's phenomenon,** propranolol is traditionally particularly harmful. Nonetheless, in a prospective study, low-dose propranolol or metoprolol did not exaggerate primary Raynaud's phenomenon.[7]

In **active peripheral vascular disease,** beta-blockers are generally contraindicated, although the evidence is not firm.[17,69]

RENAL DISEASE. In renal disease, there is a risk that propranolol may decrease the glomerular filtration rate. Evidence for such an effect of other beta-blockers is not firm. Ultimately beta-blockers are usually excreted by the kidneys, so that in renal failure the dose may have to be altered, especially in the case of water-soluble agents excreted by the kidneys (atenolol, acebutolol, nadolol, sotalol) or agents partially excreted such as bisoprolol. In general, agents highly metabolized by the liver can be given in an unchanged dose.

DIABETES MELLITUS. In diabetes mellitus, the risk of beta-blockade in insulin-requiring diabetics is that the symptoms of hypoglycemia might be masked. There is a lesser risk with the cardioselective agents.

Whether **diabetic nephropathy** benefits from treatment with beta-blockade is not clear. Although control of blood pressure by beta-blockers does benefit, ACE inhibitors have established themselves in diabetic nephropathy (Chapter 5).

In **hypertensive patients with diabetic nephropathy,** beta-blockade as well as ACE inhibition improve microalbuminuria and hypertension.[59] Nonetheless, beta-blockers should only be used with caution in diabetic hypertensives except in the presence of angina or in postinfarct patients.[57]

In **non-insulin-dependent diabetes,** the risk is that continued use of beta-blockade, especially with diuretics, might impair glucose tolerance. If, therefore, there is a choice between beta-blockers and other agents such as ACE inhibitors, the latter may be better.

## Side-Effects of Beta-blockers

The **three major mechanisms** are (1) smooth muscle spasm (bronchospasm and cold extremities), (2) exaggeration of the cardiac therapeutic actions (bradycardia, heart block, excess negative inotropic effect) and (3) central nervous penetration (insomnia, depression).

The **mechanism of fatigue** is not clear. When compared with pro-pranolol, however, it is reduced by use of either a cardioselective beta-blocker or a vasodilatory agent, so that both central and periph-eral hemodynamic effects may be involved. When patients are ap-propriately selected, double-blind studies show no differences be-tween a cardioselective agent such as **atenolol** and placebo.[28] This may be because atenolol is not lipid-soluble and should have lesser effects on bronchial and vascular smooth muscle than propranolol. When **propranolol** is given for hypertension, the rate of serious side-effects (bronchospasm, cold extremities, worsening of claudication) leading to withdrawal of therapy is about 10%.[28] The rate of with-drawal with atenolol is considerably lower (about 2%), but when it comes to dose-limiting side-effects, both agents can cause cold extremities, fatigue, dreams, worsening claudication, and broncho-spasm. Heart failure, although a theoretical hazard with beta-block-ade therapy, is in fact rare when the correct contraindications are observed. Clearly if beta-blockade is given to patients who are al-ready severely ill, the risk of side-effects is increased.[11]

### Central Side-effects

An attractive hypothesis is that the lipid-soluble beta-blockers (epitomized by propranolol) with their high brain penetration are more likely to cause central side-effects. An extremely detailed com-parison of propranolol and atenolol showed that the latter, which is not lipid-soluble, causes far fewer central side-effects than does propranolol.[8] On the other hand, the lipid-solubility hypothesis does not explain why metoprolol, moderately lipid-soluble, appears to interfere less with some complex psychologic functions than does atenolol and may even enhance certain aspects of psychological performance.[31]

### Quality of Life

In the first quality of life study reported in patients with hyperten-sion, propranolol induced considerably more central effects than did the ACE inhibitor captopril.[9] Atenolol with its far fewer central side-effects, however, compares favorably with the ACE inhibitor enalapril.[16] It now appears that a variety of beta-blockers, often with different fundamental properties, all leave the quality of life intact in hypertensives (p 197).

During **exercise,** beta-blockade reduces the total work possible by about 15% and increases the sense of fatigue. Vasodilatory beta-blockers may be an exception.

**Impotence** is a side-effect quite frequently complained of by mid-dle-aged men, who in any case may be prone to this problem. Most package inserts give a rate of impotence of about 1% for any given agent. In fact, problems with erection may take place in 11% of patients given a beta-blocker, compared with 26% with a diuretic and 3% with placebo.[74] Speculatively, a change of beta-blocker to a vasodilatory compound might be beneficial, coupled with reassur-ance. Alternatively, the use of very low-dose combination therapy as in bisoprolol-hydrochlorothiazide (6.25 mg) may do the trick.

## Contraindications to Beta-blockade

The absolute contraindications can be deduced from the profile of pharmacological effects and side-effects (Table 1–3). Cardiac absolute contraindications include severe bradycardia, pre-existing high-de-gree heart block, and overt left ventricular failure (unless already con-ventionally treated). Pulmonary absolute contraindications are severe asthma or bronchospasm. The central nervous system contraindica-tion is severe depression (especially for propranolol). Active periph-eral vascular disease with rest ischemia is another contraindication.[69]

**TABLE 1–3      BETA-BLOCKADE: CONTRAINDICATIONS AND CAUTIONS**

### Cardiac

**Absolute: Severe bradycardia, high-degree heart block, overt left ventricular failure** (exception: dilated cardiomyopathies already conventionally treated).

**Relative:** Treated heart failure, Prinzmetal's angina (unopposed alpha-spasm), high doses of other agents depressing SA or AV nodes (verapamil, diltiazem, digitalis, antiarrhythmic agents); in angina, avoid sudden withdrawal, danger in unreliable patient.

### Pulmonary

**Absolute: Severe asthma or bronchospasm.** No patient may be given a beta-blocker without questions for past or present asthma. Fatalities have resulted when this rule is ignored.

**Relative:** Mild asthma or bronchospasm or chronic airways disease. Use agents with cardioselectivity plus $beta_2$-stimulants (by inhalation). High ISA* also protects, but with loss of sensitivity to bronchodilator $beta_2$-stimulation.

### Central Nervous

**Absolute: Severe depression** (avoid propranolol).

**Relative:** Vivid dreams: avoid highly lipid-soluble agents (propranolol) and pindolol; avoid evening dose. Visual hallucinations: change from propranolol. Fatigue (all agents; try change of agent). If low cardiac output is cause of fatigue, try vasodilatory beta-blockers. Impotence: rare (check for diuretic use). Psychotropic drugs (with adrenergic augmentation) may adversely interact with beta-blockers.

### Peripheral Vascular, Raynaud's Phenomenon

**Absolute: Active disease:** gangrene, skin necrosis, severe or worsening claudication, rest pain.

**Relative:** Cold extremities, absent pulses, Raynaud's phenomenon. Avoid nonselective agents (propranolol, sotalol, nadolol); prefer vasodilatory agents.

### Diabetes Mellitus

**Relative:** Insulin-requiring diabetes: nonselective agents decrease reaction to hypoglycemia; use selective agents—atenolol, metoprolol (acebutolol more doubtful). Beta-blockers may increase blood sugar by 1.0–1.5 mmol/L and impair insulin sensitivity especially with diuretic cotherapy; hence caution in family history of diabetes. Adjust control accordingly.

## Overdose of Beta-Blockers

Bradycardia may be countered by intravenous atropine 1 to 2 mg; if serious, temporary transvenous pacing may be required. When an infusion is required, glucagon (2.5 to 7.5 mg/h) is the drug of choice, because it stimulates formation of cyclic AMP by bypassing the occupied beta-receptor. Logically an infusion of a PDE inhibitor, such as amrinone or milrinone, should help cyclic AMP to accumulate. Alternatively, dobutamine is given in doses high enough to overcome the competitive beta-blockade (15 µg/kg/min). In patients without ischemic heart disease, an infusion (up to 0.10 µg/kg/min) of isoproterenol may be used.

## New Beta-blockers

Of the large number of beta-blockers in development, the ideal agent for hypertension or angina might have (1) advantageous phar-

**TABLE 1–3       BETA-BLOCKADE: CONTRAINDICATIONS AND CAUTIONS**
*(Continued)*

### Renal Failure

**Relative:** In general, renal blood flow falls. Reduce doses of agents eliminated by kidney (Fig. 1–10) and several others including bisoprolol.

### Liver Disease

**Relative:** Avoid agents with high hepatic clearance (propranolol, oxprenolol, timolol, acebutolol, metoprolol). Use agents with low clearance (atenolol, nadolol, sotalol, or pindolol). If plasma proteins low, reduce dose of highly bound agents (propranolol, pindolol, bisoprolol).

### Pregnancy Hypertension

Beta-blockade increasingly used but may depress vital signs in neonate and cause uterine vasoconstriction. Labetalol and atenolol best tested. Preferred drug methyldopa.

### Surgical Operations

Beta-blockade may be maintained throughout, provided indication is not trivial; otherwise stop 24 to 48 hours beforehand. May protect against anesthetic arrhythmias. Use atropine for bradycardia, beta-agonist for severe hypotension.

### Age

Beta-blockade effective in elderly whites but not blacks; in the latter use with diuretics. Watch pharmacokinetics and side-effects in all elderly patients.

### Smoking

In hypertension, beta-blockade is less effective in reducing coronary events in smoking men.

### Hyperlipidemia

Beta-blockers may have unfavorable effects on the blood lipid profile, especially nonselective agents. Triglycerides increase and HDL-cholesterol falls. Clinical significance unknown. Vasodilatory agents, especially those with ISA, may have mildly favorable effects.

*ISA = intrinsic sympathomimetic activity

macokinetics (lipid-insolubility); (2) a high degree of cardioselectivity; and (3) long duration of action. Vasodilatory properties should be of benefit in the treatment of hypertension and severe idiopathic cardiomyopathy with CHF, but might be a disadvantage in the treatment of certain types of angina when the heart rate must be as slow as possible.

**Betaxolol (Kerlone)** is a new long-acting lipid-soluble cardioselective beta-blocker (oral dose 10 to 40 mg once daily) now available in the USA for hypertension.

**Bisoprolol (Emcor, Monocor, Zebeta)** is a highly beta$_1$-selective agent, thought to be more selective than atenolol, licensed for hypertension and angina in the UK and for hypertension in the USA. The dose is 2.5 to 20 mg once daily with an average of 10 mg. Bisoprolol 10 mg daily and atenolol 100 mg daily have similar antihypertensive effects.[52] A combination of low-dose bisoprolol and low-dose hydrochlorothiazide (**Ziac**) is now available in the USA (p 12). The proposal is that antihypertensive efficacy can be reached at doses that cause few or no side-effects.

**Bucindolol** is a vasodilatory nonselective agent under investigation for use in CHF.[38]

**Carteolol (Cartrol)** is a nonselective beta-blocker with moderate ISA, low lipid-solubility, and a half-life similar to that of atenolol.

In hypertension (for which it is licensed in the USA), the initial dose is 2.5 mg as a single daily dose, which may be increased to 10 mg daily. Because of predominant renal excretion, the dose is decreased in renal impairment.

**Carvedilol** is a compound like labetalol with alpha-mediated vaso-dilatory capacity, but longer acting. It is extensively studied in CHF.[47] Experimentally, it has remarkable antioxidant properties. In the USA, registration is being sought for hypertension and CHF.

**Celiprolol** (**Celectol** in UK) is a highly cardioselective beta-blocker with low lipid-solubility and a half-life similar to that of atenolol. The ancillary properties include beta$_2$-mediated vasodilation.[46] It is claimed to have less adverse effects on blood lipids than atenolol;[42] atenolol was, however, more effective in bringing down the diastolic blood pressure.

**Penbutolol** (**Levatol**). This agent has modest ISA, similar to acebu-tolol, but is nonselective. It is highly lipid-soluble and liver metabo-lized. In the treatment of mild to moderate hypertension, the usual initial dose is 20 mg once daily with a flat dose-response curve.

## Ultrashort-Acting Intravenous Beta-blockade

**Esmolol** (**Brevibloc**) is an ultrashort-acting beta$_1$-blocker with a half-life of 9 minutes, rapidly converting to inactive metabolites by blood esterases. It is replacing intravenous verapamil and similar agents for peri-operative supraventricular arrhythmias and hyper-tension. The dose range is 50 to 300 µg/kg/min intravenously[14] with an effective dose usually about 100 µg/kg/min. Full recovery from beta-blockade occurs within 30 minutes in patients with a normal cardiovascular system.

INDICATIONS. These are situations in which on-off control of beta-blockade is desired, as in supraventricular tachycardia in the peri-operative period, or sinus tachycardia (noncompensatory), or emer-gency hypertension in the peri-operative period (all registered uses in the USA). Other logical indications are for emergency hyperten-sion in other situations where pheochromocytoma is excluded, or in unstable angina.[50] Exploratory uses are in acute phase AMI when the hemodynamic effects of beta-blockade may be hazardous. In atrial fibrillation or flutter, esmolol combined with digoxin appeared to be as effective as verapamil with less risk of hypotension.[65]

DOSE. For **supraventricular tachycardia,** a loading dose of 500 µg/kg/min is given over 1 minute, followed by a 4 minute infusion of 50 µg/kg/min (USA package insert). If this fails, repeat loading dose and increase infusion to 100 µg/kg/min again over 4 minutes. If this fails, repeat loading dose and then infuse at rates up to 300 µg/kg/min. Thereafter, to maintain control, infuse at adjusted rate for up to 24 hours. For **peri-operative hypertension,** give 80 mg (about 1 mg/kg) over 30 seconds and infuse at 150 to 300 µg/kg/min if needed. For more gradual control of blood pressure, follow routine for supraventricular tachycardia. Higher doses are usually required for blood pressure control than for arrhythmias. Once the emergency is over, replace by conventional antiarrhythmic or antihy-pertensive drugs.

SIDE-EFFECTS AND CAUTIONS. These are those of standard beta-blockers. The drug is contraindicated in the presence of verapamil or diltiazem cotherapy (added effects on SA and AV nodes). Likewise, exercise caution with digoxin cotherapy (Fig. 1–3). Note that extravasation of the acid solution has risk of skin necrosis.

## Conclusions

Beta-blockers come closest among all cardiovascular agents to providing all-purpose therapy—licensed indications include angina, hypertension, acute stage myocardial infarction, postinfarct follow-up, arrhythmias, and certain cardiomyopathies. Two major changes in the recent clinical use of beta-blockers are, first, the realization that these agents may be effective ventricular antiarrhythmics and, second, the possible use of low doses of beta-blockers in selected patients with CHF, to counter the enhanced adrenergic drive and beta-receptor downregulation found in CHF. Beta-blockade is very effective treatment, alone or combined with other drugs, in 70% to 80% of patients with classic angina, or 50% to 70% of those with mild to moderate hypertension; elderly black hypertensives respond less well although vasodilatory beta-blockers such as labetalol may be an exception.

**Propranolol** (**Inderal**) is likely to remain the gold standard because it is still so widely used and licensed for so many different indications, including angina, acute stage myocardial infarction, postinfarct follow-up, hypertension, arrhythmias, migraine prophylaxis, anxiety states, and essential tremor. However, propranolol is not beta$_1$-selective. Being lipid-soluble, it has a high brain penetration and undergoes extensive hepatic first-pass metabolism. Central side-effects may explain its poor performance in quality of life studies. Propranolol also has a short half-life so that it must be given twice daily unless the long-acting preparation is used.

Because of the above drawbacks, we see no particular advantage for this drug unless there is the coexistence of hypertension or angina with some other condition in which experience with propranolol is greater than with other beta-blockers (eg., hypertrophic cardiomyopathy, migraine prophylaxis, or essential tremor), or unless cost is a major consideration when generic propranolol should be used.

Other **beta-blockers** are increasingly used because of specific attractive properties: cardioselectivity (atenolol, metoprolol, acebutolol, and new agents such as bisoprolol, betaxolol and celiprolol); lipid-insolubility and no hepatic metabolism (atenolol, nadolol, sotalol); long action (nadolol > sotalol > atenolol); ISA to help avoid myocardial depression (pindolol, acebutolol); added alpha-blockade to achieve more arterial dilation and to neutralize the adverse effects of beta-blockade on the blood lipid profile (labetalol, carvedilol); and superior antiarrhythmic properties (sotalol). A new combination antihypertensive agent (bisoprolol-hydrochlorothiazide) aims to combine very low doses of two types of agents while maintaining antihypertensive efficacy and minimizing side-effects. Esmolol is the best agent for intravenous use in the peri-operative period because of its extremely short half-life.

It is clear that not all of these agents will have a wide market. Every clinician should become thoroughly familiar with only a limited number of beta-blocking agents, one of which must be cardioselective. Where side-effects are encountered, they can sometimes be avoided by a switch to another beta-blocker. Generally, if one agent in adequate dose will not work, nor will another; nor should one beta-blocker be added to another in the hope of improved therapeutic response, with the exception sometimes of a better response to vasodilatory beta-blockers, especially in black hypertensives. Probably smokers also respond better to the vasodilatory agents. *As concluded in previous editions of this book, in clinical practice the differences between existing beta-blockers are often relatively slight and hardly justify the vast commercial pressures applied in competitive promotion. In specific patients, ancillary properties such as cardioselectivity, long half-life, and vasodilation may be required.*

# References

*For references from Second Edition, see Opie et al. (1991)*

1.  Opie LH, Sonnenblick EH, Kaplan NM, Thadani U. Beta-blocking agents. In: Opie LH (ed), Drugs for the Heart, Third Edition. WB Saunders Company, Philadelphia, 1991, pp 1–25.

## References from Third Edition

2. Abernethy DR, Arendt RM, Greenblatt DJ. Am Heart J 1985; 109:1120–1125.
3. APSI Investigators. J Am Coll Cardiol 1990; 15:214A.
4. Barer DH, Cruickshank JM, Ebrahim SB, Mitchell JRA. Br Med J 1988; 296:737–741.
5. Brodsky MA, Allen BJ, Luckett CR, et al. Am Heart J 1989; 118:272–280.
6. Carlsen JE, Kober L, Heeboll-Nielsen NC. Drug Investigation 1989; 1:29–33.
7. Coffman JD, Rasmussen HM. Circulation 1985; 72:466–470.
8. Conant J, Engler R, Janowsky D, et al. J Cardiovasc Pharmacol 1989; 13:656–661.
9. Croog SH, Levine S, Testa MA, et al. N Engl J Med 1986; 314:1657–1664.
10. DeCesare N, Bartorelli A, Fabbiocchi F, et al. Am J Med 1989; 87:15–21.
11. Douglas-Jones AP, Baber NS, Lee A. Eur J Clin Pharmacol 1978; 14:163–166.
12. El-Tamimi H, Davies GJ, Kaski J-C, et al. Am J Cardiol 1989; 64:717–724.
13. Gerstenblith G, Ouyang P, Achuff SC, et al. N Engl J Med 1982; 306:885–889.
14. Gorczynski RJ, Quon CY, Krasula RW, et al. In: Scriabine A (ed). New Drugs Annual: Cardiovascular Drugs, Vol 3. Raven Press, New York, 1985, pp 99–119.
15. Guazzi M, Fiorentini C, Polese A, et al. Br Heart J 1975; 37:1235–1245.
16. Herrick A, Waller P, Berkin K, et al. Am J Med 1989; 86:421–426.
17. Hiatt WR, Stoll S, Nies AS. Circulation 1985; 72:1226–1231.
18. Hjalmarson A, Elmfeldt D, Herlitz J, et al. Lancet 1981; 2:823–827.
19. Holland Interuniversity Nifedipine/Metoprolol Trial (HINT) Research Group. Br Heart J 1986; 56:400–413.
20. ISIS-1 Group. Lancet 1986; 2:57–65.
21. Kostis JB, Lacy CR, Krieger SD, et al. Am Heart J 1984; 108:1131–1136.
22. Kostis JB, Rosen RC. Circulation 1987; 75:204–212.
23. Kraus ML, Gottlieb LD, Horwitz RI, Anscher M. N Engl J Med 1985; 313:905–909.
24. Kugiyama K, Yasue H, Horio Y, et al. Circulation 1986; 74:374–380.
25. Peart I, Bullock RE, Albers C, Hall RJC. Br Heart J 1989; 61:521–528.
26. Quyyumi AA, Crake T, Wright CM, et al. Br Heart J 1987; 57:505–511.
27. Robertson RM, Wood AJJ, Vaughn WK, Robertson D. Circulation 1982; 65:281–285.
28. Simpson WT. Postgrad Med J 1977; 53 (Suppl 3): 162–167.
29. Stone PH, Gibson RS, Glasser SP, et al. Circulation 1989; 80 (Suppl II): II-267.
30. Strauss WE, Parisi AF. Ann Intern Med 1988; 109:570–581.
31. Streufert S, DePadova A, McGlynn T, et al. Am Heart J 1988; 116:311–315.
32. Van den Meiracker AH, Man in 't Veld AJ, Ritsema van Eck HJ, et al. Circulation 1988; 78:957–968.
33. Walter P, Neil-Dwyer G, Cruickshank JM. Br Med J 1982; 284:1661–1664.

## New References

34. ASIS Group—Andrews TC, Fenton T, Toyosaki N, et al. for the Angina and Silent Ischemia Study Group (ASIS). Subsets of ambulatory myocardial ischemia based on heart rate activity. Circadian distribution and response to anti-ischemic medication. Circulation 1993; 88:92–100.
35. ASIST study (The Atenolol Silent Ischemia Study)—Pepine CJ, Cohn PF, Deedwania PC, et al. for the ASIST Study Group. Effects of treatment on outcome in mildly symptomatic patients with ischemia during daily life. Circulation 1994; 90:762–768.
36. Barnett DB. Beta-blockers in heart failure: a therapeutic paradox. Lancet 1994; 343:557–558.
37. Bristow MR, Hershberger RE, Port JD, Rasmussen R. Beta$_1$ and beta$_2$ adrenergic receptor-mediated adenylate cyclase stimulation in nonfailing and failing human ventricular myocardium. Mol Pharmacol 1989; 35:295.
38. Bristow MR, O'Connell JB, Gilbert EM, et al. Dose-response of chronic beta-blocker treatment in heart failure from either idiopathic dilated or ischemic cardiomyopathy. Circulation 1994; 89:1632–1642.
39. Collins R, Peto R, MacMahon S, et al. Blood pressure, stroke, and coronary heart disease. Part 2, short-term reductions in blood pressure: overview of randomised drug trials in their epidemiological context. Lancet 1990; 335:827–838.
40. Colucci WS, Ribeiro JP, Rocco MB, et al. Impaired chronotropic response to exercise in patient with congestive heart failure. Role of postsynaptic beta-adrenergic desensitization. Circulation 1989; 80:314–323.
41. Cruickshank JM, Lewis J, Moore V, Dodd C. Reversibility of left ventricular hypertrophy by differing types of antihypertensive therapy. J Human Hypertens 1992; 6:85–90.
42. Dujovne CA, Eff J, Ferraro L, et al. Comparative effects of atenolol versus celiprolol on serum lipids and blood pressure in hyperlipidemic and hypertensive subjects. Am J Cardiol 1993; 72:1131–1136.
43. ESVEM study—Mason JW for the Electrophysiologic Study Versus Electrocardiographic Monitoring. A comparison of seven antiarrhythmic drugs in patients with ventricular tachyarrhythmias. N Engl J Med 1993; 329:452–458.

44. Frishman WH, Bryzinski BS, Coulson LR, et al. A multifactorial trial design to assess combination therapy in hypertension: treatment with bisoprolol and hydrochlorothiazide. Arch Intern Med 1994, 154:1461–1468.

45. Frishman WH, Burris JF, Mroczek WJ, et al. First-line therapy option with low-dose bisoprolol fumarate and low-dose hydrochlorothiazide in patients with stage I and stage II systemic hypertension. J Clin Pharmacol 1994, in press.

46. Frohlich ED, Ketelhut R, Kaesser UR, et al. Hemodynamic effects of celiprolol in essential hypertension. Am J Cardiol 1991; 68:509–514.

47. Gilbert EM, Olsen SL, Renlund DG, Bristow MR. Beta-adrenergic receptor regulation and left ventricular function in idiopathic dilated cardiomyopathy. Am J Cardiol 1993; 71:23C–29C.

48. Hausdorff WP, Caron MG, Lefkowitz RJ. Turning off the signal: desensitization of beta-adrenergic receptor function. FASEB 1990; 4:2881–2889.

49. Henry JA, Cassidy SL. Membrane stabilising activity: a major cause of fatal poisoning. Lancet 1986; 1:1414–1417.

50. Hohnloser SH, Meinertz T, Klingenheben T, et al., for the European Esmolol Study Group. Usefulness of esmolol in unstable angina pectoris. Am J Cardiol 1991; 67:1319–1323.

51. Juul-Moller S, Edvardsson N, Jahnmatz B, et al. Double-blind trial of aspirin in primary prevention of myocardial infarction in patients with stable chronic angina pectoris. Lancet 1992; 340:1421–1425.

51A. Kennedy HL, Brooks MM, Barker AH, et al., for the CAST Investigators. Beta-blocker therapy in the Cardiac Arrhythmia Suppression Trial. Am J Cardiol 1994; 74:674–680.

52. Leeman M, van de Borne P, Collart F, et al. Bisoprolol and atenolol in essential hypertension: effects on systemic and renal hemodynamics and on ambulatory blood pressure. J Cardiovasc Pharmacol 1993; 22:785–791.

53. Lichstein E, Hager WD, Gregory JJ, et al., for the Multicenter Diltiazem Post-Infarction Research Group. Relation between beta-adrenergic blocker use, various correlates of left ventricular function and the chance of developing congestive heart failure. J Am Coll Cardiol 1990; 16:1327–1332.

54. Materson BJ, Reda DJ, Cushman WC, et al. Single-drug therapy for hypertension in men. A comparison of six antihypertensive agents with placebo. N Engl J Med 1993; 328:914–921.

55. Medical Research Council Working Party: Medical Research Council trial of treatment of mild hypertension: principal results. Br Med J 1985; 291:97–104.

56. Nadazdin A, Davies GJ. Investigation of therapeutic mechanisms of atenolol and diltiazem in patients with variable-threshold angina. Am Heart J 1994; 127:312–317.

57. National High Blood Pressure Education Program Working Group report on hypertension in diabetics. Hypertension 1994; 23:145–158.

58. Opie LH. Adverse cardiovascular drug interactions. In: Schlant RC, Alexander RW (eds), The Heart (8th edition). McGraw-Hill, New York, 1994, 1971–1985.

59. Parving H-H, Andersen AR, Smidt UM, Svendsen PA. Early aggressive antihypertensive treatment reduces rate of decline in kidney function in diabetic nephropathy. Lancet 1983; 1:1175–1178.

60. Pfeffer MA, Braunwald E, Moye LA, et al. Effect of captopril on mortality and morbidity in patients with left ventricular dysfunction after myocardial infarction. Results of the Survival and Ventricular Enlargement Trial. N Engl J Med 1992; 327:669–677.

61. Psaty BM, Savage PJ, Tell GS, et al. Temporal patterns of antihypertensive medication use among elderly patients. JAMA 1993; 270:1837–1841.

62. Rapaport E. Should beta-blockers be given immediately and concomitantly with thrombolytic therapy in acute myocardial infarction? Circulation 1991; 83:695–697.

63. Senior R, Imbs JL, Bory M, et al. Comparison of the effects of indapamide with hydrochlorothiazide, nifedipine, enalapril and atenolol on left ventricular hypertrophy in hypertension: A double-blind parallel study (abstr). J Am Coll Cardiol 1993; 21:57A.

64. SHEP Cooperative Research Group. Prevention of stroke by antihypertensive drug treatment in older persons with isolated systolic hypertension. Final results of the Systolic Hypertension in the Elderly Program (SHEP). JAMA 1991; 265:3255–3264.

65. Shettigar UR, Toole G, O'Came Appunn D. Combined use of esmolol and digoxin in the acute treatment of atrial fibrillation or flutter. Am Heart J 1993; 126:368–374.

66. Steinbeck G, Andresen D, Bach P, et al. A comparison of electrophysiologically guided antiarrhythmic drug therapy with beta-blocker therapy in patients with symptomatic, sustained ventricular tachyarrhythmias. N Engl J Med 1992; 327:987–992.

67. STOP study—Dahlof B, Lindholm LH, Hansson L, et al. Morbidity and mortality in the Swedish Trial in Old Patients with Hypertension (STOP-Hypertension). Lancet 1991; 338:1281–1285.

68. Teo KK, Yusuf S, Furberg D. Effects of prophylactic antiarrhythmic drug therapy in acute myocardial infarction. An overview of results from randomized controlled trials. JAMA 1993; 270:1589–1595.

69. Thadani U, Whitsett TL. Beta-adrenergic blockers and intermittent claudication. Arch Intern Med 1991; 151:1705–1707.

70. Theodorakis GN, Kremastinos DT, Stefanakis GS, et al. The effectiveness of beta-blockade and its influence on heart rate variability in vasovagal patients. Eur Heart J 1993; 14:1499–1507.

71. TIBET study—Dargie HJ, for the TIBET Study Group. Medical treatment of angina can favourably affect outcome (abstr). Eur Heart J 1993; 14 (Abstr Suppl): 304.

72. TIMI-IIB study—Roberts R, Rogers WJ, Mueller HS, et al., for the TIMI Investigators. Immediate versus deferred beta-blockade following thrombolytic therapy in patients with acute myocardial infarction. Results of the Thrombolysis in Myocardial Infarction (TIMI) II-B Study. Circulation 1991; 83:422–437.

73. Waagstein F, Bristow MR, Swedberg K, et al., for the Metoprolol in Dilated Cardiomyopathy (MDC) Trial Study Group. Beneficial effects of metoprolol in idiopathic dilated cardiomyopathy. Lancet 1993; 342:1441–1446.

74. Wassertheil-Smoller S, Oberman A, Blaufox MD, et al. The trial of antihypertensive interventions and management (TAIM) study. Final results with regard to blood pressure, cardiovascular risk, and quality of life. Am J Hypertens 1992; 5:37–44.

75. Wolfson S, Gorlin R. Cardiovascular pharmacology of propranolol in man. Circulation 1969; 40:501–511.

76. Yusuf S, Pepine CJ, Garces C, et al. Effect of enalapril on myocardial infarction and unstable angina in patients with low ejection fractions. Lancet 1992; 340:1173–1178.

## Book Chapter

77. Frishman WH, Sonnenblick EH. Beta-adrenergic blocking drugs. In: Schlant RC, Alexander RW (eds), The Heart, Arteries and Veins, Eighth Edition. McGraw-Hill, New York, 1994, 1271–1290.

# 2  Nitrates

U. Thadani ◆ L. H. Opie

*"As often true in matters of the heart, absence (nitrate-free intervals) makes the heart grow fonder (more nitrate responsiveness)."*[17]

## Mechanism of Action in Angina

In 1933 Sir Thomas Lewis held that the effect of amyl nitrite was probably due mainly to its powerful dilation of the coronary vessels, rather than to its effect in lowering the blood pressure, as had originally been suggested by Lauder Brunton in Scotland in 1867. As time went on, the important role of nitrate-induced venodilation came to be recognized. Currently, emphasis is on the endothelial-derived relaxation factor (EDRF), now known to be nitric oxide (NO•). Nitrates provide an exogenous source of NO• in the vascular cells, thereby inducing coronary vasodilation even when endogenous production of NO• is impaired by coronary artery disease. Chronic use of nitrates produces tolerance, a significant clinical problem still not fully understood. The main focus of current clinical work is on strategies to minimize or prevent the development of tolerance. The major proposal is that a nitrate-free or -low interval allows blood levels to fall and thereby to restore nitrate responsiveness.

### Vasodilatory Effects, Coronary and Peripheral

A distinction must be made between antianginal and coronary vasodilator properties. Nitrates dilate large coronary arteries and arterioles greater than 100 μm in diameter[38] to: (1) redistribute blood flow along collateral channels and from epicardial to endocardial regions and (2) relieve coronary spasm and dynamic stenosis, especially at epicardial sites,[1] including the coronary arterial constriction induced by exercise.[5] Thereby exercise-induced myocardial ischemia is relieved.[44A] Thus, nitrates are "effective" vasodilators for angina; dipyridamole and other vasodilators acting more distally in the arterial tree are not, rather having the risk of diverting blood from the ischemic area—a "coronary steal" effect.

The peripheral hemodynamic effects of nitrates, originally observed by Lauder Brunton, cannot be ignored. Nitrates do reduce the afterload, but especially the preload of the heart (Fig. 2–1). Hence, nitrates are now being used not only to treat angina pectoris but also to unload the heart in left ventricular (LV) failure and in selected cases of early-phase myocardial infarction.

### Reduced Oxygen Demand

Nitrates increase the venous capacitance, causing pooling of blood in the peripheral veins and thereby a reduction in venous return and in ventricular volume. There is less mechanical stress on the myocardial wall and the myocardial oxygen demand is reduced. Furthermore, a modest fall in arterial pressure also reduces the oxygen demand, although this benefit is offset by a reflex increase in heart rate. The tachycardia can be attenuated by concurrent beta-blockade.

ACTION OF NITRATES ON CIRCULATION

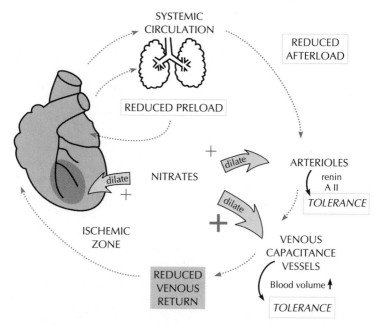

FIGURE 2–1.  Schematic diagram of effects of nitrate on the circulation. The major effect is on the venous capacitance vessels with additional coronary and peripheral arteriolar vasodilatory benefits. Fig. copyright L.H. Opie.

### Vascular Receptors

The cellular mechanism of these vascular effects may be as follows. An intact vascular endothelium is required for the vasodilatory effects of some vascular active agents (thus acetylcholine physiologically vasodilates but constricts when the endothelium is damaged). Nitrates vasodilate whether or not the endothelium is intact. The postulated but unidentified "nitrate receptor" is therefore likely to be situated on the myocyte rather than on the endothelium. Nitrates, after entering the vessel wall, are eventually converted by an unknown enzymatic mechanism[38] to nitric oxide (NO•), which is thought to stimulate guanylate cyclase to produce cyclic GMP (Fig. 2–2). Calcium in the vascular myocyte falls either by inhibition of calcium ion entry or by promotion of calcium exit and vasodilation results. Sulfhydryl (SH) groups are required for the formation of NO• and the stimulation of guanylate cyclase. Nitroglycerin powerfully dilates when injected into an artery, an effect that is probably limited in man by reflex vasoconstriction in response to concurrent preload reduction.[1] Hence nitrates are better venous than arteriolar dilators. The beneficial effect of nitrates in congestive heart failure (CHF) chiefly depends on venodilation.

### Antiplatelet Effect

A modest inhibitory effect on platelet aggregation can be found in patients with stable or unstable angina or recent AMI.[31,44] The failure of nitrates to alter the prognosis of patients with AMI in two megatrials (Chapter 5) suggests that this potential antithrombotic effect is not of crucial clinical significance when nitrates are given concurrently with aspirin.

## Pharmacokinetics of Nitrates

**Nitroglycerin (glyceryl trinitrate)**, the prototype nitrate, is absorbed from skin and oral mucosa and, less readily, from the gut.

NITRATE MECHANISM

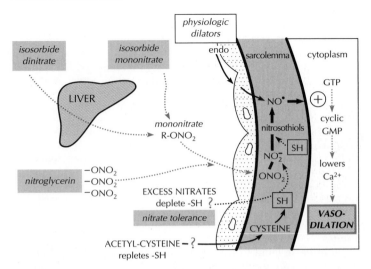

**FIGURE 2–2.** Effects of nitrates in generating NO˙ and stimulating guanylate cyclase to cause vasodilation. Note role of cysteine cascade in stimulating guanylate cyclase. Previously SH depletion was thought to explain nitrate tolerance. Note that mononitrates bypass hepatic metabolism. SH = sulfhydryl; GTP = guanosine triphosphate; GMP = guanosine monophosphate. (For further details, see Harrison and Bates;[38] Fung and Bauer[35]). Fig. copyright L.H. Opie.

There are five types of preparations: tablets, sprays, ointments, patches, and vials for intravenous infusion.

**Sublingual nitroglycerin tablets (Nitrostat;** others) have incomplete bioavailability, but clinical effects start within a minute or two and last up to an hour (Table 2–1); peak blood levels occur at 2 minutes, and the elimination half-life is 7 minutes.

**Nitroglycerin spray (Nitrolingual)** releases 0.4 mg per dose, and the vial contains 200 doses. Pharmacokinetically, equal doses of the spray and nitroglycerin tablets have equipotent effects.

**Oral nitroglycerin (Nitroglycerin SR capsules, Nitroglyn extended-release capsules).** These cannot be chewed nor taken sublingually. Poor bioavailability. No efficacy data for chronic use.

**Nitroglycerin extended-release buccal tablets (Nitrogard)** are placed under the lip or in the buccal pouch. Antianginal efficacy persists for 3 to 5 hours after a 3 mg tablet. Inadequate data on efficacy for chronic use after second and third doses given 5 hours apart.

**Nitroglycerin ointment (Nitrol, Nitro-Bid ointment 2%)** is slower in its onset of action. The antianginal effect is sustained for up to 7 hours (manufacturer's data), the amount of nitroglycerin absorbed depending on the surface area covered. The manufacturers suggest an initial dose of 7.5 mg spread over 6 × 6 inches or 15 × 15 cm, once in the morning and then 6 hours later, with a top dose of 20 mg twice daily. There is, however, no proof of efficacy during chronic use.

**Nitroglycerin patches (Nitrodur, Nitrodisc, Transderm-Nitro, Deponit, Minitran,** others) contain nitroglycerin in a reservoir or matrix and give plasma levels that are fairly constant from 2 to 24 hours or longer. The nitroglycerin content of the patches is variable, and the amount delivered is dependent upon the surface area covered by the patch.[1] For effort angina, intermittent therapy with the patch off at night is now standard. Initial doses are 0.2 to 0.4 mg/hour, up to 0.8 mg/hour or 10 mg/12 hours.[3]

**Intravenous nitroglycerin (Tridil, Nitro-Bid IV)** is given after dilution by infusion with a large and variable percentage adsorbed onto polyvinylchloride (PVC) tubing. The plasma half-life is about 3 minutes. Almost all hemodynamic effect is lost after 48 hours of continuous infusion (manufacturer's data).

**Isosorbide dinitrate** in tablet form (**Isordil, Sorbitrate**) is absorbed from the oral mucosa and gut, with slower onset and longer action than for nitroglycerin. After liver metabolism, the active mononitrate metabolites are ultimately excreted by the kidney, with a half-life of about 4 to 6 hours. Significant accumulation of intact isosorbide dinitrate occurs in plasma after 4 times daily dosing at 30 mg, 60 mg and 120 mg for 1 week.[1] The elimination half-life is about 60 minutes after a sublingual dose, and 4 hours after oral dosing. Metabolites of isosorbide dinitrate (i.e., 2- and 5-mononitrates) also contribute to its action with longer half-lives, up to 3 and 6 hours respectively. The efficacy of the first dose is sustained for 6 to 8 hours, but the antianginal duration of peak effects are attenuated during 3 or 4 times a day therapy.[1,26] Inadequate efficacy data for slow-release and sustained-release forms (**Isordil, Tembids, Sorbitrate SA**).[50]

**Intravenous isosorbide dinitrate** (not in the USA), like nitroglycerin, is lost to the infusion set. The elimination half-life is 18 to 139 minutes.[27]

**Mononitrate** tablets (**Monoket, Ismo, Imdur**) are logical successors to isosorbide dinitrate, because the latter's activity depends on hepatic conversion to mononitrates (Fig. 2–2). Thus with mononitrates the potentially variable effect of liver metabolism can be avoided; mononitrates have a high bioavailability with less variation in their effect when there is a fixed dose. Plasma levels of isosorbide-5-mononitrate reach their peak between 1/2 and 2 hours after the administration of the standard formulation (Monoket, Ismo) and the elimination half-life is 4 to 6 hours. After the first 20 mg dose the clinical efficacy lasts for 6 to 8 hours and correlates with the plasma concentration.[19] In the case of the slow-release formulation (**Imdur**), the plasma level peaks at 4 hours and the clinical efficacy is up to 12 hours after the 120 and 240 mg doses.

Mononitrates are excreted by the kidney, partially unchanged and partially as an inactive glucuronide metabolite. As with all nitrates, tolerance remains a problem when inappropriate dosing regimens are used.[50]

## Short-Acting Nitrates for Acute Effort Angina

**Sublingual nitroglycerin** is very well established in the initial therapy of angina of effort, yet may be ineffective, frequently because the patient has not received proper instruction. When angina starts, the patient should rest in the sitting position (standing promotes syncope, lying enhances venous return and heart work) and take sublingual nitroglycerin (0.3 to 0.6 mg) every 5 minutes until the pain goes or a maximum of 4 to 5 tablets have been taken. **Nitroglycerin spray** is an alternative mode of oral administration, which is more acceptable to some patients.

**Isosorbide dinitrate** may be given **sublingually** (5 mg) to abort an anginal attack and then exerts antianginal effects for about 1 hour. Because the dinitrate requires hepatic conversion to the mononitrate, the onset of antianginal action (mean time 3.4 minutes) must be slower than with nitroglycerin (mean time 1.9 minutes), so that the manufacturers of the dinitrate recommend sublingual administration of this drug only if the patient is unresponsive to or intolerant of sublingual nitroglycerin. After **oral** ingestion, hemodynamic and antianginal effects persist for several hours.[1] Single doses of isosorbide dinitrate confer longer protection against angina than can single doses of sublingual nitroglycerin (see Table 2–1).

(Isosorbide mononitrate is not available as a sublingual preparation for acute relief of angina).

# Long-Acting Nitrates for Angina Prophylaxis

Long-acting nitrates are not continuously effective if regularly taken over a prolonged period, unless allowance is made for a nitrate-free or -low interval.

**Isosorbide dinitrate** (oral preparation) is frequently given for the prophylaxis of angina. An important question is whether regular therapy with isosorbide dinitrate gives long-lasting protection against angina. Improvement in exercise tolerance for up to 3 hours during acute and for up to 5 hours during sustained therapy with isosorbide dinitrate has been reported.[1] In a crucial placebo-controlled study, exercise duration improved significantly for 6 to 8 hours after single oral doses of 15 to 120 mg isosorbide dinitrate, but for only 2 hours when the same doses were given repetitively 4 times daily.[1] Marked tolerance to the antianginal effects of 30 mg 4 times daily can develop during sustained therapy,[12] despite much higher plasma isosorbide dinitrate concentrations during sustained than during acute therapy.[1] Even treatment with 30 mg isosorbide dinitrate 3 times daily with the last dose at 6 pm produced progressive tolerance towards the second and third dose of the drug, so that exercise duration improved only transiently for 2 to 3 hours after the first and second doses.[26] Thus the total duration of antianginal action was only 6 hours. With the extended-release formulation of isosorbide dinitrate (**Tembids**), eccentric twice-daily treatment with a 40 mg dose administered in the morning and 7 hours later was not superior to placebo in a large multicenter study.[50] This result is in contrast to that of Silber et al.[18] who on the basis of ST-changes during exercise recommended two daily eccentric doses of Tembids; duration of exercise was not reported. Currently eccentric dosing schedules of the ordinary formulation of isosorbide dinitrate are recommended to avoid tolerance.[12] The *existing data are inadequate* to make definite recommendations regarding either the exact dose or the dosing schedule.[50]

**Mononitrates** have been compared with dinitrates in only a few clinical trials. The mean incidence of attacks of angina and use of nitroglycerin during the mononitrate therapy was lower than during medication with slow-release dinitrate or with placebo.[1] On the whole, the dosage and effects of mononitrates are similar to those of isosorbide dinitrate. Nitrate tolerance, likewise a potential problem,[1,19,20,21] can be prevented or minimized when rapid-release preparations (**Monoket, Ismo**) are given twice daily in an eccentric pattern with doses spaced by 7 hours.[47,53] Using the slow-release preparation (**Imdur**), patients in the active arm received either 30 mg, 60 mg, 120 mg or 240 mg once daily. Only the latter two doses improved exercise times at 4 and 12 hours after administration, even after 42 days of daily use.[29] These high doses were reached by titration over 7 days. A daily dose of 30 mg or 60 mg, often used in Europe, was ineffective.

**Transdermal nitroglycerin patches** are designed to permit the timed release of nitroglycerin over a 24-hour period. Despite initial claims of 24-hour efficacy, almost all recent studies have failed to show prolonged improvement.[51] The problem does not lie in premature patch exhaustion.[42] The decisive study was a multicenter FDA-monitored trial evaluating chronic patch therapy in 562 patients, using patches which delivered up to 105 mg of nitroglycerin over a 24-hour period. There was no improvement in treadmill exercise duration measured at 4 and 24 hours after patch application when compared with placebo.[55] Furthermore, in a British trial on 427 men, 5 mg nitroglycerin patches had no antianginal effect and actually decreased the quality of life as judged by the psychosocial score.[4] However, eccentric dosage schedules of patches do work[3] apparently without rebound at night in patients receiving concurrent beta-blockade.[34,39] In patients with unstable anginal syndromes, a coronary event can rarely be precipitated in the nitrate-free period.[22]

**TABLE 2–1**   NITRATE PREPARATIONS: DOSES, PREPARATIONS, AND DURATION OF EFFECTS

| COMPOUND | ROUTE | PREPARATION AND DOSE | DURATION OF EFFECTS AND COMMENTS |
|---|---|---|---|
| Amyl nitrite | Inhalation | 2–5 mg | 10 sec–10 min; for diagnosis of LV outflow obstruction in hypertrophic cardiomyopathy |
| Nitroglycerin (trinitrin, TNT, glyceryl trinitrate) | (a) Sublingual tablets | 0.3–0.6 mg up to 1.5 mg | Peak blood levels at 2 min; t 1/2 7 min; for acute therapy of effort or rest angina |
| | (b) Spray | 0.4 mg/metered dose, as needed | Similar to tablets at same dose. |
| | (c) Ointment | 2%; 6 × 6 ins or 15 × 15 cm or 7.5–40 mg | Apply 2 × daily; 6 h intervals; effect up to 7 h after first dose. No efficacy data for chronic use. |
| | (d) Transdermal patches | 0.2–0.8 mg/h patch on for 12 h, patch off for 12 h. | Effects start within 1–2 h, last 8–12 h during intermittent therapy. Not effective during continuous patch-on therapy. |
| | (e) Oral; sustained release | 2.5–13 mg 1–2 tablets 3 × daily | 4–8 h after first dose; no efficacy data for chronic therapy. |
| | (f) Buccal | 1–3 mg tablets 3 × daily | Effects start within minutes and last 3–5 h. No efficacy data for second or third doses during chronic therapy. |
| | (g) Intravenous infusion | 5–200 µg/min (care with PVC) Tridil 0.5 mg/ml or 5.0 mg/ml Nitro-bid IV 5 mg/ml | In unstable angina, increasing doses are often needed to overcome tolerance. High-concentration solutions contain propylene glycol; cross-reacts with heparin. |

| Drug | Route | Dose | Comments |
|---|---|---|---|
| **Isosorbide dinitrate** (= sorbide nitrate); Isordil | (a) Sublingual | 2.5–15 mg | Onset 5–10 min, effect up to 60 min |
| | (b) Oral tablets | 5–80 mg 2–3× daily | Up to 8 h (first dose; then tolerance) with 3× or 4× daily doses; 2× daily 7 h apart may be effective but data inadequate. |
| | (c) Spray | 1.25 mg on tongue | Rapid action 2–3 min |
| | (d) Chewable | 5 mg as single dose | Exercise time raised for 2 min–2.1/2 h. |
| | (e) Oral; slow-release | 40 mg once or 2× daily | Up to 8 h (first dose; 2x daily not superior to placebo)[50] |
| | (f) Intravenous infusion | 1.25–5.0 mg/h (care with PVC) | May need increasing doses for unstable angina at rest |
| | (g) Ointment | 100 mg/24 h | Not effective during continuous therapy |
| **Isosorbite-5-monotrate** | Oral tablets | 20 mg 2× day (7 h apart) | 12–14 h after chronic dosing for 2 weeks |
| | | 120–240 mg 1× daily (slow release) | Efficacy up to 12 h after 6 weeks |
| **Pentaerythritol tetranitrate** | Sublingual | 10 mg as needed | No efficacy data |
| **Erythrityl tetranitrate** | (a) Sublingual | 5–10 mg as needed | No efficacy data |
| | (b) Oral | 10–30 mg 3× daily, chew before swallowing | No efficacy data |

For references, see previous editions and text.

IV = intravenous, PVC = polyvinylchloride tubing.

TABLE 2–2      INTERVAL THERAPY FOR EFFORT ANGINA BY ECCENTRIC
NITRATE DOSAGE SCHEDULES DESIGNED TO AVOID TOLERANCE

| PREPARATION | DOSE | REFERENCE |
|---|---|---|
| Isosorbide dinitrate | 30 mg at 7 am, 1 pm* | 50 |
| Isosorbide mononitrate | 20 mg at 8 am and 3 pm | 47 |
| (Robins-Boehringer- | | 49 |
| Wyeth-Ayerst; | | 53 |
| Pharma-Schwarz) | | |
| Isosorbide mononitrate, | 120–240 mg daily | 29 |
| extended-release | | |
| (Key, Astra) | | |
| Transdermal nitrate | 7.5 –10 mg per 12 h | 3 |
| patches | patches removed after | |
| | 12 h | |
| Phasic release | 15 mg, most released | 11† |
| nitroglycerin patch | in first 12 h | |

* efficacy of second dose not established; no data for other doses.

† no data for other doses.

**Nitroglycerin paste** may be used for nocturnal angina or angina
at rest. Clearly, its nocturnal use cannot be combined with eccentric
therapeutic schedules, which work by providing a nocturnal nitrate-
free interval (see Table 2–2). For convenience, nitroglycerin paste is
applied to the skin of the chest. In AMI, it can be wiped off in the
event of an adverse reaction.

## Limitations: Side-effects and Nitrate Failure

SIDE-EFFECTS. The most common side-effect is the development of
headaches and the most serious side-effect is hypotension (Table
2–3). Sometimes the headaches pass over while antianginal efficacy
is maintained; yet often headaches lead to loss of compliance. Concomitant aspirin may protect from the headaches and from coronary
events. In chronic lung disease, arterial hypoxemia may result from
vasodilation and increased venous admixture. Occasionally, prolonged high-dose therapy can cause methemoglobinemia (Table
2–3).

FAILURE OF NITRATE THERAPY. With short-acting preparations, the most
common causes of failure are noncompliance (headaches), loss of
potency of the tablets, and incorrect timing (nitrates are more effective if taken before the expected onset of anginal pain). Sometimes
the diagnosis may be wrong, because nitrates also relieve the pain
of esophageal spasm and, sometimes, renal or biliary colic. Nitrates
may be less effective than expected owing to tachycardia, so that
combination with beta-blockade gives better results.

During therapy with long-acting preparations, two of the chief
causes of failure are (1) the development of tolerance, treated by
decreasing the frequency of drug administration until there is a
nitrate-free interval (see p 43); and (2) worsening of the underlying
disease process.

MANAGEMENT OF APPARENT FAILURE OF NITRATE THERAPY. Exclude poor
compliance (headaches), tolerance, and then step up therapy (Table
2–4) while excluding aggravating factors such as hypertension, thyrotoxicosis, atrial fibrillation or anemia.

## Nitrates for Mixed Angina and Silent Ischemia

**Mixed** or **double-component angina** means the combination of
nocturnal and effort angina. In a double-blind comparison of a beta-

**TABLE 2–3          PRECAUTIONS AND SIDE-EFFECTS IN USE OF NITRATES**

**Precautions**
Nitroglycerin tablets should be kept in *airtight containers.* Nitrate sprays are inflammable.

**Common Side-Effects**
**Headaches** frequently limit dose. Arterial tolerance may exceed that on the veins. Therefore, headaches may pass over while antianginal venous efficacy is sustained.[35] Headaches often respond to aspirin. Facial flushing. Sublingual nitrates may cause halitosis.

**Serious Side-Effects**
**Syncope** and **hypotension** from reduction of preload and afterload; alcohol or cotherapy with vasodilators may enhance. Treat by recumbency. **Tachycardia** frequent, but unexplained **bradycardia** occasionally arises in acute myocardial infarction. Hypotension may cause cerebral ischemia. Prolonged high dosage can cause **methemoglobinemia** (nitrate ions can oxidize hemoglobin to methemoglobin); treat by intravenous methylene blue (1–2 mg/kg). High-dose intravenous nitrates can induce **heparin resistance.**

**Contraindications**
In angina caused by **hypertrophic obstructive cardiomyopathy,** nitrates may exaggerate outflow obstruction and are contraindicated except for diagnosis. **Acute inferior myocardial infarction** with right ventricular involvement; fall in filling pressure may lead to hemodynamic and clinical deterioration.

**Relative Contraindications**
In **cor pulmonale** and arterial hypoxemia, nitrates decrease arterial $O_2$ tension by venous admixture. Although **glaucoma** is usually held to be a contraindication, there is no objective evidence to show any increase in intraocular pressure (possible exception: amyl nitrite).[1] **Cardiac tamponade** or constrictive pericarditis or tight mitral stenosis; the already compromised diastolic filling may be aggravated by reduced venous return.

**Tolerance**
Shown experimentally and clinically. Continuous therapy and high-dose frequent therapy leads to tolerance that eccentric dosage may avoid. Cross-tolerance established.

**Withdrawal Symptoms**
Established in munition workers, in whom withdrawal may precipitate symptoms and sudden death. Some evidence for a similar clinical syndrome. Therefore, only gradually discontinue long-term nitrate therapy. Recurrence of anginal pain in nitrate-free intervals during sustained therapy in some patients, but uncommon with beta-blocker cotherapy.

blocker (atenolol 100 mg daily), a calcium antagonist (nifedipine 20 mg 3 times daily), and isosorbide mononitrate (40 mg twice daily), the beta-blocker was best overall, although equal control of nocturnal ST-segment changes was achieved by all three agents. Pain relief was similar with nifedipine and isosorbide.[13]

In **silent myocardial ischemia,** although nitrates are effective electrocardiographically,[13] there is the same risk of development of tolerance as with overt angina, as judged by a study with transdermal nitroglycerin.[8]

TABLE 2–4    PROPOSED STEP-CARE FOR ANGINA OF EFFORT

1. **General:** History and physical examination to exclude valvular disease, anemia, hypertension, thromboembolic disease, thyrotoxicosis, and heart failure. Check risk factors for coronary artery disease (smoking, hypertension, blood lipids, diabetes). Must stop smoking. Give aspirin if not contraindicated.

2. **Intermittent nitrates,** short ± long-acting (eccentric doses) as needed to control pain. Combination therapy (next section) often introduced here.

3. **Combination nitrate therapy** with (1) beta-blocker (if not already used); or (2) calcium antagonist (preferably verapamil or diltiazem or long-acting dihydropyridine).

4. **Triple therapy.** Long-acting nitrates plus beta-blockers plus calcium antagonists. Use with caution when therapy with two agents ineffective.

5. **Consider bypass surgery** after failure to respond to medical therapy or for left main stem lesion or for triple vessel disease, especially if reduced LV function. Even response to medical therapy does not eliminate need for investigation.

6. **PTCA** may be attempted at any stage in selected patients, especially for highly symptomatic single vessel disease.

7. **Bepridil,** an atypical calcium antagonist, may as a last resort replace a standard agent (diltiazem, verapamil, dihydropyridine). Risk of torsades de pointes mandates monitoring QT-interval and exclusion of hypokalemia.

When using **prophylactic long-acting nitrates** in a dose schedule known to avoid tolerance, intermittent short-acting nitrates are still added as needed.

## Nitrates for Unstable Angina at Rest

*"The one setting in which intermittent nitrate therapy does not have a role is the treatment of the hospitalized patient with unstable ischemic symptoms with or without myocardial infarction."*[14]

In the therapy of unstable angina, it is presumed that upward titration of the dose of intravenous nitrate can overcome tolerance,[52] as also in the case of AMI.[43] Nonetheless, the manufacturers warn that continuous use of nitroglycerin leads to almost complete loss of hemodynamic effect (blood pressure reduction) within 48 hours. Nitroglycerin is preferred to isosorbide dinitrate, as it has a more rapid onset and offset of action.

**Intravenous nitroglycerin** is very effective in the management of pain in patients with unstable angina, although there is surprisingly little objective evidence of such efficacy in properly controlled trials. Intravenous therapy allows more rapid titration to an effective dose and the use of nitroglycerin rather than isosorbide dinitrate permits rapid reversal of hemodynamic effects if an adverse reaction occurs. The usual initial starting dose is 5 to 10 μg/min, which can be titrated up to 200 μg/min or occasionally higher up to 1,000 μg/min, depending on the clinical course and aiming at the relief of anginal pain. In patients who are already pain-free, the aim is a fall of mean blood pressure by 10%, the infusion being maintained for up to 36 hours.[1] A problem in dosing is that nitroglycerin is readily absorbed (40% to 80%) by PVC tubing, but not onto polyethylene or glass. **Nitrostat infusion sets** use nonabsorbent materials. The result is that the calculated dose will in fact be delivered to the patient, so that substantially lower doses than in many published series will be effective.

**Intravenous isosorbide dinitrate** (not in the USA), infused in patients with repetitive episodes of angina at rest at a rate of 1.25 to 5.0 mg/hour, relieves pain and reduces the incidence of ischemic episodes as judged by spontaneous ST-deviations[1] with few side-effects. Why the intravenous route is so much more effective than the oral route is not well understood. However, the blood levels are almost $10\times$ higher for equivalent doses given intravenously than when given orally,[1] stressing the poor bioavailability of oral isosorbide dinitrate, due to extensive presystemic metabolism.

**Nitrate patches** and **nitroglycerin ointment** are still frequently used in unstable angina at rest despite any good evidence that the development of tolerance can be avoided. As there is no role for intermittent nitrate therapy in unstable angina, eccentric dosage schedules cannot be used. Intravenous therapy, which can be titrated upwards as needed, is far better for control of pain.

INTERACTION WITH HEPARIN.   In patients receiving both drugs, the dose of heparin required is often higher than anticipated; i.e., there is **heparin resistance.**[41] The problem lies in the propylene glycol used in some intravenous nitroglycerin formulations (eg., Nitro-Bid IV, Tridil 25 to 100 mg). The dose of nitroglycerin required to produce heparin resistance is relatively high ($> 350$ μg/min).

INTRACORONARY NITROGLYCERIN.   This is often used to avoid coronary spasm during PTCA. Some nitrate solutions contain high potassium that may precipitate ventricular fibrillation.

## Acute Myocardial Infarction

SUBLINGUAL NITROGLYCERIN.   When the patient presents with acute prolonged ischemic-type pain in the emergency room, it is often not possible to know whether the diagnosis is unstable angina or early phase AMI. While setting up the intravenous line, sublingual nitroglycerin is often given against ischemic pain. These agents do, however, have the risk of excess hypotension and occasional unexpected bradycardia. Hence intravenous therapy with slow dose titration is preferable.

INTRAVENOUS NITROGLYCERIN.   Although nitrates are often given intravenously at the onset of AMI, there is ongoing controversy about their possible long-term benefit. Several small studies have suggested that intravenous nitrates reduce mortality,[23] acting by reduction of infarct size, lessened infarct expansion, improved LV remodeling, and fewer infarct-related complications.[43] On the other hand, the recent megatrials in AMI, such as ISIS-4[40] and GISSI-3,[37] have shown that routine nitrates do not improve the average case when added to thrombolytic therapy and aspirin. The difference probably lies in the fact that the small series studied more acutely ill patients with more compromised LV function, whereas these two megatrials included low-risk patients. Also, the dose of mononitrate chosen in the ISIS-4 study (**Imdur** 60 mg daily) was probably too low to have had the desired effects.[29] The choice of intravenous nitroglycerin for the first 24 hours in GISSI-3 was probably better, and it was titrated to reduce the blood pressure and followed by prolonged intermittent patch therapy. Nonetheless, there was no obvious benefit.[37]

*At present it would seem prudent to limit the use of intravenous nitrates in AMI to those complicated patients* with ongoing anginal pain, for large anterior infarcts when LV end-diastolic pressure is invariably elevated and would benefit from unloading, for those with LV failure (combined with ACE inhibition, see below) or severe hypertension, or when the differential diagnosis between early transmural AMI and Prinzmetal's angina is not clear. Initial low-dose therapy is required to avoid excess hypotension (blood pressure $< 90$ mmHg). Nitroglycerin 5 μg/min is increased by 5 to 20 μg/min every 5 to 10 minutes to a ceiling of 200 μg/min (using standard intravenous

PVC sets with glass bottles) until the mean blood pressure is reduced by 10% in normotensives and by 30% in hypertensives.[43] The infusion is maintained for 24 hours[37] or longer.[43] It is not clear whether prolonging the nitrate infusion beyond 12 hours, when the blood pressure effect ceases, achieves benefit on LV size as claimed by Jugdutt.[43] The major danger is hypotension, when the infusion must be stopped abruptly and restarted at 5 μg/min. Otherwise, to discontinue, taper down. When doses of 200 μg/min fail to reduce the blood pressure, there is nitrate resistance and the infusion should be abandoned.[43] After the acute phase, oral nitroglycerin can be given at doses titrated to reduce the blood pressure by 10% for 6 weeks,[43] or transdermal nitroglycerin patches (off at night) used as in GISSI-3.[37]

**Combination therapy** by ACE inhibition with early intravenous nitroglycerin followed by intermittent nitroglycerin patches was successfully used in GISSI-3 to reduce mortality by 17% (2P < 0.003), a substantial figure that cannot be ignored. This combination merits further evaluation. At present it would appear to be the therapy of choice for clinically evident LV failure in the acute stage.

INTRAVENOUS LINSIDOMINE. In a large European study,[33] this new NO• donor followed by molsidomine for 12 days was ineffective in reducing mortality. These data further argue against the routine use of nitrates in AMI.

## Congestive Heart Failure

Both short- and long-acting nitrates are used as unloading agents in the relief of symptoms in acute and chronic heart failure. Their dilating effects are more pronounced on veins than on arterioles, so they are best suited to patients with raised pulmonary wedge pressure and clinical features of pulmonary congestion.

In **acute pulmonary edema** from various causes, including AMI, nitroglycerin can be strikingly effective, with some risk of precipitous falls in blood pressure and of tachycardia or bradycardia. Sublingual nitroglycerin in repeated doses of 0.8 to 2.4 mg every 5 to 10 minutes can relieve coarse rales and dyspnea within 15 to 20 minutes, with a fall of LV filling pressure and a rise in cardiac output.[1] Intravenous nitroglycerin, however, is usually a better method to administer nitroglycerin, as the dose can be rapidly adjusted upward or downward depending upon the clinical and hemodynamic response. Doses required may be higher than the maximal use for AMI (i.e., above 200 μg/min[43]). Little has been reported on the combination of nitrates with conventional therapy in acute pulmonary edema.

In **severe CHF,** nitrates may be used as the sole vasodilator agent,[1] or added to ACE inhibitors[45] or hydralazine. Combination of high-dose isosorbide dinitrate (60 mg 4 times daily) plus hydralazine, better than placebo in decreasing mortality, was nonetheless inferior to an ACE inhibitor in severe CHF (VeHeFT-II trial, p 115). Dinitrate-hydralazine may, therefore, be chosen when a patient cannot tolerate an ACE inhibitor, while nitrates without hydralazine are selected for relief of pulmonary symptoms.

In **mild CHF,** already treated by an ACE inhibitor and diuretics, added isosorbide dinitrate in eccentric doses did not help.[56]

**Nitrate tolerance** remains a problem. Intermittent dosing, designed to counter periods of expected dyspnea (at night, anticipated exercise), is one sensible policy. Escalating doses of nitrates provide another short-term solution.[46] A third solution is cotherapy with ACE inhibitors or hydralazine or both possibly to blunt nitrate tolerance.[35]

**Nitrate patches** have given variable results in CHF. Tolerance is inevitable with sustained-release patches.[6] Of note is that **intravenous nitroglycerin** (6.4 μg/kg/min) produces tolerance with continuous but not with interrupted infusions.[10] Nonetheless, as expected, the pulmonary capillary pressure is elevated during the nitrate-free interval—not a desirable situation.

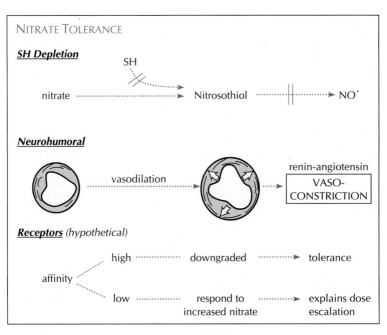

**FIGURE 2–3.** Current proposals for mechanism of nitrate tolerance. The SH depletion hypothesis is shown in Fig. 2–2. Neurohumoral activation is thought to occur as a result of nitrate-induced vasodilation, possibly involving reflex arterial constriction and impaired renal blood flow. Although nitrate receptors are still hypothetical, downgraded high-affinity receptors (responding to low concentrations of nitrates) and maintained activity of low-affinity receptors (responding to increased concentrations of nitrates) could explain the mechanism of dose escalation. Fig. copyright L.H. Opie.

## Nitrate Tolerance

As already outlined, nitrate tolerance often limits nitrate efficacy. Thus, longer-acting nitrates, while providing higher and better-sustained blood nitrate levels, paradoxically often seem to lose their efficacy with time. This is the phenomenon of nitrate tolerance. The mechanisms involved have remained elusive.[35]

**Vascular sulfhydryl depletion** is the classical theory. SH groups, derived from cysteine, are required for the intracellular formation of NO•, the active moiety stimulating guanylate cyclase (Fig. 2–2). Hypothetically, excess NO• formation depletes intracellular SH groups. Sulfhydryl donors, such as **acetylcysteine** or **methionine,** may counteract tolerance either by providing SH groups, or by forming extracellular thiols, which could enter the vascular cells to stimulate guanylate cyclase.[35] In human volunteers, acetylcysteine gives some protection against nitrate tolerance in veins but not in medium-sized arteries.[28] Similar studies on patients with angina using effort tolerance as an end-point are lacking.

The current **neurohumoral hypothesis** (Fig. 2–3) proposes that venous dilation leads to compensatory vasoconstriction, probably in part the result of activation of the renin-angiotensin and adrenergic systems.[35] In CHF, plasma catecholamines and renin activity increase during a prolonged nitroglycerin infusion, and atrial natriuretic peptide levels decrease.[32] Possibly, marked venous dilation induced by nitrates could cause a reflex arterial vasoconstriction with a reduction in renal perfusion and function.[35] Intravascular volume might increase as fluid shifts from the extravascular compartment in response to venodilation.[32]

Hypothetically, **high- and low-affinity nitrate receptors** might exist. Some evidence suggests that it is not always the absolute nitrate levels that cause vasodilation, but rather a sudden increase in levels. According to the receptor theory, the high-affinity receptors might first be downgraded, leaving low-affinity receptors to interact with the rising blood nitrate levels.

## Prevention of Nitrate Tolerance

DOSING SCHEDULES.  **Interval dosing** with eccentric doses is the simplest and most reliable procedure (Fig. 2–3).[15,50] In effort angina, many studies now show that tolerance can be avoided by interval dosing, which may explain why some nitrate efficacy seems to be kept during chronic sustained oral therapy (seesaw blood levels) in contrast to loss of efficacy with nitrate patches (sustained blood levels). **Rapidly increasing blood nitrate levels** may overcome tolerance.[49] For example, with established nitrate tolerance, sublingual nitrate can still have some therapeutic effect, albeit diminished.[15,51] During treatment of unstable angina or CHF, some propose that dose escalation may be a short-term maneuver to bypass tolerance.[46,52] In early phase AMI, only modest dose escalation is needed.[43] Occasionally there is total nitrate resistance (blood pressure will not fall).[43]

MONONITRATES AND TOLERANCE.  Eccentric twice-daily doses, spaced by 7 hours, with 20 mg of rapid-release formulation of isosorbide mononitrate (**Monoket, Ismo**) or once-daily treatment with 120 or 240 mg of the extended-release formulation of mononitrate (**Imdur**) prevents tolerance and is not associated with any rebound increase in nocturnal angina nor any deterioration of exercise performance each morning prior to administration of the morning dose.[29,47,50,53] These dosing schedules nonetheless increase exercise for a period of only 12 to 14 hours after the morning dose and leave patients unprotected at night and during the early hours of the morning.[50,53]

OTHER PROPOSALS TO AVOID TOLERANCE.  Phasic delivery systems are a logical development to achieve therapeutic benefit with nitrate patches even when left on for 24 hours.[11] Definitive studies with different doses are still lacking.

**Sulfhydryl donors,** such as N-acetylcysteine, only achieve partial reversal of tolerance.[10,35]

**Angiotensin-converting enzyme inhibitors** are logical in the prevention of renin-induced vasoconstriction, especially in CHF; there is no evidence that captopril with SH groups is more protective than enalapril without.[35] Sometimes the ACE inhibitor does not work.[30,32]

**Hydralazine** is logical, especially in CHF, to overcome the impaired renal perfusion thought to contribute to nitrate tolerance.[35] Concomitant use of hydralazine and isosorbide dinitrate could explain the benefit of this regime in CHF despite the chronic use of doses of isosorbide that should have evoked tolerance.[35] In angina, it is much less likely that renal perfusion could be critical and, furthermore, hydralazine-induced tachycardia could be undesirable.

**Diuretics** have been tried (with variable success) because water and sodium retention may occur during nitrate tolerance.[35]

## Nitrate Cross-Tolerance

Short- and long-acting nitrates are frequently combined. In patients already receiving isosorbide dinitrate, addition of sublingual nitroglycerin gives a further small (10%) therapeutic effect.[1] Logically, tolerance to long-acting nitrates should cause cross-tolerance to short-acting nitrates, as shown for the capacitance vessels of the forearm,[1] coronary artery diameter[9] and on exercise tolerance during intravenous nitroglycerin therapy.[24] Cross-tolerance to sublingual nitroglycerin (no change in blood pressure, heart rate) is proposed as a simple clinical test for nitrate tolerance.[2]

### Tolerance: Summary of Evidence

Present data do not give assurance that cotherapy with sulfhydryl donors, ACE inhibitors, hydralazine or diuretics can prevent tolerance. Rather only the nitrate-free or -low interval works consistently.

## Step-care for Angina of Effort

A full history and physical examination is required to exclude a host of remediable factors (Table 2–4), not forgetting aortic stenosis that may be occult in the elderly. Risk factors must be managed and aspirin given. Nitrates remain the basis of symptomatic control of angina. Various combinations of short- and long-acting nitrates with beta-blockers and/or calcium antagonists are the successive choices, with bepridil as a last ditch stand. PTCA and bypass surgery are taken as escape routes when coronary anatomy is appropriate. There are no long-term outcome studies on the benefits of nitrates alone in angina pectoris.

## Combination Therapy for Angina

Existing data are inadequate to evaluate the overall efficacy of the combination of nitrates plus beta-blockers or calcium antagonists, when compared with optimal therapy by any one agent alone.[50]

**Beta-blockade and nitrates** are, nonetheless, usually combined in the therapy of angina (Table 2–4). Both beta-blockers and nitrates decrease the oxygen demand, and nitrates increase the oxygen supply; beta-blockade cancels the tachycardic effect of nitrates. Beta-blockade tends to increase heart size, and nitrates to decrease it. Anginal patients receiving beta-blockers are better able to withstand pacing-stress when nitroglycerin is added,[1] and patients already receiving beta-blockade respond no less well than others to nitroglycerin or isosorbide dinitrate.[1,50] Furthermore, it is of interest that isosorbide dinitrate, when added to propranolol in a standard noneccentric dose (mean 90 mg/day) for 3 weeks, reduced the number of symptomatic anginal attacks when compared with propranolol alone.[1]

**Calcium antagonists and short-acting nitroglycerin** are commonly combined. In a double-blind trial of 47 patients with effort angina, verapamil 80 mg 3 times daily decreased the use of nitroglycerin tablets by 25% and prolonged exercise time by 20%.[1]

**Calcium antagonists and long-acting nitrates** are also often given together. Yet, there are no studies evaluating the objective benefits of current eccentric dosing schedules of long-acting nitrates plus calcium antagonists.[50] Long-acting nitrates are more readily combined with verapamil or diltiazem rather than with nifedipine, because of the powerful and sometimes excessive pre- and afterload reduction achieved by the latter combination. In contrast, nifedipine and all other dihydropyridines combine better with beta-blockers.

**Nitrates, beta-blockers, and calcium antagonists** may also be combined as triple therapy, frequently deemed to be "maximal." Triple therapy may be no more effective or even less effective than any two of the components,[25] possibly because of excess hypotension. Triple therapy should not be automatic when dual therapy fails because of individual variations among patients, so that some will tolerate one type of combination therapy better than another. Thus various combinations of dual therapy should first be explored.

*Bepridil* is an atypical calcium antagonist (pp 3–36) that is a logical choice when the patient is refractory to conventional triple therapy and not suited for revascularization.[48] To hold off torsades de pointes, hypokalemia and excessive QT prolongation must be avoided.

## New Antianginal Agents

None of these are yet approved for use in the USA or UK.

**Molsidomine** acts by release of vasodilatory metabolites such as SIN-1 formed during first-pass liver metabolism. These metabolites bypass the cysteine-dependent metabolic cascade and, therefore, should provide substantial protection from tolerance. However, strict comparisons with nitrates are not yet available. In a dose of 2 mg 3 times daily, this agent is widely used in Germany. In the ESPRIM post-AMI study,[33] the daily dose was 16 mg.

**Pirisidomine** is a NO⋅ donor and under evaluation for the treatment of angina pectoris.

**Linsidomine,** given intravenously, is slightly less effective than intravenous isosorbide dinitrate in relief of unstable angina.[36]

**Nicorandil** is a nicotinamide nitrate, acting chiefly by dilation of the large coronary arteries, as well as by reduction of pre- and afterload. It has a double cellular mechanism of action, acting both as a potassium channel activator and having a nitrate-like effect,[16] which may explain why experimentally it causes less tolerance than nitrates. It is widely used as an antianginal agent in Japan in a dose of 10 to 20 mg 12-hourly.[7] In the USA, however, nicorandil 10 or 20 mg twice daily was not superior to placebo in patients with stable effort angina.[54]

## Summary

Nitrates act by venodilation and relief of coronary vasoconstriction (including that induced by exercise) to ameliorate anginal attacks. Their unloading effects also benefit patients with CHF and high LV filling pressures. Some newer nitrate preparations are not a substantial advance over the old, especially not the nitrate patches, which clearly predispose to tolerance by sustained blood nitrate levels. Mononitrates, now available in the USA, are an advance over dinitrates because they eliminate variable hepatic metabolism on which the action of the dinitrates depends, and because the dose schedule required to avoid tolerance has been well studied. Yet with all nitrate preparations the fundamental problem of potential tolerance remains. The mechanism of such tolerance seems increasingly complex. During the treatment of effort angina by isosorbide dinitrate or mononitrate, substantial evidence suggests that eccentric doses with a nitrate-free interval go far to avoid tolerance.

For unstable angina at rest, a nitrate-free interval is not possible, and short-term treatment for 24 to 48 hours with intravenous nitroglycerin is frequently effective with, however, higher and higher doses often required to overcome tolerance. In AMI, the use of intravenous nitrates for selected and more ill patients must be differentiated from the failure of fixed-dose nitrates in mass trials. Yet the combination of an ACE inhibitor with first intravenous and then oral nitrates gave a 17% mortality reduction in one of these megatrials. It is suggested that intravenous nitrates be reserved for specific, more complicated patients, including those receiving ACE inhibitors in the acute phase. During the treatment of CHF, tolerance also develops, so that nitrates are best reserved for specific problems such as acute LV failure, nocturnal dyspnea, or anticipated exercise. Two new antianginal agents, pirsidomine and nicorandil, are still undergoing evaluation.

# References

*For references from Second Edition, see Thadani and Opie (1991)*

1.  Thadani U, Opie LH. Nitrates. In: Opie LH (ed), Drugs for the Heart, Third Edition. WB Saunders Company, Philadelphia, 1991, 26–41.

## References from Third Edition

2.  Amidi M, Shaver JA. Circulation 1989; 80 (Suppl II):II–214.
3.  DeMots H, Glasser SP. J Am Coll Cardiol 1989; 13:786–793.
4.  Fletcher A, McLoone P, Bulpitt C. Lancet 1988; 2:4–8.
5.  Gage JE, Jess DM, Murakami T, et al. Circulation 1986; 73:865–876.
6.  Lindvall K, Eriksson SV, Lagerstrand L, Sjogren A. Eur Heart J 1988; 9:373–379.
7.  Meany TB, Richardson P, Camm AJ. Am J Cardiol 1989; 63:66J-70J.
8.  Nabel EG, Barry J, Rocco MB, et al. Am J Cardiol 1989; 63:663–669.
9.  Naito H, Matsuda Y, Shiomi K, et al. Am J Cardiol 1989; 64:565–568.
10. Packer M, Lee WH, Kessler PD, et al. N Engl J Med 1987; 317:799–804.
11. Parker JO. Eur Heart J 1989; 10 (Suppl A):43–49.
12. Parker JO, Farrell B, Lahey KA, et al. N Engl J Med 1987; 316:1440–1444.
13. Quyyumi AA, Crake T, Wright CM, et al. Br Heart J 1987; 57:505–511.
14. Reichek N. Eur Heart J 1989; 10 (Suppl A):7–10.
15. Rudolph W, Dirschinger J, Reiniger G, et al. Eur Heart J 1988; 9 (Suppl A):63–72.
16. Sakai K. Am J Cardiol 1989; 63:2J-10J.
17. Schaer DH, Buff LA, Katz RJ. Am J Cardiol 1988; 61:46–50.
18. Silber S, Vogler AC, Krause K-H, et al. Am J Med 1987; 83:860–870.
19. Thadani U, Prasad R, Hamilton SF, et al. Am J Cardiol 1987; 59:756–762.
20. Thadani U, Bittar N, Doyle R, et al. Circulation 1989; 80 (Suppl II):II-215.
21. Thadani U, Friedman R, Jones JP, et al. Circulation 1989; 80 (Suppl II):II-216.
22. Waters DD, Juneau M, Gossard D, et al. J Am Coll Cardiol 1989; 13:421–425.
23. Yusuf S, Collins R, MacMahon S, Peto R. Lancet 1988; 1:1088–1092.
24. Zimrin D, Reichek N, Bogin KT, et al. Circulation 1988; 77:1376–1384.

## New References

25. Akhras F, Jackson G. Efficacy of nifedipine and isosorbide mononitrate in combination with atenolol in stable angina. Lancet 1991; 338:1036–1039.
26. Bassan MM. The daylong pattern of the antianginal effect of long-term three times daily administered isosorbide dinitrate. J Am Coll Cardiol 1990; 16:936–940.
27. Bogaert MG. Clinical pharmacokinetics of nitrates. Cardiovasc Drugs Ther 1994; 8:693–700.
28. Boesgaard S, Iversen HK, Wroblewski H, et al. Altered peripheral vasodilator profile of nitroglycerin during long-term infusion of N-acetylcysteine. J Am Coll Cardiol 1994; 23:163–169.
29. Chrysant SG, Glasser SP, Bittar N, et al. Efficacy and safety of extended-release isosorbide mononitrate for stable effort angina pectoris. Am J Cardiol 1993; 72:1249–1256.
30. Dakak N, Makhoul N, Flugelman MY, et al. Failure of captopril to prevent nitrate tolerance in congestive heart failure secondary to coronary artery disease. Am J Cardiol 1990; 66:608–613.
31. Diodati J, Theroux P, Latour J-G, et al. Effects of nitroglycerin at therapeutic doses on platelet aggregation in unstable angina pectoris and acute myocardial infarction. Am J Cardiol 1990; 66:683–688.
32. Dupuis J, Lalonde G, Lemieux R, Rouleau JL. Tolerance to intravenous nitroglycerin in patients with congestive heart failure: role of increased intravascular volume, neurohumoral activation and lack of prevention with N-acetylcysteine. J Am Coll Cardiol 1990; 16:923–931.
33. ESPRIM (European Study of Prevention of Infarct with Molsidomine (ESPRIM) Group. The ESPRIM trial: short-term treatment of acute myocardial infarction with molsidomine. Lancet 1994; 344:91–97.
34. Fox KM, Dargie HJ, Deanfield J, Maseri A on behalf of the Transdermal Nitrate Investigators. Avoidance of tolerance and lack of rebound with intermittent dose titrated transdermal glyceryl trinitrate. Br Heart J 1991; 66:151–155.
35. Fung H-L, Bauer JA. Mechanisms of nitrate tolerance. Cardiovasc Drugs Ther 1994; 8:489–499.
36. Giraud T. Unstable angina: A multicenter comparative study of linsidomine and isosorbide dinitrate (abstr). J Am Coll Cardiol 1994; 23:289A.
37. GISSI-3 (Gruppo Italiano per lo Studio della Sopravvivenza nel'Infarto Miocardico). GISSI-3: effects of lisinopril and transdermal glyceryl trinitrate singly and together on 6-week mortality and ventricular function after acute myocardial infarction. Lancet 1994; 343:1115–1122.
38. Harrison DG, Bates JN. The nitrovasodilators. New ideas about old drugs. Circulation 1993; 87:1461–1467.

39. Holdright DR, Katz RJ, Wright CA, et al. Lack of rebound during intermittent transdermal treatment with glyceryl trinitrate in patients with stable angina on background beta-blocker. Br Heart J 1993; 69:223–227.

40. ISIS-4 Fourth International Study of Infarct Survival. Ferguson JJ. Meeting highlights. Circulation 1994; 89:545–547.

41. Jaffrani NA, Ehrenpreis S, Laddu A, Somberg J. Therapeutic approach to unstable angina: Nitroglycerin, heparin, and combined therapy. Am Heart J 1993; 126:1239–1242.

42. James MA, Papouchado M, Jones JV. Attenuation of nitrate effect during an intermittent treatment regimen and the time course of nitrate tolerance. Eur Heart J 1991; 12:1266–1272.

43. Jugdutt BI. Nitrates in myocardial infarction. Cardiovasc Drugs Ther 1994; 8:635–646.

44. Lacoste LL, Theroux P, Lidon R-M, et al. Antithrombotic properties of transdermal nitroglycerin in stable angina pectoris. Am J Cardiol 1994; 73:1058–1062.

44A. Mahmarian JJ, Fenimore NL, Marks GF, et al. Transdermal nitroglycerin patch therapy reduces the extent of exercise-induced myocardial ischemia: Results of a double-blind, placebo-controlled trial using quantitative thallium-201 tomography. J Am Coll Cardiol 1944; 24:25–32.

45. Mehra A, Ostrzega E, Shotan A, et al. Persistent hemodynamic improvement with short-term nitrate therapy in patients with chronic congestive heart failure already treated with captopril. Am J Cardiol 1992; 70:1310–1314.

46. Mehra A, Ostrzega E, Shotan A, et al. Overcoming early nitrate tolerance with escalating oral dose of isosorbide dinitrate in chronic heart failure (abstr). J Am Coll Cardiol 1993; 21:252A.

47. Parker JO and the Isosorbide-5-Mononitrate Study Group. Eccentric dosing with isosorbide-5-mononitrate in angina pectoris. Am J Cardiol 1993; 72:871–876.

48. Singh BN for the Bepridil Collaborative Study Group. Comparative efficacy and safety of bepridil and diltiazem in chronic stable angina pectoris refractory to diltiazem. Am J Cardiol 1991; 68:306–312.

49. Thadani U, Bittar N. Effects of 8:00 a.m. and 2:00 p.m. doses of isosorbide-5-mononitrate during twice-daily therapy in stable angina pectoris. Am J Cardiol 1992; 70:286–292.

50. Thadani U, Lipicky RJ. Short and long-acting oral nitrates for stable angina pectoris. Cardiovasc Drugs Ther 1994; 8:611–623.

51. Thadani U, Lipicky RJ. Ointments and transdermal nitroglycerin patches for stable angina pectoris. Cardiovasc Drugs Ther 1994; 8:625–633.

52. Thadani U, Opie LH. Nitrates for unstable angina. Cardiovasc Drugs Ther 1994; 8:719–726.

53. Thadani U, Maranda CR, Amsterdam E, et al. Lack of pharmacologic tolerance and rebound angina pectoris during twice-daily therapy with isosorbide-5-mononitrate. Ann Intern Med 1994; 120:353–359.

54. Thadani U, Strauss W, Glasser SP, et al. Evaluation of antianginal and anti-ischemic efficacy of nicorandil: results of a multicenter study (abstr). J Am Coll Cardiol 1994; 23:267A.

55. Transdermal Nitroglycerin Cooperative Study. Acute and chronic antianginal efficacy of continuous twenty-four-hour application of transdermal nitroglycerin. Am J Cardiol 1991; 68:1263–1273.

56. Wieshammer S, Hetzel M, Hetzel J, et al. Lack of effect of nitrates on exercise tolerance in patients with mild to moderate heart failure caused by coronary disease already treated with captopril. Br Heart J 1993; 70:17–21.

## Book

57. Thadani U, Opie LH (eds). Nitrates Updated. Current Use in Angina, Ischemia, Infarction and Failure. Kluwer Academic Publishers, Boston, 1995.

# NOTES

# 3 Calcium Channel Antagonists (Calcium Entry Blockers)

L.H. Opie ◆ W.H. Frishman ◆ U. Thadani

Calcium antagonists remain among the most commonly used agents for angina and hypertension, acting chiefly by vasodilation and reduction of the peripheral vascular resistance. This simple concept has seemingly become complex with the introduction of a whole range of second-generation agents, as well as long-acting formulations of the existing first-generation "patriarchs," nifedipine, verapamil, and diltiazem. Furthermore, reservations have arisen about the contribution of coronary artery spasm to several anginal syndromes, including rest and unstable angina, with a corresponding downgrading of the role of coronary vasodilation by calcium antagonist therapy.

Yet in reality, the situation with calcium antagonists has become simpler rather than more complex. First, the creation of effective and truly long-acting formulations of the first-generation agents has led to a situation where differences in subjective side-effects are no longer crucial. Second, there is an increasing realization that agents structurally related to nifedipine (the group of **dihydropyridines** or **DHPs**) can be separated from the **non-DHPs,** such as verapamil and diltiazem. The major differences between these groups are (1) the greater vascular selectivity of the DHPs versus the greater myocardial selectivity of the non-DHPs and (2) the clinically evident inhibitory effect on the SA and AV nodes of the non-DHPs. The latter agents, verapamil and diltiazem, more closely resemble the beta-blockers in their therapeutic spectrum and will be considered before the DHPs. In a third group is bepridil, a nonselective calcium antagonist.

## Pharmacological Properties

### Calcium Channels: L- and T-types

The most important property of all calcium antagonists is selectively to inhibit the inward flow of charge-bearing calcium ions when the calcium channel becomes permeable or is "open." Previously, the term "slow channel" was used, but now it is realized that the calcium current travels much faster than previously believed, and that there are at least two types of calcium channels, L and T. The conventional calcium channel, long known to exist, is termed the **L-channel,** which is blocked by calcium antagonists and increased in activity by catecholamines. The **T-type channel** appears at more negative potentials than the L-type and probably plays an important role in the initial depolarization of sinus and AV nodal tissue. The function of the L-type is to admit the substantial amount of calcium ions required for initiation of contraction via calcium-induced calcium release from the sarcoplasmic reticulum (Fig. 3–1). Specific blockers for T-type calcium channels are not available, but could be expected to inhibit the sinus and AV nodes profoundly.

## Ca²⁺ Movements

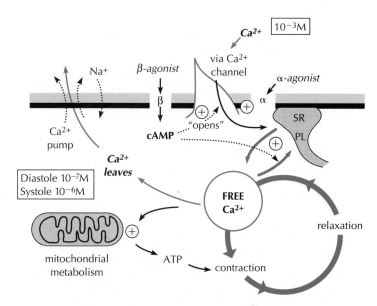

**FIGURE 3–1.** Role of calcium channel in regulating myocardial cytosolic calcium ion movements. cAMP = cyclic AMP; SR = sarcoplasmic reticulum; PL = phospholamban; β = beta-adrenergic receptor; α = alpha-adrenergic receptor. Fig. copyright L.H. Opie.

**Cellular Mechanism: Beta-blockade Versus Calcium Antagonists.** Both these categories of agents are used for angina and hypertension, yet there are important differences in their subcellular mode of antagonists relax vascular and (to a much lesser extent) other smooth muscle (Fig. 3–2). Calcium antagonists "block" the entry of calcium through the calcium channel in both smooth muscle and the myocardium, so that less calcium is available to the contractile apparatus. The result is vasodilation and a negative inotropic effect; the latter is usually modest due to the unloading effect of peripheral vasodilation.[68]

Beta-blockade has contrasting effects on smooth muscle and on the myocardium. Whereas it tends to promote smooth muscle contraction, beta-blockade impairs myocardial contraction. A fundamental difference lies in the regulation of the contractile mechanism by calcium ions in these two tissues. In the myocardium, calcium ions interact with troponin C to allow actin-myosin interaction; beta-stimulation enhances the entry of calcium ions and the rate of their uptake into the sarcoplasmic reticulum, so that calcium ion levels rise and fall more rapidly. Hence both contraction and relaxation are speeded up as cyclic AMP forms under beta-stimulation. Furthermore, a higher cytosolic calcium ion concentration at the time of systole means that the peak force of contraction is enhanced. Beta-blockade opposes all these effects.

In **smooth muscle** (Fig. 3–2), calcium ions regulate the contractile mechanism independently of troponin C. Interaction of calcium with calmodulin forms calcium-calmodulin, which then stimulates myosin light chain kinase (MLCK) to phosphorylate the myosin light chains to allow actin-myosin interaction and, hence, contraction. Cyclic AMP inhibits the MLCK. Beta-blockade, by lessening the formation of cyclic AMP, removes the inhibition on MLCK activity and, therefore, promotes contraction in smooth muscle, which explains why asthma may be precipitated. In addition, a further postulate is that beta-blockade may facilitate coronary vasoconstriction.[50]

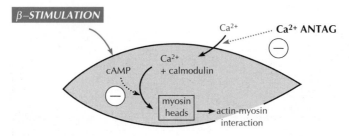

**SMOOTH MUSCLE**
*beta-blockade contracts*

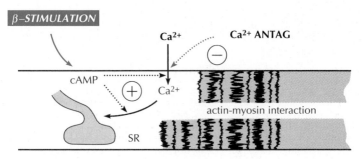

**HEART MUSCLE**
*beta-blockade inhibits contraction*

FIGURE 3–2. Proposed comparative effects of beta-blockade (BB) and calcium antagonists ($Ca^{2+}$ antag) on smooth muscle and myocardium. The opposing effects on vascular smooth muscle are of critical therapeutic importance. MLCK = myosin light chain kinase; SR = sarcoplasmic reticulum. Fig. copyright L.H. Opie.

## Classification of Calcium Antagonists

### The Dihydropyridines

The dihydropyridines (DHPs) all bind to the same sites on the alpha$_1$-subunit (the N sites), thereby establishing their common property of calcium channel antagonism (Fig. 3–3). To a different degree, they exert a greater inhibitory effect on vascular smooth muscle than on the myocardium, conferring the property of **vascular selectivity** (Table 3–1). Thus, their major therapeutic effect can be expected to be by peripheral or coronary vasodilation. There is nonetheless still the potential for **myocardial depression,** particularly in the case of agents with less selectivity and in the presence of prior myocardial disease and/or beta-blockade. For practical purposes, effects on the SA and AV nodes can be ignored.

**Nifedipine** is the prototype of the DHPs. In the fast-acting capsule form, originally available, it rapidly vasodilated to relieve severe hypertension and to terminate attacks of coronary spasm. The peripheral vasodilation led to rapid reflex adrenergic activation with tachycardia, as well as stimulation of the renin-angiotensin system (Fig. 3–4). Such intermittent adrenergic activation may explain why the short-acting DHPs have had undesirable long-term effects of aggravating congestive heart failure (CHF)[49] and failure to achieve the expected regression of left ventricular hypertrophy[60] despite short-term benefits, such as an increased LV ejection fraction in patients with CHF, and a drop in blood pressure.

Hence, the introduction of truly long-acting compounds such as

## Ca²⁺ Channel Binding sites

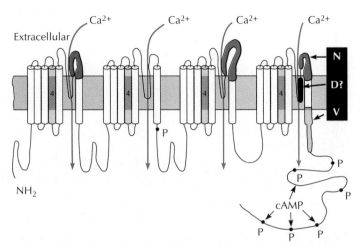

**FIGURE 3–3.** Proposed molecular model of calcium channel $alpha_1$-subunit with binding sites for nifedipine (N), diltiazem (D), and verapamil (V). It is thought that all DHPs bind to the same site as nifedipine. For details, see Kalasz et al., FEBS 1993; 331:177. For details of verapamil binding, see Striessnig et al., Proc Natl Acad Sci USA 1990; 87:9108. For details of diltiazem binding, see Watanabe et al.[83] Arrows radiating from cyclic AMP (cAMP) indicate sites of phosphorylation which act to increase the opening probability of the calcium channel. Note entry of calcium ions through the pore between segments 5 and 6 of each of the four domains. Fig. copyright L.H. Opie.

amlodipine or the extended-release formulations of nifedipine (GITS, CC) has led to substantially fewer symptomatic side-effects. A less intermittent and more sustained peripheral vasodilation is still associated with some modest neurohumoral activation.[67] Two residual side-effects of note are headache, as for all arteriolar dilators, and ankle edema, caused by precapillary dilation.

The second-generation DHPs are distinguished either by a longer half-life, as in the case of amlodipine, or by greater vascular selectivity, as in the case of all the other second-generation compounds (Table 3–1). **Vascular selectivity,** although seemingly a substantial advance, does not automatically translate into clinical benefits. For example, the most vascular selective compound of all, nisoldipine (1000:1 selectivity; not available in USA or UK), is only poorly antianginal in the short-acting formulation[79] and appears to exaggerate

**TABLE 3–1      RELATIVE VASCULAR SELECTIVITY OF VARIOUS ANTAGONISTS**

| APPROXIMATE DEGREE OF SELECTIVITY | HUMAN TISSUE | DRUG |
|---|---|---|
| 1000 | yes | nisoldipine |
| 100 | no | felodipine, isradipine, lacidipine, nicardipine, nitrendipine |
| 10 | yes | amlodipine, nifedipine |
| 7 | no | diltiazem |
| 1 | yes | diltiazem[a] |
| 1 | yes | verapamil |

Data sources: Godfraind et al.[56]

[a] For effects of diltiazem and verapamil on contractile force in the human papillary muscle, see Bohm et al., Am J Cardiol 1990; 65:1039; for comparative effects in patients, see Ferrari et al., Cardiovasc Drugs Ther 1994; 8:565.

## ISCHEMIC HEART: Ca²⁺ ANTAGONIST EFFECTS

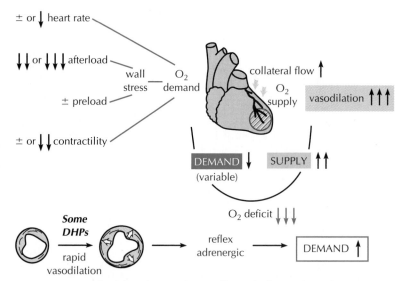

**FIGURE 3–4.** Mechanisms of anti-ischemic effects of calcium channel antagonists. Note that the rapid arteriolar vasodilation resulting from the action of some dihydropyridines (DHPs) may increase myocardial oxygen demand by reflex adrenergic stimulation. Fig. copyright L.H. Opie.

rather than improve heart failure.[41] A rapid decrease in blood pressure may precipitate **pro-ischemic effects.**[42] In contrast, when given in the extended-release form, nisoldipine benefits effort angina.[55]

A promising group of compounds appears to be those with medium degrees (about 100:1) of vascular selectivity, such as felodipine, isradipine, and nicardipine. Modest myocardial depression may contribute to antianginal effects.

Thus, among the DHPs, the two chief distinguishing properties are the duration of action and the degree of vascular selectivity.

### The Non-Dihydropyridines

Verapamil and diltiazem bind to two different sites on the alpha₁-subunit of the calcium channel, yet have many properties in common with each other (Fig. 3–5). The first and most obvious distinction from the DHPs is that verapamil and diltiazem both act on nodal tissue, being therapeutically effective in supraventricular tachycardias. Both tend to decrease the sinus rate. Both inhibit myocardial contraction more than the DHPs or, put differently, are less vascular selective. These properties, added to peripheral vasodilation, lead to substantial reduction in the myocardial oxygen demand. Such "oxygen conservation" confers properties on these compounds which make them much closer than the DHPs to the beta-blockers, with whom they share a similar spectrum of therapeutic activity. An important exception is the almost total lack of effect of verapamil and diltiazem on standard types of ventricular tachycardia, perhaps because they do not modify myocardial tissue levels of the arrhythmogenic compound, cyclic AMP.

The modest effects of these agents on the SA node compared with the AV node can be explained as follows. The pharmacologically relevant interaction of these agents with the calcium channel in nodal tissue is **frequency-dependent,** so that there is better access to the binding sites when the calcium channel pore is "open." During nodal re-entry tachycardia, the channel of the AV node opens more frequently, the drug binds better, and hence specifically inhibits the AV node to stop the re-entry path. This explanation appears to hold when considering the molecular binding site of verapamil (deep in

## VERAPAMIL OR DILTIAZEM MULTIPLE EFFECTS

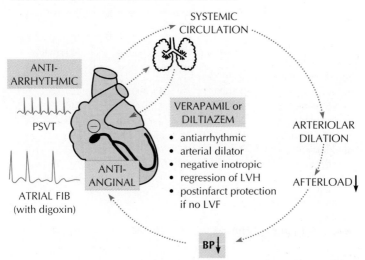

**FIGURE 3–5.** Verapamil and diltiazem have a broad spectrum of therapeutic effects. PSVT = paroxysmal supraventricular tachycardia; Atrial fib = atrial fibrillation. Fig. copyright L.H. Opie and modified from Reference 1.

the channel pore), but seems less evident in the case of diltiazem, according to the recent information that it binds more superficially in the pore.[83]

Regarding the side-effects, the non-DHPs, being less active on vascular smooth muscle, also have less vasodilatory side-effects than the DHPs—thus there is less flushing, headaches or pedal edema. Tachycardia is uncommon because of the inhibitory effects on the SA node. Left ventricular depression remains a major potential side-effect, especially in patients with pre-existing CHF. Why constipation occurs only with verapamil of all the calcium antagonists is not known.

## Major Indications for Calcium Antagonists

ANGINA PECTORIS. Common to the effects of all types of calcium antagonists is the inhibition of the L-calcium current in arterial smooth muscle, occurring at relatively low concentrations (Table 3–2). Hence coronary vasodilation is a major common property (Fig. 3–2). Although the antianginal mechanisms are many and varied, the shared effects are (1) coronary vasodilation and relief of exercise-induced vasoconstriction, and (2) afterload reduction due to blood pressure reduction (Fig. 3–4). In addition, in the case of verapamil and diltiazem, slowing of the sinus node, a decrease in exercise heart rate, and a negative inotropic effect may all contribute.

CORONARY SPASM. The role of this cause of the anginal syndromes has undergone revision. Once seen as a major contributor to pain in rest angina, coronary spasm is now thought less likely to explain the rest component of mixed angina (angina both at rest and on effort). The basis for this change of opinion is that beta-blockade has been shown to be more effective than nifedipine in four studies in mixed angina.[40,48,66,75] Also, in silent ischemia, detected by continuous ECG monitoring, nifedipine has not been conspicuously successful, and in one study was decidely worse than beta-blockade.[78] The role of coronary spasm in unstable preinfarction angina has also been downplayed since the finding that nifedipine, in the absence of concurrent beta-blockade, appeared to be harmful.[15] Coronary spasm remains important as a cause of angina precipitated by **cold** or **hyperventilation,** and in Prinzmetal's variant angina.

TABLE 3–2　RELATIVE EFFECTS OF THE THREE PROTOTYPICAL CALCIUM
ANTAGONISTS IN EXPERIMENTAL PREPARATIONS COMPARED
WITH THERAPEUTIC LEVELS IN MAN

| | VERAPAMIL | DILTIAZEM | NIFEDIPINE |
|---|---|---|---|
| Therapeutic level in man | | | |
| ng/ml | 80–400 | 50–300 | 15–100 |
| molecular weight | 455 | 415 | 346 |
| molar value | $2–8 \times 10^{-7}$ M | $1–7 \times 10^{-7}$ M | $0.3–2 \times 10^{-7}$ M |
| protein binding | about 90% | about 85% | about 95% |
| molar value, corrected for protein binding | $2–8 \times 10^{-8}$ M | $1–5 \times 10^{-8}$ M | $0.3–1 \times 10^{-8}$ M |
| Slowing of sinus rate by 20% (isolated atria) | $10^{-6}$ M | $10^{-8}$ M | $10^{-5}$ M |
| Negative inotropic effect, human papillary muscle | $6 \times 10^{-7}$ M | $6 \times 10^{-7}$ M | $10^{-7}$ M |
| Human coronary artery contraction, 50% inhibition | similar to above or lower | similar to above | $10^{-8}$ M |
| VSM contraction (portal vein) | $4 \times 10^{-7}$ M | $6 \times 10^{-7}$ M | $4 \times 10^{-8}$ M |
| Vascular selectivity | | | |
| animals | 1.4 | 7 | 14 |
| humans | 1.0 | 1.0 | 10 |

VSM = vascular smooth muscle; molar = moles per liter.

For data sources, see Table I–5 (Opie,[25] pp 50–51) with additional data from Godfraind et al.[56]

HYPERTENSION.　It is increasingly realized that the calcium antagonists are excellent antihypertensive agents and among the best for elderly and black patients (p 193). They are recommended (among others) as first-line agents by the World Health Organization, but lack of long-term outcome studies has limited their approval by the American Joint National Committee.[63] All the DHPs decrease peripheral vascular resistance, and may also have a diuretic effect. Verapamil and diltiazem are less powerful vasodilators.

SUPRAVENTRICULAR TACHYCARDIA.　Verapamil and diltiazem inhibit the AV node, which explains their effect in supraventricular tachycardias. Nifedipine and other DHPs are clinically ineffective.

POSTINFARCT PROTECTION.　In the postinfarct period, there may be important differences between DHPs and non-DHPs. Both verapamil and diltiazem gave some protection in the absence of prior left ventricular failure, whereas nifedipine does not.

POSSIBLE ADDITIONAL INDICATIONS.　Cytosolic calcium overload may be a crucial aspect of irreversible cell damage. Hence, calcium antagonists have been tried for **organ protection,** for example when added to cardioplegic solutions, in the prevention of peri-operative ischemic damage,[73] in renal protection, and in protection from cerebral ischemia. In **atherosclerosis,** calcium antagonists may inhibit the early stages of atheroma formation, without achieving regression as do the lipid-lowering agents (Table 10–4).

# Verapamil

**Verapamil (Isoptin, Calan, Verelan)**, the prototype non-DHP agent, was introduced in Europe in 1963 and more recently in the USA. Verapamil remains the calcium antagonist that has been most extensively studied experimentally and clinically. Structurally it resembles papaverine, a coronary vasodilator. As a non-DHP, it has more marked myocardial and nodal effects and less marked vasodilatory effects, so that it resembles beta-blockers in some ways. The major differences are: (1) the greater heart rate reduction with beta-blockers; (2) the use of beta-blockade in myocardial infarction and follow-up, whereas verapamil is contraindicated in early AMI and its postinfarct use is restricted to those without a prior history of heart failure; (3) peripheral vasodilation is prominent with verapamil, so that the onset of the hypotensive effect is rapid; (4) bronchospasm is not a contraindication to verapamil; (5) coronary vasodilation explains why verapamil is licensed for use in Prinzmetal's variant angina, a contraindication to beta-blockade.

## Pharmacologic Properties

**Electrophysiologically,** verapamil inhibits the action potential of the upper and middle nodal regions where depolarization is $Ca^{2+}$-mediated. Verapamil thus inhibits one limb of the re-entry circuit, which is believed to underlie most paroxysmal supraventricular tachycardias. Increased AV block and the increase in effective refractory period of the AV node explain the reduction of the ventricular rate in atrial flutter and fibrillation. On electrophysiologic grounds, one might expect verapamil not to be very effective in ventricular tachycardias except in certain uncommon forms.

**Hemodynamically,** verapamil combines arteriolar dilation with a direct negative inotropic effect (Table 3–2). The cardiac output and left ventricular ejection fraction do not increase as expected following peripheral vasodilation,[1] which may be an expression of the negative inotropic effect. Peripheral vasodilation with reflex heart rate increase generally overcomes the direct depressant effect of verapamil on the sinus node so that the heart rate is unchanged or variably altered.

PHARMACOKINETICS.  Oral verapamil takes 2 hours to act and peaks at 3 hours. Therapeutic blood levels (80 to 400 ng/ml) are seldom measured.[1] The elimination half-life is usually 3 to 7 hours, but increases significantly during chronic administration and in patients with liver or advanced renal insufficiency. Despite nearly complete absorption of oral doses, bioavailability is only 10% to 20% (high first-pass liver metabolism). Ultimate excretion of the parent compound, as well as the active hepatic metabolite norverapamil, is 75% by the kidneys and 25% by the gastrointestinal (GI) tract. Verapamil is 87% to 93% protein-bound, but no interaction with warfarin has been reported. When both verapamil and digoxin are given together, their interaction causes digoxin levels to rise, probably due to a reduction in the renal clearance of digoxin.[1]

Norverapamil is a hepatic metabolite of verapamil, which appears rapidly in the plasma after oral administration of verapamil and in concentrations similar to those of the parent compound; like verapamil, norverapamil undergoes delayed clearance during chronic dosing.

DOSE.  (Table 3–3). The usual **oral dose** of the standard preparation is 80 to 120 mg 3 times daily; large differences of pharmacokinetics among individuals mean that dose titration is required. Lower or higher doses may therefore be needed; the highest reported daily dose is 960 mg,[1] but such levels are rarely tolerated. During chronic oral dosing, the formation of norverapamil metabolites and altered rates of hepatic metabolism may mean that less frequent daily doses of verapamil are preferable;[1] for example, if verapamil has been given at a dose of 80 mg 3 times daily, then 120 mg twice daily

TABLE 3-3   FIRST-GENERATION CALCIUM CHANNEL ANTAGONISTS: SALIENT FEATURES FOR CARDIOVASCULAR USE

| AGENT | DOSE | PHARMACOKINETICS AND METABOLISM | SIDE-EFFECT AND CONTRAINDICATIONS | KINETIC AND DYNAMIC INTERACTIONS |
|---|---|---|---|---|
| **Verapamil** tablets | 240–480 mg daily in 2 or 3 doses (titrated) | Peak plasma levels with 1–2 h. Low bioavailability (10–20%), high first-pass metabolism to active norverapamil. Excretion: 75% renal, 25% GI, t½ 3–7 h. | Constipation. C/I sick sinus syndrome, digitalis toxicity, excess beta-blockade, LV failure. Care in obstructive cardiomyopathy. | Digoxin levels increase. Depression of SA, AV nodes and myocardium. Interacting drugs: beta-blockers, digoxin, disopyramide, quinidine. Carbamazepine levels rise. Cimetidine and liver disease increase blood levels. |
| SR form Verelan | Same as above, single dose, sometimes 2 doses (SR) | Peak effect 1–2 h (Isoptin SR, Calan SR) or 7–9 h (Verelan). t½ 5–12 h and 12 h (Verelan longest). | As above | As above |
| Intravenous (for PSVT or to control ventricular rate in AF or atrial flutter) | IV 5–10 mg, may repeat after 10 min. IV infusion 1 mg/min to total of 10 mg. IV infusion (if myocardial depression) 0.0001 to 0.005 mg/kg/min. | IV verapamil is rapidly metabolized in the liver with a t½ 2–5 h. Effect on AV node and PSVT within 10 min, lasting up to 6 h. | Bolus drops BP within 1–2 min, peak effect 5–12 min. C/I: Ventricular tachycardia, WPW, sick sinus syndrome, AV block, LV depression. IV beta-blocker, IV digoxin, or digoxin toxicity. | Added nodal or LV inhibition if prior IV beta-blocker or IV digoxin. To lessen hypotension, pretreat with calcium gluconate (90 mg). |

| | | | | |
|---|---|---|---|---|
| **Diltiazem** tablets | 120–360 mg daily in 3 or 4 doses | Onset time: 15–30 min. Peak time: 1–2 h. t½ 5 h. Bioavailability 45% (first-pass hepatic effect). Active metabolite accumulates. 65% GI loss. | As for verapamil but no constipation | As for verapamil, except little/no effect on digoxin levels. Cimetidine and liver disease increase blood levels. Increased propranolol levels. |
| prolonged SR, CD, XR | As above in 1 (CD, XR) or 2 (SR) doses | Slower onset, longer t½, otherwise similar. | As above | As above |
| Intravenous (for indications, see IV verapamil) | IV 0.25 mg/kg over 2 min, then 0.35 mg/kg over 2 min, then infuse at 5–15 mg/h | IV diltiazem is rapidly metabolized in the liver with t½ 4–5 h. Rates of 3, 5, 7 and 11 mg/h correspond to oral doses of 120, 180, 240 and 360 mg daily. | PSVT usually reverts within 3 min. In atrial flutter or fibrillation, heart rate reduction within 2–7 min. Hypotension may last for hours after end of infusion. | See IV verapamil. |
| **Nifedipine** capsules | 5–10 mg initial, then 10–20 mg every 4–8 h (titrated) | Poor sublingual but good gastric absorption; bite-and-swallow best for quick effect, < 10 min. High first-pass metabolisms; inactive metabolites. t½ 3 h. | Rapid vasodilation elicits reflex tachytcardia and flushing. Headache and ankle edema. C/I: severe aortic stenosis, obstructive cardiomyopathy, LV failure. | Added LV depression with beta-blockade. Avoid in unstable angina without beta-blockade. Cimetidine and liver disease increase blood levels. |
| prolonged XL, CC, LA | 30–90 mg once daily | Stable 24 h blood levels. Slow onset, about 6 h. | Few acute vasodilatory S/E headache, ankle edema. Same C/I. | As above |

BP = blood pressure; PSVT = paroxysmal supraventricular tachycardia; AF = atrial fibrillation; AF1 = atrial flutter; t½ = plasma elimination half-life; WPW = Wolff-Parkinson-White.

would be as good, especially in the treatment of hypertension.[38] Lower doses are also required in elderly patients or those with advanced renal or hepatic disease.[1]

**Slow-release preparations.** These are (1) **Calan SR** or **Isoptin SR,** which release the drug from a matrix at a rate which responds to food; and (2) **Verelan,** which releases the drug from a rate-controlling polymer at a rate not sensitive to food intake.[54] The usual dose of verapamil is 240 to 480 mg daily. The SR preparations are given once or twice daily and Verelan once daily.

**Intravenous verapamil** is discussed under Supraventricular Arrhythmias (p 64).

DOSE MODIFICATION. Start with low dose and titrate upwards. Reduce dose in severe liver disease or in the elderly, or when there is concurrent beta-blockade.

SIDE-EFFECTS. Class side-effects are those of vasodilation causing headaches, facial flushing, and dizziness. These may be lessened by the long-acting preparations. Tachycardia is not a side-effect. Constipation is specific and causes most trouble, especially in elderly patients.[1]

RARE SIDE-EFFECTS. Rare side-effects may include pain in the gums, facial pain, epigastric pain, hepatotoxicity, and transient mental confusion.

SEVERE NODAL SIDE-EFFECTS. When incorrectly given as a bolus to patients with pre-existing AV inhibition caused by disease or beta-blockade, intravenous verapamil can be fatal. In patients with sick sinus syndrome, severe asystole may result after intravenous verapamil. With oral verapamil, lesser degrees of these side-effects are possible.

MYOCARDIAL DEPRESSANT EFFECTS. A striking negative inotropic effect is seen with verapamil and other calcium antagonists in isolated preparations. Yet when correctly used, verapamil seldom causes serious cardiac depression because of the protective effects of afterload reduction. In supraventricular arrhythmias, the hemodynamic benefits of restoration of sinus rhythm usually outweigh any negative inotropic effect.[1]

CONTRAINDICATIONS TO VERAPAMIL. (Fig. 3–6, Table 3–4). Sick sinus syndrome; pre-existing AV nodal disease; excess therapy with beta-adrenergic blockade, digitalis, quinidine, or disopyramide; or myocardial depression are all contraindications especially in the intravenous therapy of supraventricular tachycardias.[1] In the **Wolff-Parkinson-White (WPW) syndrome** complicated by atrial fibrillation, intravenous verapamil is contraindicated because of the risk of anterograde conduction through the bypass tract (see pp 11–24). Verapamil is also contraindicated in ventricular tachycardia (wide QRS-complex) because of excess myocardial depression which may be lethal. An exception to this rule is exercise-induced **ventricular tachycardia.**[1] Myocardial depression, if secondary to the supraventricular tachycardia, is not a contraindication, whereas pre-existing left ventricular systolic failure is.

## Verapamil and Beta-blockers: Interactions and Combination Therapy

Special care is required when verapamil is acutely added by intravenous injection in the presence of pre-existing beta-adrenergic blockade.[1] Also, in patients with angina pectoris already receiving beta-blockers, intravenous or oral verapamil can reduce contractility, increase heart size, and cause symptomatic sinus bradycardia.[1] There may be a hepatic pharmacokinetic interaction.[1] Depending on the dose, the combination with a beta-blocker may be well tolerated or not.[1] Packer[27] has drawn attention to the possible hazards of such

VERAPAMIL or DILTIAZEM

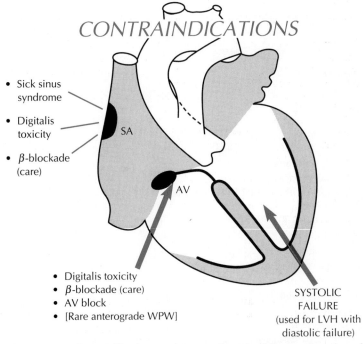

- Sick sinus syndrome
- Digitalis toxicity
- β-blockade (care)

SA

AV

- Digitalis toxicity
- β-blockade (care)
- AV block
- [Rare anterograde WPW]

SYSTOLIC FAILURE
(used for LVH with diastolic failure)

**FIGURE 3–6.** Contraindications to verapamil and diltiazem. For use of verapamil and diltiazem in patients already receiving beta-blockers, see text. WPW = Wolff-Parkinson-White syndrome. Fig. copyright L.H. Opie and modified from Reference 1.

combination therapy. In practice, clinicians can safely combine verapamil with beta-blockade in the therapy of angina pectoris or hypertension, provided that due care is taken and that the combination is avoided in elderly patients unless specific care is taken to exclude nodal disease. In angina, the combination improves myocardial function during exercise more than either agent alone.[1] Beta-blocker plus verapamil works well for hypertension, although heart rate, AV conduction and LV function may be adversely affected.[1] Similarly, with care, the combination verapamil-propranolol is used for the chronic prevention of supraventricular tachycardia.[1] To avoid any hepatic interactions, verapamil is best combined with a hydrophilic beta-blocker such as atenolol rather than one that is metabolized in the liver, such as metoprolol or propranolol.[23]

### Other Drug Interactions with Verapamil

DIGOXIN. Verapamil can interact with digitalis to increase blood digoxin levels.[1] In digitalis toxicity, rapid intravenous verapamil is *absolutely contraindicated* because it can lethally exaggerate AV block. There is no reason why, in the absence of digitalis toxicity or AV block, oral verapamil and digitalis compounds should not be combined (checking the digoxin level), because digitalis does not inhibit the inward calcium current. Experimentally, verapamil has proved effective against ventricular arrhythmias due to digitalis, but in practice intravenous verapamil should be given only with great caution to patients with digitalis poisoning, because of the risk of complete AV block.

PRAZOSIN. Verapamil has also been used combined with prazosin in hypertension, with added and possibly synergistic effects;[1] the latter may be explained by pharmacokinetic interactions.[1]

TABLE 3–4    COMPARATIVE CONTRAINDICATIONS OF VERAPAMIL, DILTIAZEM, NIFEDIPINE, AND OF BETA-ADRENERGIC BLOCKING AGENTS

| CONTRAINDICATIONS | VERAPAMIL | DILTIAZEM | NIFEDIPINE (all DHPs) | BETA-BLOCKADE |
|---|---|---|---|---|
| **Absolute:** | | | | |
| Sinus bradycardia | 0/ + | 0/ + | 0 | + + |
| Sick sinus syndrome | + + | + | 0 | + + |
| AV conduction defects | + + | + + | 0 | + + |
| WPW syndrome | + + | + + | 0 | + + |
| Digitalis toxicity with AV block* | + + | + + | 0 | + |
| Asthma | 0 | 0 | 0 | + + + |
| Bronchospasm | 0 | 0 | 0 | + + |
| Heart failure | + + | + + | + + | + + |
| Hypotension | + | + | + + | + |
| Coronary artery spasm | 0 | 0 | 0 | + |
| Raynaud's and active peripheral vascular disease | 0 | 0 | 0 | + |
| Severe mental depression | 0 | 0 | 0 | + |
| Severe aortic stenosis | + | + | + + | + |
| Obstructive cardiomyopathy | 0/ + | 0/ + | + + | + (indicated) |
| **Relative:** | | | | |
| Insulin resistance | 0 | 0 | 0 | Care |
| Adverse blood lipid profile | 0 | 0 | 0 | Care |
| Digitalis without toxicity | Care | Care | 0 | Care |
| Beta-blockade | Care | Care | Hypotension | 0 |
| Quinidine therapy | Care | Care | Care** | Care |
| Disopyramide therapy | Care | Care | 0 | Care |
| Unstable angina at rest | 0 | 0 | + + | Indicated |
| Postinfarct protection | Indicated | 0 (No LVF) | + + | Indicated |

Indicated means judged suitable for use by author (L.H. Opie), not necessarily FDA-approved.

+ + + = absolutely contraindicated; + + = strongly contraindicated; + = relative contraindication; 0 = not contraindicated; LVF = left ventricular failure

* Contraindication to rapid intravenous administration

** Nifedipine depresses blood quinidine levels with rebound upon nifedipine-withdrawal

QUINIDINE. Verapamil may adversely interact with quinidine, presumably due to the combined effect on peripheral alpha-receptors causing hypotension,[1] or by increasing quinidine levels.

DISOPYRAMIDE. The combined negative inotropic potential of verapamil and disopyramide is considerable.

ANTIEPILEPTICS AND RIFAMPIN. These induce the cytochrome system metabolizing verapamil so that its blood levels fall. Conversely, verapamil increases blood carbamazepine levels with risk of toxicity.

## Therapy of Verapamil Toxicity

There are few clinical reports on management of verapamil toxicity. Intravenous calcium gluconate (1 to 2 g) or half that dose of calcium chloride, given over 5 minutes, helps when heart failure or excess hypotension is present. If there is an inadequate response, positive inotropic or vasoconstrictory catecholamines (Fig. 6–6) are used, or else glucagon.[59] Excess AV block apparently depends less on external calcium than does hypotension or the negative inotropic effect,[1] so that intravenous atropine (1 mg) or isoproterenol is used to shorten AV conduction. A pacemaker may be needed.

## Verapamil for Chronic Stable Angina, Unstable Angina and Prinzmetal's Variant Angina

In **chronic stable effort angina,** verapamil acts by a combination of afterload reduction and a mild negative inotropic effect; there may also be an increase in the blood supply.[1] The heart rate usually stays the same or falls modestly. In several studies, verapamil has been as effective as propranolol for effort angina, or more so, and there is less risk of serious side-effects. A daily dose of verapamil (about 360 mg) is the approximate equivalent of propranolol 300 mg daily or metoprolol 200 mg twice daily or nifedipine 60 mg daily.[1]

In **unstable angina at rest** with threat of infarction, verapamil has not been tested against placebo, although licensed for this purpose in the USA. Verapamil 480 mg daily was much better than propranolol 240 mg daily in preventing recurrent chest pain; however, 7 of the 20 patients had Prinzmetal's angina, a condition for which beta-blockade is a relative contraindication.[5] Intravenous verapamil 0.002 mg/kg/min, when added to nitroglycerin, improves ECG ischemic episodes.[22]

In **silent myocardial ischemia,** together with short-lived (< 10 minutes) attacks of rest pain, verapamil in a mean daily dose of 400 mg is much better than propranolol, also in a mean dose of 300 mg.[28]

In **variant angina** (Prinzmetal's syndrome), verapamil (average daily dose 450 mg in 3 to 4 divided doses) and nifedipine (average daily dose 70 mg in 3 to 4 divided doses) were equally effective, with fewer dose-limiting side-effects with verapamil.[1] Combinations of verapamil or nifedipine with oral isosorbide dinitrate are more effective than isosorbide alone.[1] Abrupt withdrawal of verapamil may precipitate rebound angina.[52]

## Verapamil for Hypertension

Verapamil is now approved for mild to moderate hypertension in the USA. The slow-release preparations can be given once or twice daily. Although monotherapy with verapamil is claimed to be effective in nearly 90% of patients by the manufacturers, in a long-term double-blind comparative trial, mild to moderate hypertension was adequately controlled in only 45% of patients given verapamil 240 mg daily.[16] The response rate to verapamil in this study may be relatively low because the top dose was only 240 mg daily instead of 360 mg as used in some other studies. The corresponding response for hydrochlorothiazide 25 mg daily was only 25%. Adding hydrochlorothiazide to verapamil or vice versa improved the response rate to about 60%.

**Compared with beta-blockade,** verapamil doses of 240 to 360 mg daily are the approximate equivalent of propranolol 160 to 240 mg daily, labetalol 400 mg daily, and atenolol 100 mg daily (for review see Table III-6 of ref. 25). The combination of verapamil (360 mg) and propranolol (240 mg) gives better results than either agent alone, at the cost of more side-effects.[1]

For **exercising hypertensives,** verapamil reduces systolic blood pressure more than does nifedipine at similar workloads.[57]

In **black patients,** verapamil is probably better initial therapy than propranolol.[7]

**Combinations** can be with diuretics, beta-blockers, ACE inhibitors, or centrally acting agents. During combination with alpha-blockers, a hepatic interaction may lead to excess hypotension.

## Verapamil for Supraventricular Arrhythmias

For **supraventricular tachycardias,** when there is no myocardial depression, a bolus dose of 5 to 10 mg (0.1 to 0.15 mg/kg) given over 2 minutes restores sinus rhythm within 10 minutes in 60% of cases (package insert). The bolus may be repeated 10 minutes later if needed. The infusion rate after a successful bolus is 0.005 mg/kg/min for about 30 to 60 minutes, decreasing thereafter. The risk of hypotension may be countered by pretreatment with intravenous calcium gluconate (90 mg).[1] When used for uncontrolled **atrial fibrillation** with myocardial disease, verapamil is infused at a very low dose (0.0001 mg/kg/min) and titrated against the ventricular response. Otherwise verapamil may safely be given at a higher rate (0.005 mg/kg/min, increasing) or as an intravenous bolus of 5 mg (0.075 mg/kg) followed by double the dose if needed.[1]

In **atrial flutter,** the block is increased. In all supraventricular tachycardias, including atrial flutter and fibrillation, the presence of a bypass tract (WPW syndrome) contraindicates verapamil.

## Other Uses for Verapamil

In **hypertrophic cardiomyopathy,** verapamil has been the calcium antagonist best evaluated. It is licensed for this purpose in Canada. When given acutely, it lessens symptoms, reduces the outflow tract gradient, improves diastolic function, and enhances exercise performance by 20% to 25%.[1] Verapamil diminishes silent ischemia.[81] Verapamil should not be given to patients with resting outflow tract obstruction,[1] when propranolol or disopyramide, which do not vasodilate, should be safer. No long-term placebo-controlled studies with verapamil are available. In retrospective comparisons with propranolol, verapamil appeared to decrease sudden death[65] and gave better 10-year survival.[72] A significant number of patients on long-term verapamil develop severe side-effects, including SA and AV nodal dysfunction, and occasionally overt heart failure.[1]

For **ventricular tachycardia,** verapamil can be lethal. It is, therefore, *contraindicated* in standard wide complex ventricular tachycardia. However, some patients with exercise-induced ventricular tachycardia due to triggered automaticity may respond well,[1] as may young patients with idiopathic right ventricular outflow tract ventricular tachycardia (right bundle branch block and left axis deviation).

For **postinfarct protection,** verapamil is approved in Scandinavian countries when beta-blockade is contraindicated.[47,51] Verapamil 120 mg 3 times daily, started 7 to 15 days after the acute phase in patients without a history of heart failure and no signs of CHF (but with digoxin and diuretic therapy allowed) was protective and decreased reinfarction and mortality by about 25% over 18 months.

For renal protection in hypertensive insulin-dependent diabetics, verapamil reduced urinary albumin excretion.[50A]

## New Derivative of Verapamil

**Gallopamil,** available in Europe, has properties very similar to verapamil, but causing less constipation. A dose of 150 mg daily is the antianginal equivalent of verapamil 240 mg daily, both given in three divided doses.

## Summary: Verapamil

Among calcium antagonists, verapamil has the widest range of approved indications, including angina pectoris (effort, vasospastic, unstable), supraventricular tachycardias and hypertension. Compared with propranolol in the therapy of effort angina, it is at least as effective, with less risk of serious side-effects and fewer contraindications. Verapamil is now increasingly used as one of a number of early options in the therapy of hypertension. The combination with beta-blockade can be more effective than either component in the therapy of angina or hypertension, but a number of cautions and contraindications must be observed.

# Diltiazem

**Diltiazem** (**Cardizem, Dilacor** in the USA; **Tildiem** in the UK; **Herbesser** or **Tilazem** elsewhere), initially developed in Japan, is now available worldwide. Although molecular studies show that there are different binding sites for each of the three major calcium antagonists (nifedipine, diltiazem and verapamil), in clinical practice, diltiazem and verapamil have somewhat similar therapeutic spectra and contraindications, so that these agents are combined in some classifications of calcium antagonists, as the non-DHPs or "heart rate slowing" agents.[85] Both agents have frequency-dependent inhibition of the AV node. Although there are few good comparative studies, a common clinical impression is that diltiazem seems more active than verapamil on the sinus node, so that it is more likely to decrease the heart rate, whereas verapamil may be more active on the AV node. Clinically, diltiazem is used for the same spectrum of disease as is verapamil: angina pectoris, hypertension, and supraventricular arrhythmias. Of these, angina and hypertension are approved in the USA, with only the intravenous form approved for supraventricular tachycardias. Diltiazem has a low side-effect profile, similar to or possibly better than that of verapamil, specifically the incidence of constipation is much lower (Table 3–5). There are no strictly comparable clinical studies to establish that diltiazem is less cardiodepressant than verapamil, as is often thought to be the case. One study on isolated human cardiac tissue suggests similar cardiac depression (Table 3–1). New slow-release preparations are now available in the USA to allow once-daily dosing.[80A]

## Pharmacologic Properties

PHARMACOKINETICS. Following oral administration of diltiazem, over 90% is absorbed, but bioavailability is about 45% (first-pass hepatic metabolism). The onset of action is within 15 to 30 minutes (oral), with a peak at 1 to 2 hours. The elimination half-life is 4 to 7 hours; hence, dosage every 6 to 8 hours of the short-acting preparation is required for sustained therapeutic effect. The therapeutic plasma concentration range is 50 to 300 ng/ml. Protein binding is 80% to 86%. Diltiazem is acetylated in the liver to deacyldiltiazem (40% of the activity of the parent compound), which accumulates with chronic therapy. Unlike verapamil and nifedipine, only 35% of diltiazem is excreted by the kidneys (65% by the GI tract).

DOSE. For all varieties of angina, the dose of diltiazem is 120 to 360 mg, usually in 4 daily doses of the short-acting formulation. Yet a single 120 mg dose improves exercise tolerance for 8 hours.[1]

**Slow-release preparations: Cardizem SR** permits twice-daily

**TABLE 3–5**  SOME SIDE-EFFECTS OF THE THREE PROTOTYPICAL CALCIUM ANTAGONISTS AND LONG-ACTING DIHYDROPYRIDINES

| | VERAPAMIL (%) | DILTIAZEM (%) | DILTIAZEM XR OR CD (%) | NIFEDIPINE CAPSULES (%) | NIFEDIPINE XL (%) | AMLODIPINE (%) | FELODIPINE ER (%) |
|---|---|---|---|---|---|---|---|
| Facial flushing | 6–7 | 0–3 | 0–1 | 6–25 | 0 | 2 | 4–8 |
| Headaches | 6 | 4–9 | < placebo | 7–34 | 16* | < placebo | 11–19[+] |
| Tachycardia | 0 | 0 | 0 | low–25 | 0 | 0 | 1–2 |
| Lightheadedness, dizziness | 7 | 6–7 | 0 | 3–12 | 4 | 5 | 6 |
| Constipation | 34 | 4 | 1–2 | 0 | 3 | 0 | 0 |
| Ankle edema, swelling | 6 | 6–10 | 2–3 | 1–8 | 10–30 | 10 | 14–36 |
| Provocation of angina | 0 | 0 | 0 | low–14 | 0 | 0 | 0 |

Data sources from Opie[25] (p 197). For nifedipine XL, diltiazem XR, and felodipine ER, see package inserts.

For amlodipine, mean values of 6 trials on 2573 patients calculated from Osterloh.[26] See also Omvik et al.[64]

N.B. Side-effects are dose-related; no strict comparisons exist except for nifedipine versus diltiazem.

\* vs 10% in placebo

[+] vs 12% in placebo

< = less than

doses. For once-daily use, **Dilacor XR** is licensed in the USA for hypertension and **Cardizem CD** for hypertension and angina.

**Intravenous diltiazem** (approved for arrhythmias, not hypertension) is given as 0.25 mg/kg over 2 minutes with ECG and blood pressure monitoring; then if the response is inadequate, the dose is repeated as 0.35 mg/kg over 2 minutes. Acute therapy is usually followed by an infusion of 5 to 15 mg/hr.

SIDE-EFFECTS. Normally side-effects of the standard preparation are few and limited to headaches, dizziness, and ankle edema in about 6% to 10% of patients (Table 3–5). With high-dose diltiazem (360 mg daily), constipation may also be found. When the extended-release preparation (Dilacor XR) is used for hypertension, the side-effect profile is similar to placebo. When used for angina or hypertension (Cardizem CD), bradycardia and first degree AV block are reported (each about 3%). In the case of intravenous diltiazem, side-effects should resemble those of intravenous verapamil, including hypotension and the possible risk of asystole and high-degree AV block when there is pre-existing nodal disease. In postinfarct patients with pre-existing poor LV function, mortality is increased by diltiazem, not decreased.[24] Occasionally, severe skin rashes such as exfoliative dermatitis are found.

CONTRAINDICATIONS. Contraindications resemble those of verapamil (Fig. 3–6, Table 3–4)—pre-existing marked depression of the sinus or AV node, hypotension, myocardial failure and the WPW syndrome. Use in nodal disease may require a pacemaker. Postinfarct, LV failure with an ejection fraction below 40% is a clear contraindication.[24]

DRUG INTERACTIONS. Unlike verapamil, the effect of diltiazem on the **blood digoxin** level is often slight or negligible.[33]

COMBINATION WITH BETA-BLOCKERS AND OTHER DRUGS. Diltiazem plus beta-blocker may be used for angina with risk of excess bradycardia or hypotension. In some studies the combination was no more effective than diltiazem itself, presumably because of the bradycardia already induced by diltiazem.[1] In patients with coronary artery spasm, the combination of beta-blocker plus diltiazem has no obvious advantage over diltiazem alone.[1] Occasionally diltiazem plus nifedipine is used for refractory coronary artery spasm.[30] **Diltiazem plus long-acting nitrates** may lead to excess hypotension.[1]

DILTIAZEM OVERDOSE. Treat as for verapamil (p 63).

## Diltiazem for Ischemic Syndromes

In **chronic stable effort angina,** the combination of vasodilation, reduced heart rate during exercise, and a modest negative inotropic effect seems very desirable.[80A] The efficacy of diltiazem in chronic angina is at least as good as propranolol, and the dose is titrated from 120 to 360 mg daily (Table 2–5[25]). The drug is generally safe with little effect on the PR-interval in the absence of pre-existing nodal disease, and severe subjective side-effects are unusual.

No studies compare diltiazem with placebo in **unstable angina at rest.** However, the properties of diltiazem should be ideal—coronary vasodilation and bradycardia, with only a modest negative inotropic effect. In comparison with beta-blockade (propranolol), diltiazem is at least as good, or possibly even better.[1] Different results probably reflect different population groups, with varying degrees of coronary spasm as a cause of the short-lived attacks of anginal pain at rest. However, diltiazem has not been tested against placebo.

In **Prinzmetal's variant angina,** diltiazem 240 to 360 mg/day reduces the number of episodes of pain. At doses of 240 mg daily, 30% of patients become pain-free, and the frequency of angina is reduced in the remaining majority.[1]

In **AMI without Q-waves,** diltiazem 360 mg daily may help to prevent early reinfarction, starting 24 to 72 hours after the onset[1] (the incorrect use of a one-tailed P-test brings about statistical doubt).

**Postinfarct diltiazem** has no overall benefit; retrospective analysis suggests harm with previous LV failure and benefit in those without.[24]

## Diltiazem for Hypertension

In a large multicenter VA study, diltiazem was the best among five agents (atenolol, thiazide, doxazosin, and captopril) in reducing blood pressure, and was especially effective in elderly white patients and in black patients.[63]

In another excellently designed multicenter trial on nearly 300 patients, monotherapy by diltiazem-SR (180 mg twice daily) reduced the diastolic blood pressure to below 90 mmHg in 57% of patients.[4] Blood pressure started to fall after 1 week and a full effect was reached at 3 to 4 weeks. **Combination with hydrochlorothiazide** (12.5 mg daily) gave a 68% response, and with 25 to 50 mg about 75%.[4] However, the combination of diltiazem 360 mg and thiazide 50 mg daily increased blood sugar by 13 mg/dL and plasma cholesterol by 8 mg/dL, so that caution is required in diabetics, in whom diltiazem monotherapy and/or low-dose thiazide (12.5 mg daily) should be much safer.

Long-term outcome studies, as in the case of other calcium antagonists, are still lacking.

## Antiarrhythmic Properties of Diltiazem

*The electrophysiological properties of diltiazem closely resemble those of verapamil.* The main effect is a depressant one on the AV node; the functional and effective refractory periods are prolonged by diltiazem. Diltiazem can be used for the elective as well as prophylactic control (90 mg 3 times daily) of most supraventricular tachyarrhythmias (oral diltiazem not approved for this use in the USA or UK). A particularly useful combination for termination of paroxysmal supraventricular tachycardia is single oral dose diltiazem (120 mg) and propranolol (160 mg), which usually works within 20 to 40 minutes.[1] Diltiazem is unlikely to be effective (and is contraindicated) in ventricular arrhythmias except in those complicating coronary artery spasm or in those few in whom verapamil works. In chronic atrial fibrillation, diltiazem (usual dose 240 mg daily) added to digoxin improves control of ventricular rate.[33] As for verapamil, the presence of a bypass tract (WPW syndrome) is a contraindication to diltiazem.

## Cardiac Transplantation

Following cardiac transplantation, diltiazem acts prophylactically to limit the development of coronary atheroma, acting independently of blood pressure reduction.[70]

## Diltiazem: Summary

Diltiazem, with its properties of peripheral vasodilation and a modest negative inotropic effect and nodal inhibition, is increasingly seen as having hemodynamic advantages in the therapy of angina pectoris. In the therapy of hypertension, it is well-tolerated, and performs well when compared with other categories of drugs. In the intravenous form, it is now approved in the USA for supraventricular tachycardias. The incidence of side-effects (usually low) will depend on the dose and the underlying state of the sinus or AV node and the myocardium, as well as any possible cotherapy with beta-blockers.

# Nifedipine, The Prototypical DHP

The major actions of the DHPs can be simplified to one: arteriolar dilation. Their direct negative inotropic effect is usually outweighed by arteriolar unloading effects (Fig. 3–4), except in patients with CHF.

**Nifedipine** was first introduced in Europe (**Adalat**) and is now widely used in the USA (**Procardia, Procardia XL, Adalat CC**). It is very successful in treating severe hypertension, Prinzmetal's variant angina, Raynaud's phenomenon, and other syndromes produced by arterial vasoconstriction. Nifedipine's action on isolated coronary smooth muscle is 10 or 12 times more powerful than that of verapamil, although in clinical practice nifedipine is only marginally better for coronary spasm.[1]

Lacking a clinically significant effect against the AV node, nifedipine is ineffective against supraventricular arrhythmias, and the combination with beta-blocking agents is theoretically less hazardous than with verapamil or diltiazem.

## Pharmacologic Properties

PHARMACOKINETICS. Nifedipine (capsule form) is almost fully absorbed after an oral dose, reaching peak blood values within 20 to 45 minutes, with a half-life of 3 hours. Almost all circulating nifedipine is broken down by hepatic metabolism by the cytochrome P-450 system to inactive metabolites (high first-pass metabolism). The hypotensive effect starts within 20 minutes of swallowing a capsule and within 5 minutes of bite-and-swallow dose. The duration of action is 4 to 6 hours in some studies, and up to 8 hours in others, especially when combined with other antihypertensives. The longer-acting slow-release preparation (**Procardia XL**) gives 24-hour stable blood levels of about 20 to 30 ng/ml, within the therapeutic range (Table 3–2). With a core-coat system (**Adalat CC**), the blood levels over 24 hours are more variable, yet with comparable control of the blood pressure.

DOSE. In **effort angina,** the usual total dose of nifedipine capsules is 30 to 90 mg daily (i.e., 1 to 3 capsules 3 times daily), which translates into 30 to 90 mg of Procardia XL (Adalat CC is not licensed in the USA for angina). Dose-titration is important to avoid precipitation of ischemic pain in some patients. In **cold-induced angina** or in **coronary spasm,** the doses are similar and capsules allow the most rapid onset of action. In **hypertension,** standard doses are 30 to 60 mg once daily of Procardia XL or Adalat CC. In **severe hypertension,** one 10 mg capsule (bite-and-swallow) usually brings down the blood pressure within 20 to 60 minutes. However, the drug is not licensed in the USA for this purpose.

DOSE MODIFICATION. In the elderly or in severe liver disease, doses must be reduced.

CONTRAINDICATIONS AND CAUTIONS (Fig. 3–7). These are tight aortic stenosis or obstructive hypertrophic cardiomyopathy (danger of exaggerated pressure gradient), severe myocardial depression (added negative inotropic effect), clinically evident heart failure, and unstable angina with threat of infarction (in the absence of concurrent beta-blockade). Relative contraindications are subjective intolerance to nifedipine, previous adverse reactions, and pre-existing tachycardia. In **pregnancy,** nifedipine should only be used if the benefits are thought to outweigh the risk of embryopathy (experimental; pregnancy category C).

MINOR SIDE-EFFECTS. Overall the drug is safe when the above contraindications are observed. On the other hand, especially with the capsules, unpleasant subjective reactions are relatively common, resulting from peripheral vasodilation and including flushing, dizziness, headaches, and palpitations. Such side-effects may occur in nearly 40% of patients given short-acting nifedipine. Sometimes angina may be precipitated about 30 minutes after the dose,[1] the mechanism presumably being reflex tachycardia or coronary underperfusion. The bilateral ankle edema of nifedipine is distressing to patients but is not due to cardiac failure; if required, it can be treated by conventional diuretics or an ACE inhibitor. Nifedipine itself has

## Dihydropyridine Contraindications

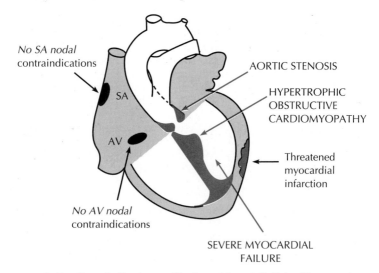

FIGURE 3–7. Contraindications to dihydropyridines (nifedipine-like agents) are chiefly obstructive lesions such as aortic stenosis or hypertrophic obstructive cardiomyopathy. Unstable angina (threatened infarction) is a contraindication unless combined nifedipine plus beta-blockade therapy is used or unless (rarely) coronary spasm is suspected. Fig. copyright L.H. Opie and reproduced from reference 25.

a mild diuretic effect. The incidence of subjective vasodilatory side-effects is higher with nifedipine capsules than with verapamil or diltiazem. With extended-release nifedipine preparations (Procardia XL), the manufacturers claim that side-effects are restricted to headache (nearly double that found in controls) and ankle edema (dose-dependent, 10% with 30 mg daily, 30% with 180 mg daily). The low incidence of acute vasodilatory side-effects, such as flushing and tachycardia, is because of the slow rate of rise of blood DHP levels.[35]

SEVERE SIDE-EFFECTS. In patients with LV depression, the direct negative inotropic effect can be a serious problem. Occasionally, side-effects compatible with the effects of excess hypotension and organ underperfusion have been reported: myocardial ischemia or even infarction, retinal and cerebral ischemia, and renal failure.[1]

RARE SIDE-EFFECTS. These include muscle cramps, myalgia, hypokalemia (via diuretic effect), and gingival swelling.

METABOLIC PROFILE. Nifedipine has no effect on the blood lipid profile. Although precipitation of diabetes mellitus was reported in earlier studies with capsules, the drug is in fact metabolically neutral or may even lessen insulin resistance.

DRUG INTERACTIONS. Cimetidine inhibits the hepatic P-450 enzyme system thereby increasing blood levels of nifedipine. **Volatile anesthetics** interfere with the myocardial calcium regulation and have inhibitory effects additional to those of nifedipine.

REBOUND AFTER CESSATION OF NIFEDIPINE THERAPY. In patients with vasospastic angina, abrupt cessation of therapy by nifedipine capsules may markedly increase the frequency and duration of attacks.[1,61] In effort angina, the evidence for rebound is less convincing.

COMBINATION WITH BETA-BLOCKERS AND OTHER DRUGS. In patients with reasonable LV function, nifedipine may be freely combined with beta-blockade (Fig. 3–8), provided that excess hypotension is guarded against. In LV depression, the added negative inotropic effects may precipitate overt heart failure. For unstable angina at

## Ca²⁺ Antagonists Versus β-Blockade

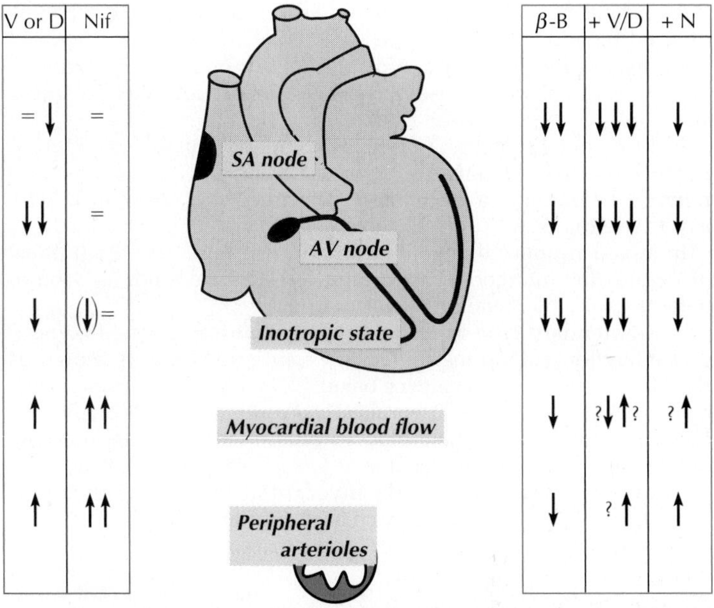

FIGURE 3–8.   Proposed hemodynamic effects of calcium antagonists, singly or in combination with beta-blockade. Note that some of these effects are based on animal data and extrapolation to man needs to be made with caution. V = verapamil; D = diltiazem; N = nifedipine; BB = beta-blockade. Fig. copyright L.H. Opie and modified from Reference 1.

rest, nifedipine, if used, must be combined with a beta-blocker (metoprolol was used in the HINT study[15]). In the therapy of angina caused by spasm, nifedipine may be combined with nitrates. In the therapy of hypertension, nifedipine may be combined with diuretics, beta-blockers, methyldopa, or ACE inhibitors. Combination with prazosin may lead to adverse hypotensive interactions, so a test dose is required.[1] Occasionally nifedipine and diltiazem have been combined with frequent side-effects.[30]

### Nifedipine for Ischemic Syndromes

In **chronic stable angina,** nifedipine is consistently better than placebo. Nifedipine with metoprolol or atenolol[1] is more effective in effort angina than either agent alone, while the beta-blocker is marginally superior as monotherapy. Nifedipine causes a modest reflex increase in heart rate, which may be dose-dependent to limit the antianginal effect. Aggravation of angina may occur through this mechanism, so that the problem should be less with the extended-release preparations. Furthermore, the absence of any significant direct negative inotropic effect may also be a disadvantage in the therapy of angina of effort. *Combination with beta-blockade is logical therapy,* giving better antianginal efficacy than nifedipine or beta-blockade alone in some[1] but not all studies.

A recent long-term outcome study (not yet published in full) in 1,682 patients with chronic stable angina found that combination treatment was better in reducing hard end-points than either treatment given singly. There was no placebo group. The hard end-points were cardiac death, acute myocardial infarction, and unstable angina.[46] The patients were treated either by nifedipine (20 mg retard preparation twice daily) or by atenolol (50 mg twice daily) or by a combination. The latter reduced hard end-points by about 30%

compared with each agent singly. A greater blood pressure reduction with the combination could perhaps be the explanation.

In **smokers with effort angina,** nifedipine is much less effective than in nonsmokers,[12] a fact which might have obscured the benefit of nifedipine in some trials.

In **angina precipitated by cold,** nifedipine is preferable to propranolol,[29] presumably because it relieves reflex coronary vasoconstriction.

In **Prinzmetal's angina** (vasospastic angina), nifedipine 40 to 80 mg in 3 to 4 divided daily doses, up to 120 mg daily gives consistent relief.[1,30] Nifedipine is even more effective when combined with isosorbide dinitrate.[1]

In **mixed angina** (combined effort and rest angina, without threat of myocardial infarction), nifedipine capsules were not as good as beta-blockade by atenolol.[66]

In the **standard type of unstable angina** with threatened myocardial infarction, nifedipine by itself is contraindicated, as shown by the HINT study,[15] but achieves benefit when added to pre-existing beta-blockade (see p 7). Theoretically, results may be obtained by the triple combination beta-blocker plus nifedipine plus nitrates,[1] taking care to avoid hypotension.

In **threatened and very early myocardial infarction,** nifedipine is contraindicated because of increased mortality.[1]

**Postinfarct,** nifedipine prophylaxis carries no benefit.[13]

## Nifedipine for Hypertension

In **systemic hypertension,** nifedipine and other DHPs are increasingly used. Due to the intermittent vasodilation and reflex adrenergic discharge of the shorter-acting forms, frequent dosing is required. Nifedipine capsules are not licensed for hypertension in the USA. Procardia XL and Adalat CC are, however, approved and the dose is initially 30 mg once daily up to 90 mg daily.

For **severe hypertension** (DBP > 120 mmHg), nifedipine capsules 10 mg (bite-and-swallow), which can be repeated once after 30 to 60 minutes, are widely used. Although nifedipine is quicker and cheaper than sodium nitroprusside infusion,[8] it is not licensed for severe hypertension in the USA (rather use intravenous nicardipine). Although the first dose is often effective, a sustained hypotensive effect frequently requires additional treatment by a combination of agents.

There are no outcome studies on the long-term effects of nifedipine in hypertension.

## Other Uses of Nifedipine

In **hypertrophic cardiomyopathy,** nifedipine may have two opposing effects: peripheral vasodilation could exaggerate resting outflow tract obstruction (hence **hypertrophic obstructive cardiomyopathy** is a *contraindication*), whereas benefit presumably results from enhanced diastolic relaxation. The combination of nifedipine and propranolol reduces peak systolic and end-diastolic pressures, the peripheral resistance, and the outflow gradient.[1]

In **CHF,** nifedipine is being used less and less, unless hypertension is the basis. In standard cases of CHF, nifedipine is harmful.[49]

In **chronic hypertensive heart failure,** nifedipine (20 mg 4 times daily) seems better than verapamil (160 mg 3 times daily) in reducing symptoms and pulmonary wedge pressure.[1]

In **severe aortic regurgitation,** nifedipine reduces the need for valve replacement compared with digoxin.[71]

In **primary pulmonary hypertension,** nifedipine is better than hydralazine, yet the high doses used require careful management.[69]

In **acute pulmonary edema** caused by hypertension, nifedipine 10 mg sublingually is effective.[1]

In **coronary atheroma** in the INTACT study,[17] nifedipine 20 mg 4 times daily given for 3 years decreased the development of new lesions on angiography. Overall noncardiac mortality was increased in the nifedipine group, possibly due to the small number of patients, so that larger trials are required to show any true patient benefit.

### Nifedipine Poisoning

In one case there was hypotension, SA and AV nodal block, and hyperglycemia.[14] Treatment was by infusions of calcium and dopamine.

### Nifedipine: Summary

Nifedipine is a widely used and powerful arterial vasodilator with few serious side-effects and is now part of the accepted therapy of effort- or cold-induced angina and of hypertension. However, in unstable angina at rest, nifedipine should not be used as monotherapy, although it is effective when added to pre-existing beta-blockade. Nifedipine, like verapamil and diltiazem, is especially useful in patients with contraindications to beta-blockade such as bronchospasm, diabetes mellitus, or active peripheral vascular disease. Contraindications to nifedipine are few (apart from severe aortic stenosis, obstructive cardiomyopathy, or LV failure), and combination with beta-blockade is usually simple. Vasodilatory side-effects are common and can be reduced by the use of prolonged release preparations, although headache and edema remain problems.

## Second-Generation DHP Calcium Antagonists

### Amlodipine

The major specific advantage of amlodipine (**Norvasc; Istin** in UK) compared with nifedipine is the slower onset of action and the much longer duration of activity (Table 3–6). It binds to the nifedipine (N) site, as do other DHPs. However, the charged nature of the molecule means that its binding is not entirely typical, with very slow association and dissociation,[62] so that the channel block is slow in onset and offset.

Regarding **pharmacokinetics** the absorption is also slow, with peak blood levels being reached after 6 to 12 hours and followed by extensive hepatic metabolism to inactive metabolites. The plasma levels increase during chronic dosage probably because of the very long half-life. The elimination half-life is 35 to 48 hours, increasing slightly with chronic dosage.[3] In the **elderly,** the clearance is reduced and the dose may need reduction.[3]

Regarding **drug interactions,** no effect on digoxin levels has been found, nor is there any interaction with cimetidine.

In **hypertension,** as initial monotherapy, amlodipine 2.5 to 5 mg daily was effective in 56% of patients, while 73% responded to 5 to 10 mg daily.[9] Ambulatory monitoring has demonstrated 24-hour efficacy of 5 mg amlodipine. In comparative studies, amlodipine was equipotent to hydrochlorothiazide or atenolol. Amlodipine 5 mg was the antihypertensive equivalent of nifedipine tablets 20 mg twice daily, and caused fewer vasodilatory symptoms.[43] A mean dose of 9 mg of amlodipine is superior to verapamil in a mean dose of 320 mg.[21]

In **angina pectoris,** amlodipine 10 mg was more effective than placebo, and its antianginal effect persisted for 24 hours.[11] Amlodipine in a mean dose of 7.7 mg is at least as effective as nadolol 105 mg, judged by exercise parameters 24 hours after the last dose.[32]

For **ischemic episodes,** amlodipine 10 mg daily reduces combined ST-changes and symptomatic angina.[44]

In **Prinzmetal's angina,** amlodipine 5 mg daily lessens symptoms and ST-changes.[83]

TABLE 3-6  SECOND-GENERATION CALCIUM CHANNEL ANTAGONISTS: SALIENT FEATURES FOR CARDIOVASCULAR USE

| AGENT | DOSE | PHARMACOKINETICS AND METABOLISM | SIDE-EFFECT AND CONTRAINDICATIONS | INTERACTIONS AND PRECAUTIONS |
|---|---|---|---|---|
| Amplodipine | 5–10 mg once daily | t max 6–12 h. Extensive but slow hepatic metabolism, 90% inactive metabolites. 60% renal. t½ 35–50 h. Steady state in 7–8 days. | As for nifedipine XL. In CHF, amplodipine does not lead to deterioration in NYHA Class II or III. | Prolonged t½ up to 56 h in liver failure. Reduce dose. Cimetidine increases blood levels. |
| Felodipine SR | 5–10 mg once daily. Reduce dose in elderly | t max 3–5 h. Complete hepatic metabolism (P-450) to inactive metabolites, 75% renal loss. t½ 22–27 h. | As for nifedipine XL. May directly stimulate myocardium. | As for nifedipine XL. Cimetidine increases and anticonvulsants decrease blood levels via hepatic metabolism. |
| Isradipine | 2.5–10 mg twice daily | t max 2 h. Complete hepatic metabolism to inactive metabolites, 75% renal, 25% GI loss. t½ 8.4 h. Food delays absorption. | As for nifedipine. Also, animal data show inhibitory effect on sinus node so that tachycardia should be less. C/I: sick sinus syndrome | As for nifedipine but greater effects on sinus node. Propranolol bioavailability increases. |

| | | | | |
|---|---|---|---|---|
| **Nicardipine** capsules | 20–40 mg 3× daily | Rapid absorption. High first-pass saturable effect; plasma clearance may be limited by hepatic blood flow. Peak time 1 h. Hepatic metabolites 60% renal, 35% GI. Increasing dose disproportionately increases blood level. | As for nifedipine, except for less cardiodepression. | As for nifedipine. Cimetidine or liver disease increases blood levels. |
| SR Intravenous | 30–60 mg 2× daily 5–15 mg/h. | As above. t½ 9 h. High first-pass metabolism inactivates drug possibly in proportion to liver blood flow. BP starts to fall within 10 min. | As above. Excess hypotension if beta-blockade plus anesthesia. C/I: severe aortic stenosis, obstructive cardiomyopathy. | As above. Caution in liver disease. |
| **Nimodipine** | 60 mg every 4 h. | t max 0.6 h. High first-pass metabolism to inactive metabolites. Short effective t½ 1–2 h. | As for nifedipine capsules. Cerebroselective claim. | As for nifedipine capsules. Cimetidine and hepatic disease increases blood levels. |

t max = time to peak blood level; t½ = plasma elimination half-life; SR = slow release.

In **diabetic hypertensives,** lipid metabolism and diabetic control, as well as microalbuminuria, are unaltered while the blood pressure falls.[86]

The major **side-effect** is peripheral edema, occurring in about 10% of patients at 10 mg daily (see Table 3–5). In women there is more edema (15%) than in men (6%). Next in significance are dizziness (3% to 4%) and flushing (2% to 3%). Tachycardia has not been reported and headache (same as placebo) seems less than with other DHPs, although there are no strict trials. Compared with verapamil, edema is more common but headache and constipation are less so.[26] Compared with diltiazem, fatigue is more common, with no other significant differences.[26] Compared with placebo, headache is not increased (package insert). In a quality of life study in hypertensives, amlodipine decreased rather than increased headache, while overall quality of life was similar to that on enalapril.[64]

**In summary,** the very long half-life of amlodipine makes it an effective once-a-day antihypertensive and antianginal agent, setting it apart from many of the other agents, which are either twice or thrice daily. Nonetheless, the introduction of extended-release preparations of nifedipine and felodipine has narrowed these differences between amlodipine and the others.

## Felodipine

Felodipine (**Plendil**) has specifically been developed to be more vascular selective than nifedipine. Of interest and relevance to its possible use in CHF is new evidence that felodipine has some calcium channel agonist properties with a positive inotropic effect.[45,67] For **hypertension,** the dose is 2.5 to 5 mg twice daily; higher doses (10 mg b.d.) are more effective, but less well tolerated.[6] The extended-release preparation (**Plendil ER**) allows once-daily dosing. As monotherapy, it is approximately as effective as nifedipine.[2] Felodipine is also the basis of a large outcome study in Scandinavia (HOTS—Hypertension Outcome of Treatment Study) in which the aim is to compare blood pressure reduction to different diastolic levels, such as 90, 85 or 80 mmHg. Felodipine, like other DHPs, combines well with beta-blockers. As a third-line agent after beta-blockers and diuretics, felodipine is equal in effect to minoxidil[37] and better than hydralazine.[6] In **angina pectoris** (not a licensed indication in the USA), felodipine 5 to 10 mg given acutely can improve exercise time for 10 to 12 hours.[36] Felodipine has also been well studied in **vasospastic angina** caused by hyperventilation.[39]

The high vascular selectivity of felodipine has led to extensive testing in **CHF,** yet providing no proof of any sustained benefit.[34] Felodipine is under study in the large Ve-HeFT-3 trial in which it will be added to conventional therapy for heart failure.

## Isradipine

Isradipine (**DynaCirc**) has a medium-duration half-life (Fig. 3–9). It is particularly well tested for experimental antiatherogenic effects. In the current MIDAS study, isradipine was better than a thiazide in curbing carotid changes. It is licensed for hypertension in the USA. Side-effects are similar to other DHPs except that the incidence of ankle edema may be less than expected.[57A]

In **mild to moderate hypertension,** isradipine 2.5 to 5 mg twice daily compares well with hydrochlorothiazide and diltiazem and is superior to propranolol and prazosin. Isradipine may cause less ankle edema than felodipine.[57A] An important finding relates to the antihypertensive mechanism of isradipine (up to 20 mg twice daily), which may be (at least in part) explained by repetitive post-dose natriuresis and diuresis.[18] This is probably a class effect. In **effort angina,** isradipine 10 mg twice daily increases exercise time for 8 but not 12 hours after the first dose.[80]

**Interactions with digoxin** are negligible.

## Nicardipine

Nicardipine (**Cardene**) has many similarities to nifedipine, including the proposed indications and the short duration of action (Table 3–6). Claimed advantages over nifedipine are (1) less of a negative inotropic effect, so that nicardipine may be more vascular-specific with a relatively greater effect on arterial smooth muscle,[19] and (2) water-solubility without light-sensitivity, so that intravenous administration is easier.

**Stable angina pectoris** and **hypertension** are the two approved indications in the USA. The dose is titrated upward from 20 to 40 mg 3 times daily (package insert). In **hypertension,** the package insert acknowledges that the peak hypotensive effect at 1 to 2 hours post-dose is much more than at trough blood levels 6 to 8 hours post-dose, so that the blood pressure should be checked at both times. A slow-release preparation (**Cardine SR**) allows twice-daily dosing and lessens peak-trough variations.

**Intravenous nicardipine** is indicated for the treatment of hypertension when oral treatment is not feasible or not desirable. In a double-blind trial, 67 of 73 patients responded rapidly.[82] The dose is 5 to 15 mg/h with an average maintenance dose of 8 mg/h for severe hypertension, and 3 mg/h for postoperative hypertension. Aortic stenosis is a contraindication.

In summary, a similar series of indications, contraindications, side-effects, and beneficial drug combinations can be anticipated with nicardipine as with nifedipine. The pharmacokinetics are similar. However, in contrast to nifedipine capsules, it is registered for use in both angina and hypertension in the USA. Unlike nifedipine, it is not light-sensitive, so that an intravenous form is now available for use in severe, urgent hypertension.

## Nimodipine

Nimodipine (**Nimotop**) is licensed to reduce morbidity and mortality in **subarachnoid hemorrhage.** The dose in the USA is 60 mg (2 capsules) every 4 hours for 21 days, starting within 96 hours of aneurysmal subarachnoid hemorrhage, irrespective of evidence for coronary vascular spasm. In the UK, the dose is 1 to 2 mg/h by central catheter starting as soon as possible and continuing for 5 days. It does not simply act as a vasodilator.[20] The major side-effect is hypotension. In **early ischemic stroke,** a dose of 120 mg daily in divided doses, added to standard therapy, reduced mortality at 4 weeks in male patients.[10] In **migraine,** nimodipine is as effective as verapamil or nifedipine, but side-effects may be less (cerebroselectivity).

## Other Agents

**Nisoldipine** (**Baymycard**) is extremely vascular selective (Table 3–1). Thus far, however, it is not licensed for hypertension nor for angina in the USA or UK. Trials with the short-acting preparation in effort angina have been disappointing;[79] efficacy is, however, achieved by the extended-release formulation.[55] In Europe, nisoldipine is undergoing clinical trials for use in ischemic **postinfarct LV dysfunction.**

**Nitrendipine** (**Baypress**) is of medium duration of action and has vascular selectivity comparable to that of felodipine. It is not registered for use in the USA. In Europe, it is undergoing large-scale testing as part of a trial in systolic hypertension in the elderly (Syst-Eur).

# Combined Sodium-Calcium Blockade

Combined channel blockade should yield a drug that is effective against ventricular arrhythmias as well as angina, in contrast to other calcium antagonists.

## NEW DHPs: COMPARATIVE PROPERTIES

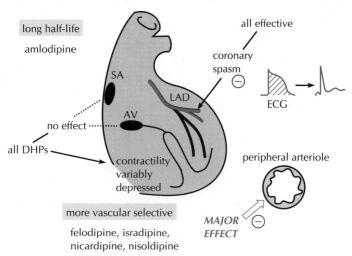

FIGURE 3–9.    Comparative properties of new DHPs. Fig. copyright L.H. Opie.

### Bepridil

This compound (**Vascor**) is a nonspecific calcium channel antagonist[77] with added sodium channel inhibition and a Class I antiarrhythmic effect. It may also inhibit repolarizing potassium currents, thereby prolonging the QT-interval. Bepridil is very long-acting (elimination half-life = 42 hours). It differs from the other calcium antagonists in having only mild antihypertensive properties. The antianginal mechanisms remain unclear but may include a reduction of the rate-pressure product on exercise.[76] Patients refractory to diltiazem may respond to bepridil.[76] It is approved for use in angina (200 to 400 mg once daily) when conventional treatment has failed. The latter restriction is because of the risk of QT-prolongation and torsades de pointes (Fig. 8–8). Therefore, to avoid torsades, hypokalemia must be guarded against and special care taken in the presence of other drugs that may prolong the QT-interval, such as sotalol and amiodarone. Furthermore, the drug is contraindicated in patients with a history of serious ventricular tachycardia or congenital QT-prolongation. It may, however, be combined with propranolol.[53] Thus far its antiarrhythmic potential has received less attention than its proarrhythmic risks.

## Additional or Experimental Uses of Calcium Antagonists

In **Raynaud's phenomenon,** nifedipine is well tested and can be taken either prophylactically or acutely (sublingual or bite-and-swallow) at the start of the attack. Diltiazem is also well documented, with suggestive data for verapamil.

In **progressive systemic sclerosis** (scleroderma), nifedipine may relieve both the associated Raynaud's and coronary artery spasm.

In **peripheral vascular disease,** calcium antagonists are poorly tested. Logically they should benefit most when spasm is the major component, as in severe disease associated with excess cigarette smoking or when intermittent claudication is precipitated by cold.

In **restenosis following coronary angioplasty,** a meta-analysis suggests a 30% reduction by calcium antagonists.[58]

In **chronic renal failure,** nisoldipine (and by implication other DHPs) may prevent progression, acting by inhibition of renal calcinosis.

In **acute renal failure,** nifedipine given prophylactically may prolong the ischemic time, hence being of possible use in renal transplantation.

In **Conn's syndrome,** inhibition of release of aldosterone makes DHPs logical agents for the treatment of hypertension.

In **primary pulmonary hypertension,** high doses (nifedipine 240 mg or diltiazem 720 mg daily) may be tested cautiously after lower initial doses.[69] Benefit is seldom sustained.

In **exercise-induced asthma,** nifedipine and verapamil are mild bronchodilators.

In **LV diastolic heart failure** with maintained systolic function, verapamil improved congestive symptoms.[74]

In **migraine,** verapamil (80 mg 4 times daily) has been well studied, nifedipine and diltiazem are not. Nimodipine and **flunarizine** are also effective, the latter acting perhaps in part through antihistaminic mechanisms.

In **reperfusion "stunning"** in dogs, nifedipine or verapamil given 30 minutes after onset of reperfusion lessened "stunning."[31]

# References

*For references from Second Edition, see Opie (1991)*

1.  Opie LH. Calcium Channel Antagonists (Calcium Entry Blockers). In: Opie LH (ed), Drugs for the Heart, Third Edition. WB Saunders Company, Philadelphia, 1991, pp 42–73.

*References from Third Edition*

2.  Aberg H, Lindsjo M, Morlin B. Drugs 1985; 29 (Suppl 2):117–123.
3.  Abernethy DR. Am Heart J 1989; 118:1100–1103.
4.  Burris JF, Weir MR, Oparil S, et al. JAMA 1990; 263:1507–1512.
5.  Capucci A, Bassein L, Bracchetti D, et al. Eur Heart J 1983; 4:148–154.
6.  Co-operative Study Group. Drugs 1987; 34 (Suppl 3):139–148.
7.  Cubeddu LX, Aranda J, Singh B, et al. JAMA 1986; 256:2214–2221.
8.  Franklin C, Nightingale S, Mamdani B. Chest 1986; 90:500–503.
9.  Frick MH, McGibney D, Tyler HM, et al. J Cardiovasc Pharmacol 1988; 12 (Suppl 7):S76-S78.
10. Gelmers HJ, Gorter K, de Weerdt CJ, Wiezer HJA. N Engl J Med 1988; 318:203–207.
11. Glasser SP, West TW. Am J Cardiol 1988; 62:518–522.
12. Hanet C, Rousseau MF, Vincent M-F, et al. Am J Cardiol 1987; 59:1035–1040.
13. Held PH, Yusuf S, Furberg CD. Br Med J 1989; 299:1187–1192.
14. Herrington DM, Insley BM, Weinmann GG. Am J Med 1986; 81:344–346.
15. HINT Research Group (Holland Interuniversity Nifedipine/Metoprolol Trial). Br Heart J 1986; 56:400–413.
16. Holzgreve H, Distler A, Michaelis J, et al. Br Med J 1989; 299:881–886.
17. INTACT study—Lichtlen PR, Hugenholtz P, Rafflenbeul W, and the INTACT group. Lancet 1990; 335:1109–1113.
18. Krusell LR, Jespersen LT, Schmitz A, et al. Hypertension 1987; 10:577–581.
19. Lambert CR, Pepine CJ. Am J Cardiol 1989; 64:8H–15H.
20. Langley MS, Sorkin EM. Drugs 1989; 37:669–699.
21. Lorimer AR, Smedsrud T, Walker P, Tyler HM. J Cardiovasc Pharmacol 1988; 12 (Suppl 7):S89–S93.
22. Mauri F, Mafrici A, Biraghi P, et al. Eur Heart J 1988; 9 (Suppl N):158–163.
23. McLean AJ, Knight R, Harrison PM, et al. Am J Cardiol 1985; 55:1628–1629.
24. Multicenter Diltiazem Postinfarction Trial Research Group. N Engl J Med 1988; 319:385–392.
25. Opie LH. Clinical Use of Calcium Antagonist Drugs. Kluwer Academic Publishers, Boston, 1990.
26. Osterloh I. Am Heart J 1989; 118:1114–1120.
27. Packer M. N Engl J Med 1989; 320:709–718.
28. Parodi O, Simonetti I, Michelassi C, et al. Am J Cardiol 1986; 57:899–906.
29. Peart I, Bullock RE, Albers C, Hall RJC. Br Heart J 1989; 61:521–528.
30. Prida XE, Gelman JS, Feldman RL, et al. J Am Coll Cardiol 1987; 9:412–419.
31. Przyklenk K, Ghafari GB, Eitzman DT, Kloner RA. J Am Coll Cardiol 1989; 13:1176–1183.
32. Singh S, Doherty J, Udhoji V, et al. Am Heart J 1989; 118:1137–1138.
33. Steinberg JS, Katz RJ, Bren GB, et al. J Am Coll Cardiol 1987; 9:405–411.

34. Tan LB, Murray RG, Littler WA. Br Heart J 1987; 58:122–128.

35. Van Harten J, Van Brummelen P, Zeegers RRECM, et al. Br J Clin Pharmacol 1988; 25:709–717.

36. Verdecchia P, Gatteschi C, Benemio G, et al. Eur Heart J 1989; 10:70–76.

37. Wathan CG, MacLeod D, Tucker L, Muir AL. Eur Heart J 1986; 7:893–897.

38. Wicker P, Roudaut R, Gosse P, Dallocchio M. Am J Cardiol 1986; 57:83D–86D.

## New References

39. Ardissino D, Savonitto S, Zanini P, et al. Ability of calcium-entry blockade by felodipine to disclose different pathogenetic mechanisms behind hyperventilation-induced myocardial ischemia in men. Am J Cardiol 1990; 66:1304–1308.

40. Ardissino D, Savonitto S, Egstrup K, et al. Transient myocardial ischemia during daily life in rest and exertional angina pectoris and comparison of effectiveness of metoprolol versus nifedipine. Am J Cardiol 1991; 67:946–952.

41. Barjon J-N, Rouleau J-L, Bichet D, et al. Chronic renal and neurohumoral effects of the calcium entry blocker nisoldipine in patients with congestive heart failure. J Am Coll Cardiol 1987; 9:622–630.

42. Baumgart D, Ehring T, Heusch G. A proischemic action of nisoldipine: Relationship to a decrease in perfusion pressure and comparison to dipyridamole. Cardiovasc Res 1993; 27:1254–1259.

43. Bremner AD, Fell PJ, Hosie J, et al. Early side-effects of antihypertensive therapy: Comparison of amlodipine and nifedipine retard. J Human Hypertens 1993; 7:79–81.

44. CAPE Investigators—Deanfield JE for the CAPE Investigators. Amlodipine reduces the total ischemic burden of patients with coronary disease: Double-blind, Circadian Anti-ischemic Program in Europe (CAPE) Trial (abstr). J Am Coll Cardiol 1994; 23:53A.

45. Cheng C-P, Noda T, Norlander M, et al. Comparison of effects of dihydropyridine calcium antagonists on left ventricular systolic and diastolic performance. J Pharmacol Exp Ther 1994; 268:1232–1241.

46. Dargie HJJ, for the TIBET Study Group. Medical treatment of angina can favourably affect outcome (abstr). Eur Heart J 1993; 14 (Abstract Suppl):304.

47. DAVIT-II study—Danish Study Group on Verapamil in Myocardial Infarction. Effect of verapamil on mortality and major events after acute myocardial infarction (The Danish Verapamil Infarction Trial II—DAVIT-II). Am J Cardiol 1990; 66:779–785.

48. DeCesare N, Bartorelli A, Fabbiocchi F, et al. Superior efficacy of propranolol versus nifedipine in double-component angina, as related to different influences on coronary vasomotility. Am J Med 1989; 87:15–21.

49. Elkayam U, Amin J, Mehra A, et al. A prospective, randomized, double-blind, crossover study to compare the efficacy and safety of chronic nifedipine therapy with that of isosorbide dinitrate and their combination in the treatment of chronic congestive heart failure. Circulation 1990; 82:1954–1961.

50. El-Tamimi H, Mansour M, Wargovich TJ, et al. Intravenous metoprolol enhances coronary vasoreactive response to acetylcholine in patients with chronic stable angina (abstr). Circulation 1993; 88:I–493.

50A. Fioretto P, Frigato F, Velussi M, et al. Effects of angiotensin-converting enzyme inhibitors and calcium antagonists on atrial natriuretic peptide release and action and on albumin excretion rate in hypertensive insulin-dependent diabetic patients. Am J Hypertens 1992; 5:837–846.

51. Fischer Hansen J and The Danish Study Group on Verapamil in Myocardial Infarction. Treatment with verapamil during and after an acute myocardial infarction: A review based on the Danish Verapamil Infarction Trials I and II. J Cardiovasc Pharmacol 1991; 18 (Suppl 6):S20–S25.

52. Freedman SB, Richmond DR, Kelly DT. Long-term follow-up of verapamil and nitrate treatment for coronary artery spasm. Am J Cardiol 1982; 50:711–715.

53. Frishman WH. Comparative efficacy and concomitant use of bepridil and beta-blockers in the management of angina pectoris. Am J Cardiol 1992; 69:50D–55D.

54. Frishman WH, Rosenberg A, Katz B. Calcium channel blockers in the management of systemic hypertension: The impact of sustained-release drug delivery systems. Coronary Artery Disease 1994; 5:4–13.

55. Glasser S, Ripa S, MacCarthy EP, for the Nisoldipine CC Multicenter Study Group. Efficacy and safety of extended-release nisoldipine as monotherapy for chronic stable angina pectoris (abstr). J Am Coll Cardiol 1994; 23:1A–48A.

56. Godfraind T, Salomone S, Dessy C, et al. Selectivity scale of calcium antagonists in the human cardiovascular system based on in vitro studies. J Cardiovasc Pharmacol 1992; 20 (Suppl 5):S34–S41.

57. Halperin AK, Icenogel MV, Kapsner CO, et al. A comparison of the effects of nifedipine and verapamil on exercise performance in patients with mild to moderate hypertension. Am J Hypertens 1993; 6:1025–1032.

57A. Hammond JJ, Cutler SA for the Physician's Study Group. A comparison of isradipine and felodipine in Australian patients hypertension: Focus on ankle edema. Blood Pressure 1993 205–211.

58. Hillegass WB, Ohman EM, Leimberger JD, Califf RM. A meta-analysis of randomized trials of calcium antagonists to reduce restenosis after coronary angioplasty. Am J Cardiol 1994; 73:835–839.

59. Kenny J. Treating overdose with calcium channel blockers. Br Med J 1994; 308:992–993.

60. Leenen FHH, Holliwell DL. Antihypertensive effect of felodipine associated with persistent sympathetic activation and minimal regression of left ventricular hypertrophy. Am J Cardiol 1992; 69:639–645.

61. Lette J, Gagnon RM, Lemire JG, Morissette M. Rebound of vasospastic angina after cessation of long-term treatment with nifedipine. Can Med Ass J 1984; 130:1169–1171.

62. Mason RP. Differential effect of cholesterol on membrane interaction of charged versus uncharged 1, 4-dihydropyridine calcium channel antagonists: A biophysical analysis. Cardiovasc Drugs Ther 1994, in press.

63. Materson BJ, Reda DJ, Cushman WC, et al. Single-drug therapy for hypertension in men. A comparison of six antihypertensive agents with placebo. N Engl J Med 1993; 328:914–921.

64. Omvik P, Thaulow, Herland OB, et al. Double-blind, parallel, comparative study on quality of life during treatment with amlodipine or enalapril in mild or moderate hypertensive patients: A multicentre study. J Hypertens 1993; 11:103–113.

65. Pelliccia F, Cianfrocca C, Romeo F, Reale A. Hypertrophic cardiomyopathy: long-term effects of propranolol versus verapamil in preventing sudden death in "low-risk" patients. Cardiovasc Drugs Ther 1990; 4:1515–1518.

66. Quyyumi AA, Crake T, Wright CM, et al. Medical treatment of patients with severe exertional and rest angina: Double-blind comparison of beta-blocker, calcium antagonist, and nitrate. Br Heart J 1987; 57:505–511.

67. Redfield MM, Neumann A, Tajik J, et al. Effect of long-acting oral felodipine and nifedipine on left ventricular contractility in patients with systemic hypertension: Differentiation between reflex sympathetic and direct contractile responses (abstr). J Am Coll Cardiol 1994; 23:348A.

68. Remme WJ, Krauss H, Van Hoogenhuyze DCA, Kruyssen DACM. Hemodynamic tolerability and anti-ischemic efficacy of high dose intravenous diltiazem in patients with normal versus impaired ventricular function. J Am Coll Cardiol 1993; 21:709–720.

69. Rich S, Kaufmann E, Levy PS. The effect of high doses of calcium channel blockers on survival in primary pulmonary hypertension. N Engl J Med 1992; 327:76–81.

70. Schroeder JS, Gao S-Z, Alderman EL, et al. A preliminary study of diltiazem in the prevention of coronary artery disease in heart-transplant recipients. N Engl J Med 1993; 328:164–170.

71. Scognamiglio R, Rahimtoola S, Fasoli G, et al. Nifedipine in asymptomatic patients with severe aortic regurgitation and normal left ventricular function. N Engl J Med 1994; 331:689–694.

72. Seiler C, Hess OM, Schoenbeck M, et al. Long-term follow-up of medical versus surgical therapy for hypertrophic cardiomyopathy: A retrospective study. J Am Coll Cardiol 1991; 17:634–642.

73. Seitelberger R, Zwolfer W, Huber S, et al. Nifedipine reduces the incidence of myocardial infarction and transient ischemia in patients undergoing coronary bypass grafting. Circulation 1991; 83:460–468.

74. Setaro JF, Zaret BL, Schulman DS, et al. Usefulness of verapamil for congestive heart failure associated with abnormal left ventricular diastolic filling and normal left ventricular systolic performance. Am J Cardiol 1990; 66:981–986.

75. Shapiro W, Narahara KA, Kostis JB, et al. Comparison of atenolol and nifedipine in chronic stable angina pectoris. Am J Cardiol 1989; 64:186–190.

76. Singh BN for the Bepridil Collaborative Study Group. Comparative efficacy and safety of bepridil and diltiazem in chronic stable angina pectoris refractory to diltiazem. Am J Cardiol 1991; 68:306–312.

77. Spedding M, Paoletti R. Classification of calcium channels and calcium antagonists: Progress report. Cardiovasc Drugs Ther 1992; 6:35–39.

78. Stone PH, Gibson RS, Glasser SP, et al. Comparison of propranolol, diltiazem, and nifedipine in the treatment of ambulatory ischemia in patients with stable angina. Differential effects on ambulatory ischemia, exercise performance, and anginal symptoms. Circulation 1990; 82:1962–1972.

79. Thadani U, Zellner S, Glasser S, et al. Double-blind, dose-response, placebo-controlled multicenter study of nisoldipine. A new second-generation calcium channel blocker in angina pectoris. Circulation 1991; 84:2398–2408.

80. Thadani U, Chrysant S, Gorwit J, et al. Duration of effects of isradipine during twice daily therapy in angina pectoris. Cardiovasc Drugs Ther 1994; 8:199–210.

80A. Thadani U, Glasser S. Bittar N, Beach CL, and the Diltiazem CD Study Group. Dose-reponse evaluation of once-daily therapy with a new formulation of diltiazem for stable angina pectoris. Am J Cardiol 1994; 74:9–17.

81. Udelson JE, Bonow RO, O'Gara PT, et al. Verapamil prevents silent myocardial perfusion abnormalities during exercise in asymptomatic patients with hypertrophic cardiomyopathy. Circulation 1989; 79:1052–1060.

82. Wallin JD, Fletcher E, Ram VS, et al. Intravenous nicardipine for the treatment of severe hypertension. Arch Intern Med 1989; 149:2662–2669.

83. Watanabe T, Kalasz H, Yabana H, et al. Azidobutyryl clentiazem, a new photoactivatable diltiazem analog, labels benzothiazepine binding sites in the alpha$_1$-subunit of the skeletal muscle calcium channel. FEBS 1993; 334:261–264.

84. Watanabe K, Izumi T, Miyakita Y, et al. Efficacy of amlodipine besilate therapy

for variant angina: Evaluation by 24-hour Holter monitoring. Cardiovasc Drugs Ther 1993; 7:923–928.

85.    Yusuf S, Held P, Furberg C. Update of effects of calcium antagonists in myocardial infarction or angina in light of the second Danish Verapamil Infarction Trial (DA-VIT-II) and other recent studies. Am J Cardiol 1991; 67:1295–1297.

86.    Zanetti-Elshater F, Pingitore R, Beretta-Piccoli C, et al. Calcium antagonists for treatment of diabetes-associated hypertension. Metabolic and renal effects of am-lodipine. Am J Hypertens 1994; 7:36–45.

## *Book Chapter*

87.    Frishman WH, Sonnenblick EH. Calcium channel blockers. In: Schlant RC, Alexander RW (eds), The Heart, Arteries and Veins. McGraw-Hill, New York, 1994, pp 1291–1308.

# 4 Diuretics

L.H. Opie ♦ N.M. Kaplan ♦ P.A. Poole-Wilson

*"Little benefit is to be derived from using large doses of oral diuretics to reduce blood pressure."*[29]

Diuretics have traditionally been the drug of first choice in the treatment of symptomatic heart failure, and still retain their primacy despite the lack of outcome studies. In hypertension, diuretics continue to be used as first-line therapy, albeit in much lower doses—a position supported by recent outcome studies in the elderly (p 192).

## Differing Effects of Diuretics in Heart Failure and Hypertension

In **heart failure,** diuretics are given to control pulmonary and peripheral symptoms and signs of congestion. They are standard first-line agents. To limit sodium and water retention, furosemide is often the initial drug of choice because of its efficacy, even in the presence of renal impairment that often accompanies severe heart failure. In general, diuretic doses are higher than those used in hypertension. Besides the induction of renal sodium and water loss, furosemide given to previously untreated patients with severe congestive heart failure (CHF) calls forth two opposing stimuli.[23] The vasoconstrictory renin-angiotensin system is stimulated, and there are also increased levels of vasodilatory atrial natriuretic peptide (ANP). The latter unexpected effect may explain furosemide-induced vasodilation (p 63). The natriuretic effect of the latter is limited, perhaps as a result of renin activation.[54] Hence, the addition of ACE inhibitors to offset the renin rise should be beneficial.

In **hypertension,** to exert an effect, the diuretic must provide enough natriuresis to shrink fluid volume at least to some extent. Diuretics may also work as vasodilators and in other ways. Some persistent volume depletion is required to lower the blood pressure. Therefore, once-daily furosemide is usually inadequate because the initial sodium loss is quickly reconstituted throughout the remainder of the day.[46] Thus, a longer-acting thiazide-type diuretic is usually chosen for hypertension.

## Benefit-Risk Ratio

The benefit-to-risk ratio of diuretics is very high in CHF. In contrast, the risk of standard or high doses diuretics in the therapy of mild hypertension is increasingly questioned, because of the "wrong-way" blood biochemical changes. Therefore, the time-honored role of diuretics as first-line therapy in hypertension is challenged though these agents still have an important place when given in low doses, especially in certain groups of hypertensive patients—the elderly, the obese and blacks—and those already receiving ACE inhibitors. Furthermore, the realization that low doses of diuretics can be given over prolonged periods with minimal changes in blood lipids, glucose and potassium[55] has been accompanied by a recommendation

## DIURETIC SITES OF ACTION

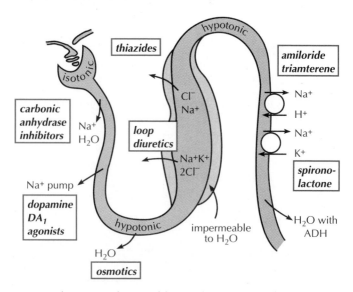

**FIGURE 4-1.** The six sites of action of diuretic agents. CA = carbonic anhydrase inhibitors. A common maximal combination, using the principle of sequential nephron blockade, is a loop diuretic plus a thiazide plus a K$^+$-sparing agent. Fig. copyright L.H. Opie and modified from Reference 1.

from the Joint National Committee[34] that diuretics as well as beta-blockers should be considered for first choice in the treatment of hypertension.

For practical purposes, the three major groups of diuretics are the loop diuretics, the thiazides, and the potassium-sparing diuretics. Each type of diuretic acts at a different site of the nephron (Fig. 4-1) leading to the concept of **sequential nephron blockade.** All but the potassium sparers must be transported to the luminal side; this process is blocked by the buildup of organic acids in renal insufficiency so that progressively larger doses are needed. Especially thiazides lose their potency as renal function falls.

## Loop Diuretics

In the therapy of CHF, a loop diuretic is often chosen as initial therapy especially when the CHF is severe. A particular advantage of loop diuretics, such as furosemide, is that increasing doses exert an increasing diuresis before the "ceiling" is reached (**high-ceiling diuretics**).

### Furosemide

Furosemide (= frusemide; **Lasix, Dryptal, Frusetic, Frusid**) is one of the standard loop diuretics for severe CHF. Furosemide is initial therapy in acute pulmonary edema and in left-sided failure of acute myocardial infarction (AMI). Relief of dyspnea even before diuresis results from venodilation and preload reduction.[1]

PHARMACOLOGIC EFFECTS AND PHARMACOKINETICS. Loop diuretics including furosemide (Fig. 4-1) inhibit the Na$^+$/K$^+$/2Cl$^-$ cotransporter concerned with the transport of chloride across the lining cells of the ascending limb of the loop of Henle (site 2). This site of action is reached intraluminally, after the drug has been excreted by the proximal tubule. The effect of the cotransport inhibition is that chloride, sodium, potassium, and hydrogen ions all remain intraluminally and are lost in the urine with the possible side-effects of hyponatremia,

**TABLE 4–1** URINARY ELECTROLYTE COMPOSITION DURING DIURESIS

| | VOLUME (ML/MIN) | pH | Na$^+$ (mM/L) | K$^+$ (mM/L) | Cl$^-$ | HCO$_3^-$ | Ca$^{2+}$ |
|---|---|---|---|---|---|---|---|
| Control | 1 | 6.0 | 50 | 15 | 60 | 1 | Variable |
| Thiazides | 3 | 7.4 | 150 | 25 | 150 | 25 | 0 |
| Furosemide | 8 | 6.0 | 140 | 10 | 155 | 1 | + |
| Triamterene | 3 | 7.2 | 130 | 5 | 120 | 15 | 0 |
| Amiloride | 2 | 7.2 | 130 | 5 | 110 | 15 | 0 |

Modified from Mudge[15] with permission. O = decreased; + = increased

hypochloremia, hypokalemia, and alkalosis. The plasma half-life of furosemide is 1.5 hours; the duration of action is 4 to 6 hours. Diuresis starts within 10 to 20 minutes of an intravenous dose and peaks 1 to 1.5 hours after an oral dose.[1]

DOSE. **Intravenous furosemide** is usually started as a slow 40 mg injection (give 80 mg slowly IV 1 hour later if needed). When renal function is impaired, as in elderly patients, higher doses are required,[1] with much higher doses for renal failure and severe CHF. **Oral furosemide** also has a wide dose range (20 to 250 mg/day or even more; 20, 40, and 80 mg tablets in the USA; in Europe, also scored 500 mg tablets). A short duration of action (4 to 5 hours) means that frequent doses are needed when sustained diuresis is required. When 2 daily doses are required, they should be given in the early morning and midafternoon to obviate nocturia and to protect against volume depletion. Once acute relief has been obtained, however, twice-daily dosage, reducing to once daily, is usually given to rest the kidneys and the patients (at night). Because of variable responses, such as a brisk initial diuresis with a residual resistant component, the dose regime must be individualized. For **hypertension,** furosemide is sometimes used as initial monotherapy with 20 mg twice daily being the approximate equivalent of hydrochlorothiazide 25 mg.[1] In healthy subjects, furosemide causes a much greater earlier (0 to 6 hours) sodium loss than does hydrochlorothiazide, but there is a later rebound with furosemide, so that the total 24-hour sodium loss may be less.[46] This observation supports the practice of giving furosemide twice daily in hypertension, as recommended by the manufacturers. In the presence of **oliguria,** as the GFR drops below 20 ml/min, from 250 mg up to 2,000 mg of furosemide may be required because of decreasing luminal excretion. Similar arguments lead to increasing doses of furosemide in **severe refractory heart failure.**

INDICATIONS. Furosemide is frequently the diuretic of choice for **severe heart failure** for three reasons: First, it induces a more acute sodium loss than other diuretics (Table 4–1); second, it is effective (in high doses) in promoting diuresis even in the presence of a low glomerular filtration rate (GFR); and third, furosemide promotes venodilation and preload reduction.[1] Similar reasons make it the initial drug of choice in **acute pulmonary edema.** After initial intravenous use, oral furosemide is usually continued as standard diuretic therapy, to be replaced by thiazides as the heart failure ameliorates. In **AMI** with clinical failure, intravenous furosemide has rapid beneficial hemodynamic effects[53] and is often combined with ACE inhibition. **Postinfarct,** a low ejection fraction is better treated by captopril than by furosemide.[20] In **hypertension,** twice-daily low-dose furosemide can be effective even as monotherapy[1] or combined with other agents. However, if thiazides do not work for hypertension, furosemide will probably not work either unless the problem is a very low GFR. In **severe hypertension,** intravenous furosemide is sometimes used, especially if fluid overload is present. In **severe renal failure,**

**TABLE 4–2** LOOP DIURETICS: DOSES AND KINETICS

| DRUG | DOSE | PHARMACOKINETICS |
| --- | --- | --- |
| 1. Furosemide (USA)<br>Frusemide (UK)<br>  = Lasix | 10–40 mg oral, 2× for BP<br>20–80 mg 2–3× for CHF<br>Up to 250–2000 mg oral or IV | Diuresis within 10–20 min;<br>Peak diuresis at 1.5 h<br>Total duration of action 4–5 h<br>Renal excretion |
| 2. Bumetanide<br>  = Bumex (USA)<br>  = Burinex (UK) | 0.5–2 mg oral 1–2× daily for CHF<br>5 mg oral or IV for oliguria<br>(not licensed for BP) | Peak diuresis 75–90 min<br>Total duration of action 4–5 h<br>Renal excretion |
| 3. Torsemide<br>  = Demadex (USA) | 5–10 mg oral 1× daily for BP<br>10–20 mg oral 1× daily or IV for CHF (up to 200 mg daily) | Diuresis within 10 min of IV dose;<br>Peak diuresis at 60 min<br>Oral peak 1–2 h<br>Oral duration of diuresis 6–8 h |

BP = blood pressure control

it is widely believed that furosemide increases the GFR, yet the subject is poorly understood.

CONTRAINDICATIONS. Anuria, although listed as a contraindication to the use of furosemide, is sometimes treated (as is oliguria) by furosemide in the hope of evoking a diuresis; first exclude dehydration and a history of hypersensitivity to furosemide or sulfonamides. Furosemide (like other sulfonamides) may precipitate or exaggerate lupus erythematosus or photosensitive skin eruptions or may cause blood dyscrasias. Furosemide should not be used intravenously when electrolytes cannot be monitored.

SIDE-EFFECTS. The risk of **hypokalemia** is greatest with high-dose furosemide, especially when given intravenously, and at the start of myocardial infarction when hypokalemia with risk of arrhythmias is common even in the absence of diuretic therapy. Carefully regulated intravenous potassium supplements may be required in these circumstances. In heart failure, digitalis toxicity may be precipitated by over-diuresis and hypokalemia. Standard oral doses of furosemide (40 to 80 mg daily), as used for the chronic therapy of heart failure and hypertension, probably cause less hypokalemia than do some thiazides (Table 4–1).[1] Clearly, much depends on the doses chosen and the degree of diuresis achieved. A lesser degree of hypokalemia than expected occurs because (1) the actual potassium concentration lost per unit volume during the diuresis is low (see Table 4–1), and (2) the short action of furosemide allows for postdiuresis correction of potassium and magnesium balance.[46] Addition of potassium supplements to furosemide therapy is neither needed nor very effective;[1,6] rather add a potassium-sparing diuretics or an ACE inhibitor.[1]

OTHER SIDE-EFFECTS. In 2,580 patients, the chief side-effects, in addition to **hypokalemia,** were **hypovolemia** and **hyperuricemia.**[1] Hypovolemia can be lessened by a low initial dose (20 to 40 mg); if hypovolemia occurs, prerenal azotemia may develop (monitor blood urea). A few patients on high-dose furosemide have developed severe hyperosmolar nonketotic **hyperglycemic states.**[1] **Atherogenic**

**blood lipid changes,** similar to those found with thiazides, may also be found with loop diuretics, although not so well documented.[1] Occasionally, gout or diabetes may be precipitated. It is not clear whether furosemide causes fewer metabolic side-effects than conventional thiazides. First principles suggest that minimizing hypokalemia should lessen the risk of glucose intolerance.[51]

Reversible dose-related **ototoxicity** (electrolyte disturbances of the endolymphatic system) can be avoided by infusing furosemide at rates not greater than 4 mg/min and keeping the oral dose below 1,000 mg daily.

In the **elderly,** vigorous diuresis may be associated with nocturia, prostatism and urinary retention.

In **nursing mothers,** furosemide is excreted in the milk with the risk of delayed closure of a patent ductus.[1]

DRUG INTERACTIONS. **Probenecid** may interfere with the effects of thiazides or loop diuretics by blocking their secretion into the urine of the proximal tubule.[1] **Indomethacin** and other nonsteroidal antiinflammatory drugs (**NSAIDs**) cause loss of response of the kidney to loop diuretics, presumably by interfering with formation of vasodilatory prostaglandins.[1] High doses of furosemide may competitively inhibit the excretion of **salicylates** to predispose to salicylate poisoning with tinnitus. **Steroid** or ACTH therapy may predispose to hypokalemia. Furosemide, unlike thiazides, does not decrease renal excretion of **lithium,** so that lithium toxicity is not a risk.[32] Loop diuretics do not alter blood digoxin levels, nor do they interact with warfarin. Recently, an interaction with **captopril** has been described. The latter decreases renal excretion of furosemide to interfere with its diuretic potency.[39] Similar effects are not found with ramipril or enalapril.[56] These observations may explain why ultralow doses of captopril appear to be better than standard doses when added to furosemide.[40]

## Bumetanide

The site of action of bumetanide (**Bumex, Burinex**) and its effects (and side-effects) are very similar to that of furosemide (Table 4–2). The onset of diuresis is within 30 minutes, with a peak at 75 to 90 minutes, and a total duration of action of 270 minutes.[1] Although it has been claimed that potassium loss may be less than that caused by furosemide while achieving a comparable loss of sodium, other studies show a powerful potassium-losing capacity.[1] In practice, as with furosemide, low-dose therapy need not occasion undue concern regarding hypokalemia as a possible side-effect, while higher doses can cause considerable electrolyte disturbances, including hypokalemia. Again, as in the case of furosemide, a combined diuretic effect is obtained by addition of a thiazide diuretic.

DOSE AND CLINICAL USES. In **CHF,** bumetanide is claimed to be effective in patients with edema resistant to furosemide, but additional studies are required to prove this point. The usual oral dose is 0.5 to 2 mg (0.5 and 1 mg tablets) with 1 mg bumetanide being equal to 40 mg furosemide;[1] other estimates are that bumetanide is $70\times$ more powerful than furosemide.[1] In **renal failure,** the comparative potency of bumetanide might be much less than 40.[1] In **acute pulmonary edema,** a single dose of 1 to 3 mg can be effective; usually it is given intravenously over 1 to 2 minutes, and the dose can be repeated at 2- to 3-hourly intervals to a maximum of 10 mg daily. In **renal edema,** the effects of bumetanide are similar to those of furosemide. In the USA, bumetanide is not approved for hypertension.

SIDE-EFFECTS AND CAUTIONS. These are rather similar to those of furosemide; ototoxicity may be less[1] and renal toxicity more. The combination with other potentially nephrotoxic drugs, such as aminoglycosides, must be avoided. In patients with renal failure, high doses have caused myalgia, so that the dose should not exceed 4 mg/day when the GFR is below 5 ml/min.[1] Patients allergic to sulfonamides may also be hypersensitive to bumetanide; however, the package insert suggests that bumetanide might be safe when allergy to furosemide develops. Whether glucose tolerance is preserved by bumetanide needs further study. In pregnancy, the risk is similar to furosemide (Category C).

SUMMARY. Until more careful studies are available on the comparison between bumetanide and furosemide, most clinicians will continue to use the agent they know best (i.e., furosemide) unless there is a specific reason for not giving furosemide (allergic reaction, ototoxicity). As furosemide is widely available in generic form, its cost is likely to be less than that of bumetanide. Nonetheless, the use of bumetanide is increasing.

## Torsemide

This recently introduced loop diuretic (**Demadex**) is much better studied than others in the therapy of **hypertension**. Although initial studies suggested that a subdiuretic daily dose of 2.5 mg was antihypertensive and free of changes in plasma potassium or glucose,[25] in the USA the only doses registered for antihypertensive efficacy are 5 to 10 mg daily. These natriuretic doses[46] decrease plasma potassium, increase uric acid, and transiently increase serum cholesterol, while the 10 mg dose mildly increases plasma glucose (package insert). The information available is not enough to state whether torsemide or other loop diuretics cause less metabolic disturbances than do thiazides in equihypotensive doses.

In **heart failure,** an intravenous dose of torsemide 10 to 20 mg initiates a diuresis within 10 minutes that peaks within the first hour. Similar oral doses (high availability) give an onset of diuresis within 1 hour and a peak effect within 1 to 2 hours, and a total duration of action of 6 to 8 hours. Higher doses cause greater diuresis with more evident potassium loss. Thereafter, in the chronic therapy of heart failure, the torsemide dose given once daily is about two-fifths that of furosemide.[35]

In **renal failure,** as in the case of other loop diuretics, the renal excretion of the drug falls as does the renal function. Yet the plasma half-life torsemide is unaltered, probably because hepatic clearance increases.[26] "Chronic use of any diuretic in renal disease has not been studied in adequate and well controlled trials" (package insert).

In **hepatic cirrhosis,** the dose is 5 to 10 mg daily, titrated upwards to a maximum of 200 mg daily. Torsemide is given with an aldosterone antagonist.

In **pregnancy,** torsemide may be relatively safe (Category B vs. Category C for furosemide).

There are no long-term outcome studies available for any of the above indications. Side-effects, cautions, and contraindications are similar to those of furosemide.

## Ethacrynic Acid

Ethacrynic acid (**Edecrin**) closely resembles furosemide in dose (25 and 50 mg tablet), duration of diuresis, and side-effects (except for more ototoxicity). The usual intravenous dose is 50 mg. Furosemide is much more widely used because it has a broader dose-response curve than ethacrynic acid, which allows easier definition of the optimal dose for a given patient.[1] However, there may be an advantage for ethacrynic acid in pregnancy (Category B; furosemide, Category C).

## Class Side-Effects of Loop Diuretics

Loop diuretics all produce a powerful and rapid natriuresis and can be used in the therapy of acute and chronic heart failure. They are also used for hepatic cirrhosis and hypertension. The important question is whether or not the loop diuretics, like the thiazides, can induce adverse metabolic changes, such as an increased plasma cholesterol, glucose and uric acid. The answer is yes—as shown by the recently FDA-approved information sheet on the new loop diuretic, torsemide, and by the available but scant information on the other loop diuretics.

HYPOKALEMIA. In the doses used for mild hypertension (furosemide 40 mg, torsemide 5 to 10 mg), hypokalemia is limited and possibly less than with hydrochlorothiazide 25 to 50 mg daily.[12] Nonetheless, it does make sense to combine a loop diuretic with a potassium-retaining agent or with an ACE inhibitor unless these are contraindicated.

HYPERGLYCEMIA. Indirect evidence suggests that diuretic-induced glucose intolerance is related to hypokalemia,[43,51] so that measures to avoid the latter should prevent the former. There are no large prospective studies on the effects of loop diuretics on insulin insensitivity or glucose tolerance in hypertensive patients. The FDA-approved package insert for torsemide claims that antihypertensive doses (5 to 10 mg) only reduce plasma potassium by 0.1 mEq/L after 6 weeks, yet the higher dose increases plasma glucose by 5.5 mg/dL (0.3 mmol/L) after 6 weeks with a further increase of 1.8 mg/dL during the subsequent year. Thus, hypokalemic and hyperglycemic effects may not seem to be tightly related. Nonetheless, an interesting proposal is that the transient postprandial fall of potassium impairs the effect of insulin at that time and hence leads to intermittent hyperglycemia.[47]

BLOOD LIPID PROFILE. Whether a loop diuretics cause blood lipid changes similar to thiazides is not known. Imperfect evidence, not citing the dose or drugs used, says "yes."[22] For torsemide, the package insert indicates that short-term treatment with doses of 5 to 20 mg daily increased plasma cholesterol by 4 to 8 mg/dL and that the changes subsided during chronic therapy over 1 year. Likewise, triglycerides rose and then reverted to normal. These transient changes are rather similar to the situation described with low-dose thiazides.

METABOLIC CHANGES—RECOMMENDATIONS. The overall evidence suggests that loop diuretics, like the thiazides, can cause dose-related metabolic disturbances. High doses used for heart failure might therefore pose problems. It makes sense to take special precautions against the hypokalemia of high-dose loop diuretics because of the link between intermittent falls in plasma potassium and hyperglycemia. A sensible start is addition of an ACE inhibitor.[42]

# Thiazide Diuretics

Thiazide diuretics (Table 4–3) remain the most widely used first-line therapy for hypertension, although increasingly other first-liners such as beta-blockers, alpha-blockers, calcium antagonists, and ACE inhibitors are taking over. Thiazides are also standard therapy for chronic CHF, when edema is modest, either alone or in combination with loop diuretics.

PHARMACOLOGIC ACTION AND PHARMACOKINETICS. Thiazide diuretics act to inhibit the reabsorption of sodium and chloride in the more distal part of the nephron (Fig. 4–1). This cotransporter is insensitive to the loop diuretics. More sodium reaches the distal tubules to stimulate the exchange with potassium, particularly in the presence of an activated renin-angiotensin-aldosterone system. Thiazides may also increase the active excretion of potassium in the distal renal tubule.[1]

**TABLE 4–3**     **THIAZIDE DIURETICS: DOSES AND DURATION OF ACTION**

| | Dose | Duration of Action (H) | Trade Name (UK-Europe) | Trade Name (USA) |
|---|---|---|---|---|
| Hydrocholoro-thiazide | 12.5–25 mg (BP); 25–100 mg (CHF) | 6–12 | Esidrex HydroSaluric | Hydro-Diuril; Esidrix; Thiuretic |
| Hydroflu-methazide | 12.5–25 mg (BP); 25–200 mg (CHF) | 2–24 | Hydrenox | Saluron; Diucardin |
| Chlorthal-idone | 12.5–50 mg | 48–72 | Hygroton | Hygroton; Hylidone |
| Metolazone | 2.5–5 mg (BP); 5–20 mg (CHF) | 18–25 | Metenix; Diulo | Zaroxolyn; Diulo |
| Bendroflu-azide = bendro-flumethi-azide | 1.25–2.5 mg⁺(BP); 10 mg (CHF) | 6–12 | Aprinox; Centyl; Urizide | Naturetin |
| Polythiazide | 1–2 mg (BP) | 24–48 | — | Renese |
| Benzthiazide | 50–200 mg | 2–18 | — | Aquatag Exna |
| Chlorothi-azide | 250–1000 mg | 6–12 | Saluric | Diuril |
| Cyclothiazide | 1–2 mg | 6–24 | — | Anhydron |
| Trichlormeth-iazide | 1–4 mg | About 24 | Fluitran (not in UK) | Meta-hydrin; Naqua |
| Cyclopen-thiazide | 0.125–0.25 mg | 6–12 | Navidrex | — |
| Indapamide | 1.25–2.5 mg (BP); 2.5–5 mg (CHF) | 16–36 | Natrilix | Lozol |
| Xipamide | 20–40 mg (BP) | 6–12 | Diurexan | — |

† See Carlsen et al.[27]

BP = Use for blood-pressure-lowering; CHF = Use for congestive heart failure.

NB: The doses given here for antihypertensive therapy are generally **LOWER** than those recommended by the manufacturers (exception: Lozol 1.25 mg is recommended).

Thiazides are rapidly absorbed from the gastrointestinal (GI) tract to produce a diuresis within 1 to 2 hours, which lasts for 6 to 12 hours in the case of the prototype thiazide, hydrochlorothiazide. Some major differences from the loop diuretics are (1) the longer duration of action; (2) the different site of action (Fig. 4–1); (3) the relatively low "ceiling" of thiazide diuretics (i.e., the maximal response is reached at a relatively low dosage); and (4) the much decreased capacity of thiazides to work in the presence of renal failure (serum creatinine > 2.0 mg/dL; GFR below 15 to 20 ml/min).[1] The fact that thiazides, loop diuretics and potassium-sparing agents all act at different tubular sites explains their additive effects (**sequential nephron block**).

DOSE AND INDICATIONS.   In **hypertension,** diuretics still appear to be the initial agent of choice in the elderly and in black patients. The thiazide doses have generally been too high. Whether lower doses

**TABLE 4–4**   SIDE-EFFECTS OF DIURETIC THERAPY FOR HYPERTENSION

**Causing withdrawal of therapy**
  Impaired glucose tolerance
  Gout
  Impotence
  Lethargy
  Nausea, dizziness, or headache
**Blood biochemical changes**
  Glucose—hyperglycemia
  Uric acid—hyperuricemia
  Urea
  Potassium—hypokalemia
  Cholesterol—rise in serum cholesterol

All effects are minimized by appropriately lower doses such as bendrofluazide 1.25 to 5 mg instead of 10 mg daily as used in the MRC trial.[14] See also McVeigh et al.,[13] Carlsen et al.,[27] Johnston et al.,[33] SHEP study,[49] and TOHM study.[55]

with fewer biochemical alterations provide full antihypertensive efficacy is still not clear. In the SHEP study,[49] chlorthalidone 12.5 mg was initially used and after 5 years, 30% of the subjects were still on this lower dose and in 16% the dose was doubled. Overall, documented biochemical changes were small, including an 0.3 mmol/L fall in potassium, a rise in serum uric acid, and small increases in glucose and serum cholesterol. These changes found after 1 year of treatment do not necessarily predict changes over a longer period. In the case of cyclopenthiazide, widely used in the UK, only 0.125 mg (the approximate equivalent of hydrochlorothiazide 8 mg) gives as much antihypertensive effect as 0.5 mg daily with fewer metabolic side-effects.[13] Higher doses are marginally more effective, with greater risks of undesirable side-effects (Table 4–4). In the case of bendrofluazide, a lower dose (2.5 to 5 mg daily) causes less metabolic side-effects than the 10 mg dose used in a large British outcome trial.[2] An even lower dose (1.25 mg) only increased urate but not blood lipids nor glucose, while the antihypertensive effect was similar.[27] With hydrochlorothiazide, the full antihypertensive effect of 12.5 mg daily may take up to 12 weeks,[1,58] and *a common error is "premature step therapy" (i.e., going on to the next step too soon).*

The **response rate in hypertension** to thiazide monotherapy is variable and may be disappointing, being only about 45% in one trial with 12.5 to 25 mg hydrochlorothiazide daily.[9] The response depends in part on the age and race of the patient and probably also on the sodium intake. Increasing the dose of hydrochlorothiazide up to a maximum of 200 mg daily may improve the response, but the risk of metabolic side-effects is unacceptably high, so that combination therapy becomes preferable rather than increasing the dose beyond 25 mg daily.

In **obesity with hypertension,** there is both increased sodium reabsorption and adrenergic activation, so that weight reduction plus either a thiazide or a beta-blocker would be logical (Chapter 7).

In **CHF,** higher doses are justified (50 to 100 mg hydrochlorothiazide daily are probably ceiling doses), while watching the plasma potassium.

CHOICE OF THIAZIDE.  It seems to matter little which of the various thiazide preparations is chosen; the majority, including hydrochlorothiazide, have an intermediate duration of action (6 to 12 hours). Preference must, however, be given to those compounds proved to be effective in low doses, such as hydrochlorothiazide, bendrofluazide, cyclopenthiazide, and chlorthalidone. In the case of the latter agent, there is also a good positive-outcome study.[49]

CONTRAINDICATIONS. These include renal edema with poor renal function, hypokalemia, ventricular arrhythmias, and cotherapy with proarrhythmic drugs. In hypokalemia (including early AMI), thiazide diuretics may precipitate arrhythmias. Relative contraindications include pregnancy hypertension, because of the risk of a decreased blood volume; moreover, thiazides can cross the placental barrier with risk of neonatal jaundice. In mild renal impairment, the GFR may fall further as thiazides decrease the blood volume.

SIDE-EFFECTS. Besides the increasingly emphasized "wrong way" metabolic side-effects, such as hypokalemia, hyponatremia, increased insulin resistance, and increased blood triglyceride and cholesterol levels, thiazide diuretics rarely cause sulfonamide-type immune side-effects including intrahepatic jaundice, pancreatitis, blood dyscrasias, angiitis, pneumonitis, and interstitial nephritis. Impotence is newly emphasized.

DRUG INTERACTIONS. **Steroids** and estrogens (eg., the contraceptive pill) may cause salt retention to antagonize the action of thiazide diuretics. **Indomethacin** and other NSAIDs blunt the response to thiazide diuretics.[1] **Antiarrhythmics** that prolong the QT-interval, such as Class IA or III agents including sotalol, may precipitate torsades de pointes in the presence of diuretic-induced hypokalemia. The **nephrotoxic effects of certain antibiotics**, such as the aminoglycosides, may be potentiated by diuretics. **Probenecid** (for the therapy of gout) and **lithium** (for mania) may block thiazide effects by interfering with thiazide excretion into the urine. Thiazide diuretics also interact with lithium by impairing renal clearance with risk of lithium toxicity.[32]

# Other Thiazide-like Agents

## Metolazone

Metolazone (**Zaroloxyn, Diulo, Metenix**) also belongs to the category of thiazide diuretics. An important additional property is that *metolazone appears to be effective even in patients with reduced renal function.*[1] There are, however, no strict studies comparing metolazone with standard thiazides in renal impairment. The duration of action is up to 24 hours. The standard dose is 5 to 20 mg once daily for CHF or renal edema and 2.5 to 5 mg for hypertension. In combination with furosemide, metolazone may provoke a profound diuresis, with the risk of excessive volume and potassium depletion.[1] Nonetheless, metolazone may be added to furosemide with care, especially in patients with renal as well as cardiac failure. The side-effect profile of metolazone closely resembles that of the ordinary thiazides.

In 17 patients with severe CHF, almost all of whom were already on furosemide, captopril and digoxin, metolazone 1.25 to 10 mg once daily was given in titrated doses; most responded by a brisk diuresis within 48 to 72 hours.[10]

**Mykrox** is a rapidly acting formulation of metolazone with high bioavailability, registered for use in hypertension only in a dose of 0.5 to 1 mg once daily. The maximum antihypertensive effect is reached within 2 weeks.

## Indapamide

Indapamide (**Lozol, Natrilix**) is a thiazide-like diuretic (albeit with a different indoline structure) with a terminal half-life of 14 to 16 hours, that lowers the blood pressure. The initial dose is 1.25 mg once daily for 4 weeks, then if needed 2.5 mg daily. In higher doses (2.5 to 5 mg), diuresis can be achieved.[1] Part of the antihypertensive action might be peripheral vasodilation.[1] Indapamide appears to be more lipid-neutral than other thiazides but is equally likely to cause hypokalemia. In **cardiac edema,** the drug has little advantage over other well-tried diuretics,[1] although approved for this purpose. As a third-line antihypertensive agent, after beta-blocker with calcium antagonist, adding indapamide 2.5 mg was as effective as adding hydrochlorothiazide 25 mg plus amiloride 2.5 mg (1/2 Moduretic tablet). Hypokalemia was somewhat more common with indapamide and hyperuricemia equally frequent in both regimes.[18] In **left ventricular hypertrophy,** indapamide 2.5 mg daily appeared to be better in inducing regression than hydrochlorothiazide 25 mg daily at equal diastolic blood pressure values.[48] In **diabetes,** indapamide is sometimes thought to be the diuretic of choice. There are no strict comparisons with low-dose thiazides concerning effects on glucose tolerance. Although indapamide is documented as reducing microalbuminuria in diabetics,[31] there are, again, no good comparisons with low-dose thiazide diuretics, which probably have a similar effect.[41]

## Metabolic and Other Side-effects of Thiazides

Many side-effects of thiazides are similar to those of the loop diuretics: electrolyte disturbances including hypokalemia, hyponatremia, hyperuricemia, the precipitation of gout and diabetes, a decreased blood volume, and alkalosis. **Atherogenic blood lipid changes** and especially impotence have recently been emphasized. **Hyponatremia** may sometimes occur in the elderly even with low diuretic doses.

HYPOKALEMIA. As in the case of loop diuretics, hypokalemia is probably an overfeared complication, especially when low doses of thiazides are used.[1] Yet many physicians remain impressed by the risk of fall in plasma potassium that may only become covert when dietary potassium decreases or intercurrent diarrhea develops. Hence the frequent choice of combination of thiazides with the potassium-retaining diuretics triamterene or amiloride. This choice in turn brings about the alternative but lesser risk that some patients will develop **hyperkalemia,** especially in the presence of renal impairment or during the concomitant use of potassium supplements or ACE inhibitors.

Whether or not diuretic therapy predisposes to serious **ventricular arrhythmias** has been a matter of dispute since at least 1986,[8,16] and the debate continues, although at a greater level of sophistication.[38,50] There can be no dispute that diuretic-induced hypokalemia can contribute to torsades de pointes and hence to sudden death, especially when there is cotherapy with agents prolonging the QT-interval.[50] The proarrhythmic risk seems much more serious in patients with pre-existing clinical coronary disease or heart failure.

In **mild to moderate hypertension,** the degree of hypokalemia evoked by low-dose thiazides seldom matters.[38]

THERAPEUTIC STRATEGIES FOR HYPOKALEMIA. Common sense says that in patients with a higher risk of arrhythmias, as in ischemic heart disease, heart failure on digitalis, or hypertension with LV hypertrophy, a potassium- and magnesium-sparing diuretic should be part of the therapy unless contraindicated by renal failure or by cotherapy with an ACE inhibitor. A potassium-sparer may be better than potassium supplementation, especially because the supplements do not avoid hypomagnesemia; yet these issues are not completely resolved. For **hypertension,** it should be considered that most combination diuretic tablets contain too much thiazide. *When ACE inhibitors are part of the therapy, potassium supplements must be avoided and potassium-sparing diuretics should be replaced by simple hydrochlorothiazide.* It must be stressed that the above proposals are based on extrapolation, albeit reasonable.

When *cost is important,* a generic thiazide may be cheaper than a potassium-sparing thiazide combination; and when hypokalemia is suspected or detected, oral potassium supplementation with a salt substitute is less expensive than KCl supplements.

HYPOMAGNESEMIA. Hypomagnesemia, like hypokalemia, is blamed for arrhythmias of QT-prolongation during diuretic therapy.[50] Animal data suggest that hypomagnesemia can be prevented by the addition of a potassium-retaining component such as amiloride to the thiazide diuretic.[1] Despite the marketing of an oral magnesium preparation (**Slow Mag**), there is only marginal evidence that such supplements avoid serious arrhythmias or decrease afterload during diuretic therapy.[24]

DIABETOGENIC EFFECTS. The thiazides provoke overt diabetes in a minority of prediabetic patients. The mechanism may be indirect via intermittent hypokalemia.[47] Patients with a familial tendency to diabetes are probably prone to the diabetogenic side-effects; thiazides, if used, should only be given in low doses, such as chlorthalidone 15 mg daily[57] and, in addition, plasma potassium should be monitored. Even a hydrochlorothiazide dose of only 25 mg daily for 4 months increased fasting glucose by 11% and fasting plasma insulin by 31%.[17] Precipitation of true hyperglycemia or frank diabetes is less common, in the order of 0.6% to 5%.[38]

URATE EXCRETION AND GOUT. Most diuretics decrease urate excretion with the risk of increasing blood uric acid and causing gout in those predisposed; thus a personal or family history of gout should limit therapy to low-dose diuretics.[33] When **allopurinol** is given for associated gout, or when the blood urate is high in association with a family history of gout, it must be remembered that the normal dose of 300 mg daily is for a normal creatinine clearance. With a clearance of only 40 ml/min, the dose drops to 150 mg daily and, for 10 ml/min down, to 100 mg every 2 days.[7] *Dose reduction is essential* to avoid serious skin reactions, which are dose-related and can even be fatal.

ATHEROGENIC CHANGES IN BLOOD LIPIDS. Thiazides may increase the total blood cholesterol by an average of 15 to 20 mg/dl[17] in a dose-related fashion, even at a low dose of 12.5 mg daily. Also the LDL-cholesterol (LDL = low density lipoprotein) and triglycerides increase even after 4 months with standard-dose hydrochlorothiazide (25 mg daily).[17] Low-dose cyclopenthiazide was without effect on cholesterol over 8 weeks.[33] In the TOMH study,[55] chlorthalidone 15 mg daily increased cholesterol levels at 1 year but not at 4 years. During prolonged standard-dose thiazide therapy a lipid-lowering diet is advisable.

HYPERCALCEMIA. Thiazide diuretics tend to retain calcium by increasing proximal tubular reabsorption (along with sodium). Especially in hyperparathyroid patients, hypercalcemia can be precipitated.[3]

IMPOTENCE. Originally impotence was unexpectedly found in the large British antihypertension trial which used a high-dose diuretic (Table 4–4). The hope was that decreasing diuretic doses would avoid this unexplained problem. In the TOMH study,[55] low-dose chlorthalidone (15 mg daily given over 4 years) increased impotence marginally, whereas in the TAIM study[52] a higher dose (25 mg daily) clearly caused impotence.

PREVENTION OF METABOLIC SIDE-EFFECTS. Reduction in the dose of diuretic is the basic step. In addition, restriction of dietary sodium, and additional dietary potassium will reduce the frequency of hypokalemia. Combination of a thiazide with a potassium-sparer lessens hypokalemia. Addition of potassium supplements seems ineffective.[6] Combination therapy of hydrochlorothiazide with an ACE inhibitor reduces the incidence of hypokalemia and hyperuricemia, and possibly also of hyperglycemia. Hence, combination therapy with hydrochlorothiazide and potassium-sparing or potassium-re-

TABLE 4–5        POTASSIUM-SPARING DIURETICS (GENERALLY ALSO SPARE
                 MAGNESIUM)

|                | DOSE        | DURATION OF ACTION | TRADE NAMES     |
|----------------|-------------|--------------------|-----------------|
| Spironolactone | 25–200 mg   | 3–5 days           | Aldactone       |
| Amiloride      | 2.5–20 mg   | 6–24 h             | Midamor         |
| Triamterene    | 25–200 mg   | 8–12 h             | Dytac, Dyrenium |

taining diuretics is frequently used. In the treatment of hypertension, standard doses of diuretics should not be combined, if possible, with other drugs with unfavorable effects on blood lipids, such as the beta-blockers, but rather with ACE inhibitors or calcium antagonists which are lipid-neutral (Table 10–2).

## Potassium-Sparing or -Retaining Diuretics

### Amiloride and Triamterene

Amiloride and triamterene inhibit the sodium proton exchanger, which is concerned with sodium reabsorption in the distal tubules and collecting tubules. Thereby potassium loss is indirectly decreased (Table 4–5). Relatively weak diuretics on their own, they are often used in combination with thiazides. Advantages are that (1) the loss of sodium is achieved without a major loss of potassium or magnesium, and (2) there is an action independent of the activity of aldosterone. Side-effects are few: hyperkalemia (a contraindication) and acidosis may seldom occur, and then mostly in those with renal disease. In particular, the thiazide-related risks of diabetes mellitus and gout have not been reported with these agents. There are suggestions that amiloride may be preferable to triamterene (the latter is excreted by the kidneys with risks of renal casts on standard doses and occasional renal dysfunction); amiloride helps to retain magnesium.[4,5] In practice, compounds with triamterene have been widely and extensively used without detectable risks, for example in the EWPHE study.[30]

### Spironolactone

Spironolactone acts on the distal tubule to inhibit $Na^+/K^+$ exchange at the site of aldosterone action. Experimentally, it inhibits the development of myocardial fibrosis in LVH. It is logical therapy in those few patients who develop heart failure or hypertension in the presence of high mineralocorticoid levels, as during prednisone therapy or as part of Conn's syndrome. *This diuretic is the agent of choice when noninsulin-dependent diabetes or gout may be present or when there is fear of their precipitation.* Spironolactone is a more powerful diuretic than amiloride or triamterene in the presence of hyperaldosteronism and probably more effective as sole agent in hypertension (strict trials are lacking). Spironolactone can be better than amiloride in remedying thiazide-induced hypokalemia. One daily dose of spironolactone is usually adequate for diuresis (25 to 100 mg); in contrast, for therapy of Conn's syndrome 100 mg or more 3 times daily with meals may be needed (food enhances bioavailability of canrenone, the hepatic metabolite). Besides hyperkalemia, potentially serious side-effects result from antitestosterone actions such as gynecomastia and impotence, particularly when large doses (> 100 mg daily) and long-term treatment are used, or in liver disease or alcoholism. Spironolactone may benefit hirsutes in females.

CANRENONE. Spironolactone becomes active by hepatic transformation to canrenone. Canrenoate potassium (not in USA) 200 mg can be given intravenously for severe cardiac or hepatic edema.

**TABLE 4–6**        **SOME COMBINATION DIURETIC AGENTS**

|  |  | DOSE | TRADE NAMES |
|---|---|---|---|
| Hydrochlorothiazide | 25 mg | 1–2 tablets/day | Dyazide |
| + triamterene | 50 mg | (up to 4 in CHF) |  |
| Hydrochlorothiazide | 50 mg | ¼–1 tablet/day | Moduretic |
| + amiloride | 5 mg | (up to 2 in CHF) |  |
| Hydrochlorothiazide | 50 mg | ¼–1 tablet/day | Maxzide |
| + triamterene | 75 mg |  |  |
| Hydrochlorothiazide | 25 mg | ½–1 tablet/day | Maxzide–25 |
| + triamterene | 37.5 mg |  |  |
| Spironolactone | 25 mg | 1–4 tablets/day | Aldactazide |
| + hydrochlorothiazide | 25 mg |  |  |
| Cyclopenthiazide | 0.25 mg | ½–1 tablet/day | Navidrex K* |
| + potassium chloride | 600 mg |  |  |
| Furosemide | 40 mg | 1–2 tablets/day | Frumil* |
| + amiloride | 5 mg |  |  |

\* Not in USA

CHF = congestive heart failure

For hypertension, see text—low doses generally preferred and high doses are **contraindicated.**

## ACE Inhibitors

Because these agents ultimately exert an antialdosterone effect, they too act as mild potassium-retaining diuretics. Combination therapy with other potassium-retainers should be avoided.

## Hyperkalemia—A Specific Risk

Amiloride, triamterene, and spironolactone may all cause hyperkalemia (serum potassium equal to or exceeding 5.5 mEq/L) especially in the presence of pre-existing renal disease, diabetes, in elderly patients during cotherapy with ACE inhibitors, or in patients receiving possible nephrotoxic agents without careful monitoring of the serum potassium. Hyperkalemia is treated by drug withdrawal, infusions of glucose-insulin, and cation exchange resins such as sodium, polystyrene sulfonate, and sometimes dialysis. Intravenous calcium chloride may be required to avoid VF.

# Combination Diuretics

Besides addition of one class of diuretic to another, the fear of hypokalemia has increased the use of potassium-retaining diuretic combinations (Table 4–6), such as **Dyazide, Maxzide, Moduretic,** and **Aldactazide.** For **heart failure,** a standard combination daily therapy might be 1 to 2 tablets of Moduretic (hydrochlorothiazide 50 mg, amiloride 5 mg), or 2 to 4 tablets of Dyazide (hydrochlorothiazide 25 mg, triamterene 50 mg), or 1 to 2 tablets of Maxzide (hydrochlorothiazide 50 mg, triamterene 75 mg). When used for **hypertension,** special attention must be given to the thiazide dose (25 mg hydrochlorothiazide in Dyazide; 50 mg in Moduretic; while Maxzide has both 25 mg and 50 mg), where the initial aim is only 12.5 mg hydrochlorothiazide. A potassium-retaining furosemide combination is available in Europe (**Frumil**).

A logical combination is that of ACE inhibitor with low-dose thiazide. Thiazide diuretics increase renin levels and ACE inhibitors decrease metabolic side-effects of thiazides (Chapter 5).

## Minor Diuretics

**Carbonic anhydrase inhibitors** such as acetazolamide (**Diamox**) are weak diuretics. They decrease the secretion of hydrogen ions by the proximal renal tubule, with increased loss of bicarbonate and hence of sodium. These agents, seldom used as primary diuretics, have found a place in the therapy of **glaucoma** because carbonic anhydrase plays a role in the secretion of aqueous humor in the ciliary processes of the eye. In **salicylate poisoning,** the alkalinizing effect of carbonic anhydrase inhibitors increases the renal excretion of lipid-soluble weak organic acids.[1]

**Calcium antagonists** of the dihydropyridine group have a direct diuretic effect that contributes to the long-term antihypertensive effect.[1,11] For example, nifedipine increases urine volume and sodium excretion and may inhibit aldosterone release by angiotensin.[1] Diuresis explains the occasional tendency to hypokalemia with high-dose nifedipine. The diuretic action is quite independent of any change in renal blood flow or glomerular filtration.

**Dopamine** has a diuretic action apart from the improvement in cardiac function and indirect diuresis that it induces. The mechanism of the diuresis, found only in conditions of fluid retention, appears to involve $DA_1$-receptors on the renal tubular cells where dopamine stimulation opposes the effects of antidiuretic hormone.[37]

## Potassium Supplements

The routine practice in many centers of giving potassium supplements with loop diuretics is usually unnecessary (Table 4–1) and leads to extra cost and loss of compliance. Addition of low-dose potassium-retaining diuretics is usually better and can often be accompanied by a lower dose of the loop diuretic. Even high doses of furosemide may not automatically require potassium replacement because such doses are usually given in the presence of renal impairment or severe CHF when renal potassium handling may be abnormal. Clearly, potassium levels need periodic checking during therapy with all diuretics. A high-potassium, low-salt diet is advised and can be simply and cheaply achieved by the use of salt substitutes. Sometimes, despite all reasonable care, problematic hypokalemia develops, especially after prolonged diuretic therapy or in the presence of diarrhea or alkalosis. Then a potassium supplement may become necessary. Persistent hypokalemia in hypertension merits investigation for Conn's syndrome.

**Potassium chloride** in liquid form is theoretically best because (1) coadministration of chloride is required to fully correct potassium deficiency in hypokalemic hypochloremic alkalosis,[1] and (2) slow-release tablets may cause GI ulceration, which liquid KCl does not.[1] The dose is variable. About 20 mEq daily are required to avoid potassium depletion and 40 to 100 mEq are required to treat potassium depletion. Absorption is rapid and bioavailability good. To help avoid the frequent GI irritation, liquid KCl needs dilution in water or another liquid and titration against the patient's acceptability. KCl may also be given in some effervescent preparations. **Slow-release potassium chloride wax-matrix tablets** (Slow-K, each with 8 mEq or 600 mg KCl; Klotrix, K-Tab, and Ten-K each contain 10 mEq KCl; Kaon-CL, 6.7 or 10 mEq KCl) are widely used and well tolerated. Nonetheless, the USA package insert cautions against their use unless liquid or effervescent potassium preparations are not tolerated. The chloride salt carries the risk of GI ulceration or bleeding, especially when GI motility is impaired (as in elderly, immobile or diabetic patients, or in the presence of scleroderma), esophageal stricture, massive left atrial enlargement, or cotherapy with anticholinergic drugs including disopyramide. To avoid esophageal ulceration, tablets should be taken with the patient upright or sitting, and with a meal or beverage, and anticholinergic therapy should be avoided. **Microencapsulated KCl** (Micro-K, 8 mEq

KCl or 10 mEq KCl) may reduce GI ulceration to only 1 per 100,000 patient years. Nonetheless, high doses of Micro-K cause GI ulcers, especially during anticholinergic therapy.[1]

**Effervescent preparations** lessen the risk of GI ulceration and those with KCl include Klorvess (20 mEq), K-Lor (20 mEq KCl per packet), K-Lyte/Cl (25 mEq per tablet), and K-Lyte/Cl 50 (50 mEq tablet). K-Lyte contains potassium bicarbonate and citrate, 25 mEq. GI intolerance frequently limits the use of these agents, which are best given with liquid meals and in relatively small doses. **Potassium gluconate** (with citrate), Bi-K 20 mEq, or Twin-K tends to minimize the GI irritative effects of the effervescent preparations but lacks chloride.

RECOMMENDATIONS. Diet is the simplest, with high-potassium low-sodium intake achieved by salt substitutes. When $K^+$ supplements become essential, KCl is preferred. The best preparation will be one well tolerated by the patient and inexpensive. "No comprehensive adequately controlled studies of the relative efficacy of the various KCl preparations in clinical settings are available."[21]

# Special Diuretic Problems

## Over-diuresis

During therapy of **edematous states,** over-vigorous diuresis is common and may reduce venous pressure and ventricular filling so that the cardiac output drops and tissues become underperfused. The renin-angiotensin axis is further activated. Probably many patients are protected against the extremely effective potent diuretics by poor compliance. Over-diuresis is most frequently seen during hospital admissions when a rigid policy of regular administration of diuretics is carried out. Sometimes the addition of ACE inhibitors to diuretics enhances the risk of over-diuresis.

**Fixed diuretic regimes** are largely unsatisfactory in edematous patients. Often intelligent patients can manage their therapy well by tailoring a flexible diuretic schedule to their own needs, using a simple bathroom scale. Knowing how to recognize pedal edema and the time course of maximal effect of their diuretic often allows a patient to adjust his own diuretic dose and administration schedule to fit in with daily activities.

Patients who may experience **adverse effects** due to over-diuresis include (1) those with mild chronic heart failure overtreated with potent diuretics; (2) patients requiring a high filling pressure, particularly those with a "restrictive" pathophysiology, as in restrictive cardiomyopathy, hypertrophic cardiomyopathy, or constrictive pericarditis; and (3) patients in early phase AMI,[1] when the problem of excessive diuresis is most commonly encountered when using potent intravenous diuretics for acute heart failure. It may be necessary to cautiously administer a "**fluid challenge**" with saline solution or a colloid preparation while checking the patient's cardiovascular status. If the resting heart rate falls, renal function improves, and blood pressure stabilizes, the ventricular filling pressure has been inadequate.[1]

## Diuretic Resistance

Repetitive diuretic administration leads to a levelling off of the effect, because (in the face of a shrunken intravascular volume) the part of the tubular system not affected reacts by reabsorbing more sodium. Additional mechanisms are an abnormally low cardiac output in patients with heart failure; prominent activation of the renin-angiotensin axis; or an electrolyte-induced resistance (Fig. 4–2). Apparent resistance can also develop when there is concomitant therapy with indomethacin or with some other NSAIDs (possible exceptions: ibuprofen, sulindac[44]) or with probenecid. The thiazide diuretics will not work well if the GFR is below 15 to 20 ml/min;[1] metolazone may

in improving symptoms, alt[  ]
treated by the diuretic.[36] The[  ]
symptomatic heart failure ha[  ]
and the use of thiazide diure[  ]
to the ceiling, which is rapid[  ]
potassium (and sometimes m[  ]
and (4) high-dose furosemide [  ]
have used combined thiazide[  ]
before high-dose furosemide.[  ]
ACE inhibitors whenever the [  ]
is a contraindication. ACE in[  ]
renin-angiotensin activation i[  ]

For **severe CHF,** when cong[  ]
toms, initial therapy is usua[  ]
renal perfusion may be impai[  ]
fashioned, helps to promote a[  ]
mide required in resistant CH[  ]
daily). Alternatively, the prin[  ]
may be used with a lower d[  ]
should be given to intermitte[  ]

**Sequential nephron block[  ]**
of a diuretic acting at a diffe[  ]
diuretic, is logical.[46] Thus, the[  ]
thiazide and digoxin improve[  ]
gestive heart failure.[28]

**ACE inhibitors** are now s[  ]
failure. In CHF, the action o[  ]
renal perfusion and vasocons[  ]
GFR lessening sodium excre[  ]
additions to diuretics. They h[  ]
by inhibiting aldosterone re[  ]
potassium and magnesium.[42]

## Summary

Diuretics are powerful the[  ]
major and serious side-effect[  ]
antihypertensive agent, altho[  ]
ily high doses (exception: c[  ]
dose in the SHEP study[49]). [  ]
the therapy of mild hyperte[  ]
in three groups of patients: th[  ]
with renal impairment also r[  ]
For most hypertensives, low[  ]
a potassium-retaining comp[  ]
be the answer. Most combin[  ]
hydrochlorothiazide, so that[  ]
12.5 mg hydrochlorothiazide[  ]
combine well with ACE inhi[  ]
ing component is not advisa[  ]

In the therapy of heart fail[  ]
is high and their use remain[  ]
vigorous diuresis; rather eac[  ]
tion with a specific cardiolog[  ]
ble defects are appropriatel[  ]
thiazide (for mild heart fail[  ]
failure). A logical practice i[  ]
of diuretic and ACE inhibit[  ]
severities of failure, increasi[  ]
switching to or combining v[  ]
The principle of sequential n[  ]
that automatic addition of [  ]
an ideal practice. Rather, th[  ]

### DIURETIC RESISTANCE IN CHF

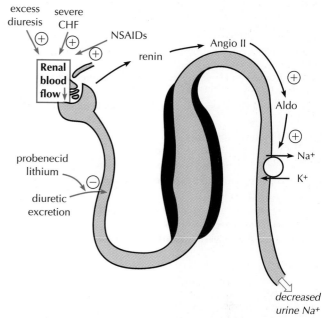

**FIGURE 4–2.** The causes of resistance to diuretics (for further details see text). Fig. copyright L.H. Opie and modified from Reference 1.

be an exception (Table 4–7). When potassium depletion is severe, diuretics will not work well for complex reasons.

Is there compliance with dietary salt restriction? Is complete bed rest required? Is the optimal agent being used, avoiding thiazide diuretics (except metolazone), when the GFR is low? Is the optimal dose being used? Are there interfering drugs or severe electrolyte or volume imbalances that can be remedied? Has the general cardiovascular status been made optimal by judicious use of unloading or inotropic drugs? *To achieve diuresis,* an ACE inhibitor may have to be added cautiously to thiazide and/or loop diuretics, or metolazone may have to be combined with loop diuretics, all following the principle of sequential nephron blockade. Sometimes spironolactone is also required. Furthermore, intravenous **dopamine** may through its action on $DA_1$-receptors help induce a diuresis acting in part by increasing renal blood flow. In outpatients, compliance and dietary salt restriction must be carefully checked, while all unnecessary drugs are eliminated. Sometimes fewer drugs work better than more (here the prime sinners are potassium supplements, requiring many daily tablets frequently not taken).

### Hyponatremia

In patients severely ill with CHF, despite an increased total body sodium, a hyponatremic state may develop from predominant water retention. The latter is caused by (1) the inappropriate release of arginine vasopressin-antidiuretic hormone, and (2) increased activity of angiotensin-II.[1] The best treatment seems to be the combination of furosemide and an ACE inhibitor (p 96); restriction of water intake is also important.

## Less Common Uses of Diuretics

Less common indications are: (1) **hypernatremia** when not due to fluid depletion; (2) intravenous furosemide in **malignant or pre-**

**TABLE 4–7**  **SOME CAUSES OF A**
**THERAPY OF CARDI**

**Incorrect use of diuretic agent**
   combination of 2 thiazides or ?
type
   use of thiazides when GFR is
   excessive diuretic dose
   poor compliance, especially ca
      supplements
**Electrolyte volume imbalance**
   hyponatremia, hypokalemia, h
   hypomagnesemia may need c
**Poor renal perfusion diuretic-in**
   cardiac output too low
   excess hypotension (vasodilat
**Excess circulating catecholamin**
   (frequent in severe congestive h
   and
      limits renal blood flow)
   correct by additional therapy
**Activation of renin-angiotensin**
   (frequent in diuretic-treated sev
   correct by ACE inhibition
**Interfering drugs**
   indomethacin and naproxen i
   probenecid and lithium inhibi
      loop diuretics

\* GFR = glomerular filtration rate b
† Pope et al.[44]

**malignant hypertension,** espe
fluid retention; (3) high-dose f
**failure** when it is hoped that
**hypercalcemia,** high-dose loo
of calcium; intravenous furose
gency treatment of severe hyp
**rogenic form of diabetes ins**
not clear, but there is a diminu
thiazide diuretics decrease the
proximal reabsorption, so tha
**calciuria** to decrease the form
diuretics increase urinary excr
of thiazides on urinary calciu
may increase bone mineraliz
hip fractures,[19] hence suggesti
thiazides in osteoporosis. The
first-line (low-dose) diuretic t
   An additional use, entirely
therapy is insufficient (diuret

## Diuretics in Step-Care

In **mild to moderate CHF,** d
There are, however, no long-t
case with the ACE inhibitors
on 123 patients with NYHA C
zide 25 mg given twice daily w

low-dose thiazide plus potassium-retaining diuretic is reasonable, except when an ACE inhibitor is used because of the anti-aldosterone effect of the latter. Today, some combination of diuretics plus ACE inhibitors would be standard therapy in mild to moderate heart failure.

## References

*For references from Second Edition, see Opie and Kaplan (1991)*

1. Opie LH, Kaplan NM. Diuretics. In: Opie LH (ed), Drugs for the Heart, Third Edition. WB Saunders Company, Philadelphia, 1991, 74–99.

*References from Third Edition*

2. Berglund G, Andersson O. Lancet 1981; 1:744–747.
3. Christensson T, Hellstrom K, Wengle B. Arch Intern Med 1977; 137:1138–1142.
4. Devane J, Ryan MP. Br J Pharmacol 1981; 72:285–289.
5. Devane J, Ryan MP. Br J Pharmacol 1983; 79:891–896.
6. Dorup I, Skajaa K, Clausen T, Kjeldsen K. Br Med J 1988; 296:455–458.
7. Hande KR, Noone RM, Stone WJ. Am J Med 1984; 76:47–56.
8. Helfant RH. Am J Med 1986; 80 (Suppl 4A):13–22.
9. Holzgreve H, Distler A, Michaelis J, et al. Br Med J 1989; 299:881–886.
10. Kiyingi A, Field MJ, Pawsey CC, Yiannikas J, et al. Lancet 1990; 335:29–31.
11. Krusell LR, Jespersen LT, Schmitz A, et al. Hypertension 1987; 10:577–581.
12. Licht JH, Haley RJ, Pugh B, et al. Arch Intern Med 1983; 143:1694–1699.
13. McVeigh G, Galloway D, Johnston D. Br Med J 1988; 297:95–98.
14. Medical Research Council Working Party on Mild to Moderate Hypertension. Lancet 1981; 2:539–543.
15. Mudge GH. In: Gilman AG, Goodman LS, Gilman AG (eds). The Pharmacological Basis of Therapeutics, 6th ed. MacMillan Publishing Co, New York, 1980, pp 892–915.
16. Papademetriou V. Am Heart J 1986; 111:1217–1224.
17. Pollare T, Lithell H, Berne C. N Engl J Med 1989; 321:868–873.
18. Poulsen L, Friberg M, Noer I, Krusell K, Pedersen OL. Cardiovasc Drugs Ther 1989; 3:141–144.
19. Ray WA, Griffin MR, Downey W, Melton LJ III. Lancet 1989; 1:687–690.
20. Sharpe N, Murphy J, Smith H, Hannan S. Lancet 1988; 1:255–259.
21. Szatalowicz VL, Arnold PE, Chaimovitz C, et al. N Engl J Med 1981; 305:263–266.
22. Weidmann P, Uehlinger DE, Gerber A. J Hypertens 1985; 3:297–306.

*New References*

23. Anand IS, Kalra GS, Harris P, et al. Diuretics as initial and sole treatment in chronic cardiac failure. Cardioscience 1991; 2:273–277.
24. Bashir Y, Sneddon JF, Staunton HA, et al. Effects of long-term oral magnesium chloride replacement in congestive heart failure secondary to coronary artery disease. Am J Cardiol 1993; 72:1156–1162.
25. Baumgart P. Torasemide in comparison with thiazides in the treatment of hypertension. Cardiovasc Drugs Ther 1993; 7:63–68.
26. Brater DC, Rudy DR, Voelker JR, et al. Pharmacokinetics and pharmacodynamics of torasemide in patients with chronic renal insufficiency—preliminary evaluation. Cardiovasc Drugs Ther 1993; 7:69–73.
27. Carlsen JE, Kober L, Torp-Pedersen C, Johansen P. Relation between dose of bendrofluazide, antihypertensive effect, and adverse biochemical effects. Br Med J 1990; 300:975–978.
28. Cheitlin MD, Byrd R, Benowitz N, et al. Amiloride improves hemodynamics in patients with chronic congestive heart failure treated with chronic digoxin and diuretics. Cardiovasc Drugs Ther 1991; 5:719–726.
29. Cranston WI, Juel-Jensen BE, Semmence AM, et al. Effects of oral diuretics on raised arterial pressure. Lancet 1963; 2:966–969.
30. EWPHE study—Amery A, Birkenhager W, Brixko P, et al. Mortality and morbidity results from the European Working Party on high blood pressure in the elderly trial. Lancet 1985; 1:1349–1354.
31. Gambardella S, Frontoni S, Lala A, et al. Regression of microalbuminuria in type II diabetic, hypertensive patients after long-term indapamide treatment. Am Heart J 1991; 122:1232–1238.
32. Jefferson JW, Kalin NH. Serum lithium levels and long-term diuretic use. JAMA 1979; 241:1134–1136.
33. Johnston GD, Wilson R, Mcdermott BJ, et al. Low-dose cyclopenthiazide in the

treatment of hypertension: A one-year community-based study. Qty J Med 1991; 78:135–143.

34. Joint National Committee. The fifth report of the Joint National Committee on detection, evaluation, and treatment of high blood pressure (JNC V). Arch Intern Med 1993; 153:154–183.

35. Kindler J. Torasemide in advanced renal failure. Cardiovasc Drugs Ther 1993; 7:75–80.

36. Kleber FX, Thyroff-Friesinger U. Ibopamine versus digoxin in the treatment of mild congestive heart failure. Cardiology 1990; 77 (Suppl 5):75–80.

37. Lokhandwala MF, Amenta F. Anatomical distribution and function of dopamine receptors in the kidney. FASEB J 1991; 5:3023–3030.

38. McInnes GT, Yeo WW, Ramsay LE, Moser M. Cardiotoxicity and diuretics: much speculation—little substance. J Hypertens 1992; 10:317–335.

39. McLay JS, McMurray JJ, Bridges AB, et al. Acute effects of captopril on the renal actions of furosemide in patients with chronic heart failure. Am Heart J 1993; 126:879–886.

40. Motwani JG, Fenwick MK, Morton JJ, Struthers AD. Furosemide-induced natriuresis is augmented by ultra low-dose captopril but not by standard doses of captopril in chronic heart failure. Circulation 1992; 86:439–445.

41. National high blood pressure education program working group report on hypertension in diabetes. Hypertension 1994; 23:145–158.

42. O'Keeffe S, Grimes H, Finn J, et al. Effect of captopril therapy on lymphocyte potassium and magnesium concentrations in patients with congestive heart failure. Cardiology 1992; 80:100–105.

43. Plavinik FL, Rodrigues CIS, Zanella MT, Ribeiro AB. Hypokalemia, glucose intolerance, and hyperinsulinemia during diuretic therapy. Hypertension 1992; 19 (Suppl II):II-26–II-29.

44. Pope JE, Anderson JJ, Felson DT. A meta-analysis of the effects of nonsteroidal anti-inflammatory drugs on blood pressure. Arch Intern Med 1993; 153:477–484.

45. Puschett JB. Clinical pharmacologic implications in diuretic selection. Am J Cardiol 1986; 57:6A–13A.

46. Reyes AJ, Leary WP. Clinicopharmacological reappraisal of the potency of diuretics. Cardiovasc Drugs Ther 1993; 7:23–28.

47. Santoro D, Natali A, Palombo C, et al. Effects of chronic angiotensin-converting enzyme inhibition on glucose tolerance and insulin sensitivity in essential hypertension. Hypertension 1992; 20:181–191.

48. Senior R, Imbs JL, Bory M, et al. Comparison of the effects of indapamide with hydrochlorothiazide, nifedipine, enalapril and atenolol on left ventricular hypertrophy in hypertension: A double-blind parallel study (abstr). J Am Coll Cardiol 1993; 21:57A.

49. SHEP Cooperative Research Group. Prevention of stroke by antihypertensive drug treatment in older persons with isolated systolic hypertension. Final results of the Systolic Hypertension in the Elderly Program (SHEP). JAMA 1991; 265:3255–3264.

50. Singh BN, Hollenberg NK, Poole-Wilson PA, Robertson JIS. Diuretic-induced potassium and magnesium deficiency: relation to drug-induced QT prolongation, cardiac arrhythmias and sudden death. J Hypertens 1992; 10:301–316.

51. Swanepoel CR. Which diuretic to use? Cardiovasc Drugs Ther 1994; 8:123–128.

52. TAIM study—Wassertheil-Smoller S, Oberman A, Blaufox MD, et al. The Trial of Antihypertensive Interventions and Management (TAIM) Study. Final results with regard to blood pressure, cardiovascular risk, and quality of life. Am J Hypertens 1992; 5:37–44.

53. Taylor SH. Diuretics in postinfarction heart failure. Cardiovasc Drugs Ther 1993; 7:885–889.

54. Thomas MR, Wright RS, Aarhus LL, et al. Chronic diuretic treatment mediates a renal resistance to the natriuretic actions of atrial natriuretic peptide in experimental mild heart failure (abstr). J Am Coll Cardiol 1994; 23:173A.

55. TOMH study—Neaton JD, Grimm RH, Prineas RJ, et al for the Treatment of Mild Hypertension Study Research Group. Treatment of mild hypertension study. Final results. JAMA 1993; 270:713–724.

56. Toussaint C, Masselink A, Gentges A, et al. Interference of different ACE inhibitors with the diuretic action of furosemide and hydrochlorothiazide. Klin Wochenschr 1989; 67:1138–1146.

57. Vardan S, Mehrotra KG, Mookherjee S, et al. Efficacy and reduced metabolic side effects of a 15-mg chlorthalidone formulation in the treatment of mild hypertension. A Multicenter study. JAMA 1987; 258:484–488.

58. Weir MR, Weber MA, Punzi HA, et al. A dose escalation trial comparing the combination of diltiazem SR and hydrochlorothiazide with the monotherapies in patients with essential hypertension. J Human Hypertens 1992; 6:133–138.

## Book

59. Kaplan NM. Clinical Hypertension, Sixth Edition. Wilkins and Wilkins, Baltimore, 1994.

# Notes

# 5 Angiotensin-Converting Enzyme Inhibitors. Contrasts with Conventional Vasodilators

L. H. Opie ◆ P. A. Poole-Wilson ◆ E. Sonnenblick
K. Chatterjee

## Introduction

Since the description in 1977 of the first angiotensin-converting enzyme (ACE) inhibitor, captopril, by the Squibb Group led by Ondetti and Cushman,[93] at least sixteen ACE inhibitors have appeared worldwide in just under 20 years. There are more and more indications with increasingly intense pharmaceutical promotion, sometimes verging on fanfare. The purpose of this chapter is to critically assess the evidence for the use and limitations of these agents, and to emphasize differences from the earlier standard vasodilator agents.

## Mechanisms of Action

### Angiotensin-II Signal Systems

Logically, ACE inhibition should work by lessening the complex and widespread effects of angiotensin-II (Table 5–1). This octapeptide is formed from its precursor, **angiotensin-I,** by the activity of the angiotensin-converting enzyme (ACE). ACE activity is found chiefly in the vascular endothelium of the lungs, but occurs in all vascular beds including the coronary arteries. Angiotensin-I originates in the liver from **angiotensinogen** under the influence of the enzyme **renin,** a protease, that is formed in the renal juxtaglomerular cells. Classic **stimuli to the release of renin** include (1) impaired renal blood flow as in ischemia or hypotension; (2) salt depletion or sodium diuresis; and (3) beta-adrenergic stimulation.

THE ANGIOTENSIN-CONVERTING ENZYME. This protease has two zinc groups of which only one participates in the high-affinity binding site that interacts with angiotensin-II or with the ACE inhibitors.[71] The converting enzyme not only converts angiotensin-I to angiotensin-II but inactivates bradykinin, hence the alternate name of **kininase.** ACE inhibition is potentially vasodilatory by decreased formation of angiotensin-II and by increased formation of bradykinin (Fig. 5–1).

ANGIOTENSIN-II RECEPTORS AND INTRACELLULAR MESSENGER SYSTEMS. Just as there are many intermediate steps between occupation of the beta-adrenoceptor and increased contractile activity of the myocardium, so there are many complex steps between occupation of the angiotensin-II receptor and ultimate mobilization of calcium with a vasoconstrictor effect in vascular smooth muscle. Activity of the **signaling system** starts when occupation of the angiotensin-II receptor stimulates the phosphodiesterase (called phospholipase C) that breaks down phosphatidylinositol bisphosphate to **inositol trisphosphate** ($IP_3$ = $InsP_3$) and **diacylglycerol** (Fig. 5–2). The latter activates a specialized enzyme, **protein kinase C,** that transfers a phosphate group from ATP to the target protein. Thus, the ultimate messengers of the **inositol signaling pathway** are, first, $IP_3$ which liberates cal-

TABLE 5–1    ACTIONS OF ANGIOTENSIN-II

| ORGAN(ELLE) | CELLULAR EFFECT | CONSEQUENCE |
| --- | --- | --- |
| Arteriolar myocyte | $IP_3$ and $Ca^{2+}$ increase | Vasoconstriction |
| Myocytes; fibrocytes | Protein kinase C stimulation | Expression of proto-oncogenes; cell growth |
| Terminal neurone | Enhanced release of NE | Enhanced vasoconstriction |
| Glomeruli[1] | Efferent arteriolar constriction, enlarges glomerular pores | Promotes microalbuminuria |
| Juxtaglomerular apparatus | Inhibits renin release | Relief of raised intraglomerular pressure |
| Adrenal cortex | Synthesis of aldosterone | Increased sodium retention and kaliuresis |
| Fibrinolysis[2] | Increase of plasminogen activator inhibitor-I | Impaired fibrinolysis |

$IP_3$ = inositol trisphosphate; NE = norepinephrine

For review, see Timmermans et al.[119]

1. Ridker et al.[108]
2. Yoshioka et al.[127]

cium from the intracellular sarcoplasmic reticulum,[29] and, second, protein kinase C which is an important growth signal.

When the vascular angiotensin-II receptors are stimulated, it is proposed that two mechanisms lead to an increased cytosolic calcium: (1) the formation of $IP_3$, and (2) a direct G-protein-mediated stimulation of the calcium channel.

In the myocardium, there are also angiotensin-II receptors that are thought to be coupled to the $IP_3$ system; yet the positive inotropic effect of this signal is variable. Rather, activation of protein kinase C is held to be a growth signal because it evokes the growth-stimulating proto-oncogenes.[83]

## Renin-Angiotensin-Aldosterone System

RENIN RELEASE. The major factors stimulating release of renin from the juxtaglomerular cells of the kidney are (Fig. 5–3): (1) increased $beta_1$-sympathetic activity; (2) low arterial blood pressure; and (3) decreased sodium reabsorption in the distal tubule, as when dietary sodium is low or during diuretic therapy. Local formation of angiotensin-II following renin release seems to explain efferent arteriolar vasoconstriction in the renal glomerulus. Thus, for example, during a state of arterial hypotension, the increased efferent arteriolar vasoconstriction resulting from increased angiotensin-II will help to preserve renal function by maintaining the intraglomerular pressure.

STIMULATION OF ALDOSTERONE BY ANGIOTENSIN-II. Angiotensin-II also stimulates the adrenal cortical cells to release the sodium-retaining hormone **aldosterone.** Hence, ACE inhibition is associated with aldosterone reduction and has potential indirect natriuretic and potassium-retaining effects. Aldosterone formation does not, however, stay fully blocked during prolonged ACE inhibitor therapy. This late rise of the aldosterone level does not appear to compromise the antihypertensive effects achieved by ACE inhibitors; nonetheless it might detract from the prolonged benefit of these agents in heart failure. Currently, added low-dose spironolactone (12.5 to 25 mg daily) is under test.

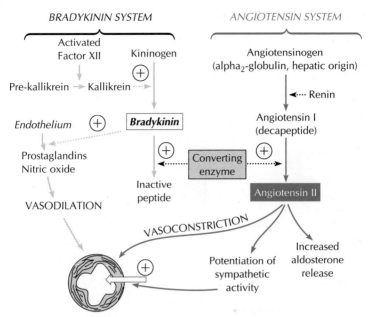

**FIGURE 5–1.**   ACE inhibitors have dual vasodilatory actions, chiefly on the renin-angiotensin system with ancillary effects on the breakdown of bradykinin. The result of the former action is the inhibition of the vasoconstrictory systems and the result of the latter is the formation of vasodilatory nitric oxide and prostacyclin. These effects of bradykinin may protect the endothelium. Fig. copyright L.H. Opie and adapted from Angiotensin-Converting Enzyme Inhibitors. Scientific Basis for Clinical Use, 2nd edition, Wiley-Liss/Authors' Publishing House, New York.

## VASCULAR AII RECEPTORS

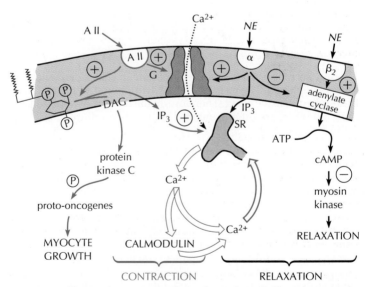

**FIGURE 5–2.**   Proposed messengers of vascular angiotensin-II receptor stimulation. A phosphodiesterase (phospholipase C) splits phosphatidylinositol into two messengers: $IP_3$ (inositol trisphosphate) and DAG (1-, 2-diacylglycerol). $IP_3$ promotes the release of calcium from the sarcoplasmic reticulum (SR), and DAG activates protein kinase C. The latter stimulates myocyte growth. Activity of the angiotensin-II receptor also helps to open the calcium channel, possibly by G-proteins (G). Norepinephrine (NE) vasodilates by beta$_2$-adrenergic stimulation and vasoconstricts via alpha-adrenergic activity. Fig. copyright L.H. Opie and adapted from Angiotensin-Converting Enzyme Inhibitors. Scientific Basis for Clinical Use, 2nd edition, Wiley-Liss/Authors' Publishing House, New York.

## RENIN-ANGIOTENSIN-ALDOSTERONE

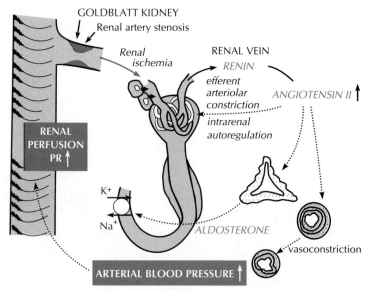

**FIGURE 5–3.** Renal ischemia (Goldblatt kidney) initiates the release of renin from the juxtaglomerular (JG) cells. Formation of angiotensin-II (1) causes efferent arteriolar constriction to maintain intraglomerular pressure and filtration, (2) stimulates the synthesis and release of sodium-retaining aldosterone, and (3) causes peripheral vasoconstriction. Renal perfusion pressure rises and there is a compensatory increase in renal blood flow. Fig. copyright L.H. Opie and adapted from Angiotensin-Converting Enzyme Inhibitors. Scientific Basis for Clinical Use, 2nd edition, Wiley-Liss/Authors' Publishing House, New York.

**FEEDBACK INHIBITION OF RENIN BY ANGIOTENSIN-II.** Angiotensin-II exerts feedback inhibition of renin secretion. Therefore renin release is suppressed both directly by angiotensin-II and indirectly by the sodium retention associated with the increased aldosterone levels.

### Sodium Status, Renin and ACE Inhibitor Efficacy

Renin secretion from the juxtaglomerular cells is enhanced by sodium depletion. The result is that ACE inhibition, in general, has a greater hypotensive effect. Therefore, in the therapy of hypertension, ACE inhibitors are often combined with either a diuretic or a low-sodium diet or both.

SALT SENSITIVITY. Why do certain individuals react adversely to a high salt intake by increasing the arterial blood pressure? In normal subjects, a high-sodium diet leads to increased tubular reabsorption of sodium, which inhibits renin release, decreasing efferent arteriolar vasoconstriction so that renal blood flow increases. Furthermore, less formation of angiotensin-II (Angio II) leads to a lower level of aldosterone, which leads to increased sodium diuresis. In nonmodulating hypertensive patients, the above sequence does not happen in response to sodium, so these patients do not modulate this control mechanism the way they should.[69] It is also proposed that such subjects may respond well to monotherapy by ACE inhibitors because decreased formation of angiotensin-II within the renal vasculature restores the renal blood flow response to the high-sodium diet.

### Autonomic Interactions of Angiotensin-II

Angiotensin-II promotes the release of norepinephrine from adrenergic terminal neurons, and also enhances adrenergic tone by central activation and by facilitation of ganglionic transmission. Furthermore, angiotensin-II amplifies the vasoconstriction achieved by

**TABLE 5–2      ACTIONS OF BRADYKININ**

| ORGAN(ELLE) | CELLULAR EFFECT | CONSEQUENCE |
|---|---|---|
| Gut | $Ca^{2+}$ mobilization | Slow contraction (brady, slow; kinin, movement) |
| Vascular endothelium | Formation of nitric oxide, prostacyclin | Vasodilation; antiplatelet aggregation;[1] endothelial protection[2] |
| Respiratory tract | Formation of prostaglandins | Cough[3] |

1. Durante et al.[49]
2. Luscher.[82]
3. Fogari et al.[58]

alpha$_1$-receptor stimulation. Thus, angiotensin-II has facilitatory adrenergic actions leading to increased activity of vasoconstrictory norepinephrine. This explains the *permissive anti-adrenergic effects* of ACE inhibitors. Vagomimetic effects could explain why tachycardia is absent despite peripheral vasodilation.[24]

The combined anti-adrenergic and vagomimetic mechanisms with better potassium retention (as a result of aldosterone inhibition) could contribute to the antiarrhythmic effects of ACE inhibitors and the reduction of sudden death in several trials in CHF.[97]

## Kallikrein-kinin System and Bradykinin

Foremost among possible alternate sites of action of ACE inhibitors is bradykinin (Fig. 5–1). This nonapeptide, originally described as causing slow contractions in the gut (*brady*, slow; *kinin*, movement), is of increasing cardiovascular importance.[82] Bradykinin is inactivated by two **kininases,** kininase I and II, the latter being identical with ACE. ACE inhibition, therefore, leads to increased local formation of bradykinin, which has major vasodilatory properties.

PROPERTIES OF BRADYKININ.   Bradykinin acts on bradykinin receptors in the vascular endothelium to promote the release of two vasodilators (Table 5–2). First, there is increased formation of nitric oxide. Second, there is increased conversion of arachidonic acid to vasodilatory prostaglandins, such as prostacyclin and PGE$_2$. The current concept is that bradykinin formation, occurring locally and thus not easily measured, can participate in the hypotensive effect of ACE inhibitors. Bradykinin formed during ACE inhibition may also protect against endothelial damage, at least in part by formation of nitric oxide and prostacyclin, both of which inhibit platelet aggregation. Is formation of bradykinin part of the reason why ACE inhibition can limit experimental cardiac hypertrophy?[80] This controversial concept is argued against by studies in which direct angiotensin-II receptor blockade, which does not involve bradykinin formation, can induce regression of cardiac hypertrophy.[73]

RENAL PROSTAGLANDINS AND BRADYKININ.   During ACE inhibition there is increased local synthesis of the active bradykinin in the kidney.[33] Such bradykinin stimulates the formation of vasodilatory prostaglandins. Indomethacin, which inhibits prostaglandin synthesis, partially reduces the hypotensive effect of ACE inhibitors. Both indomethacin and high-dose aspirin[67] may impair the effect of ACE inhibition in CHF.

## Tissue Renin-Angiotensin Systems

Although the acute hypotensive effects of ACE inhibition can clearly be linked to decreased circulating levels of angiotensin-II, during chronic ACE inhibition there is a reactive hyperreninemia

## Cardiac Renin, A II and LVH

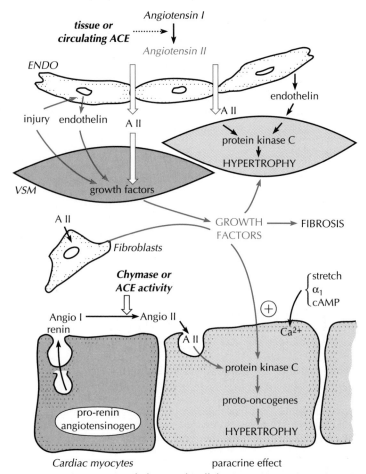

**FIGURE 5–4.** Some proposals for a multicellular interactive renin-angiotensin system involving cardiac myocytes, fibroblasts, vascular smooth muscle, and endothelium.[48] Although these systems are postulated to have an important function in regulating vascular and myocardial hypertrophy, proof of this significance is still awaited. In cardiac myocytes, a proportion of the conversion of angiotensin-I to angiotensin-II may occur independently of ACE by a chymase. GF = growth factor; alpha₁ = alpha₁-adrenergic activity; ET = endothelin receptor; other abbreviations as in Fig. 5–2. Fig. copyright L.H. Opie and adapted from Angiotensin-Converting Enzyme Inhibitors. Scientific Basis for Clinical Use, 2nd edition, Wiley-Liss/Authors' Publishing House, New York.

linked to re-emergence of circulating angiotensin-II and aldosterone. Hence, the controversial proposal is that ACE inhibitors exert their sustained antihypertensive effects by lessening formation of angiotensin-II within the target organ, acting on the tissue renin-angiotensin systems (Fig. 5–4).

## Classes of ACE Inhibitors

From the pharmacokinetic point of view, there are **three classes of ACE inhibitors** (Table 5–3). The first is represented by captopril, a compound active as it is, yet subject to further metabolism in the body to metabolites that are also active (Class I). The next category consists of the pro-drugs of which enalapril is the prototype. These are only active once converted to the diacid by hepatic metabolism (Class II). Third, in a class of its own, lisinopril is water-soluble and

**TABLE 5-3   SUMMARY OF PHARMACOLOGIC PROPERTIES, CLINICAL INDICATIONS AND DOSES OF ACE INHIBITORS**

| DRUG | ZINC LIGAND | ACTIVE DRUG | ELIM T½ (H) | HYPERTENSION (USUAL DAILY DOSE) | CHF INITIAL DOSE | CHF MAINTENANCE DOSE |
|---|---|---|---|---|---|---|
| **Class I: captopril-like** | | | | | | |
| Captopril* | SH | captopril | 4–6 | 25–50 mg 2×* | 6.25 mg | Up to 50 mg 3×* |
| **Class II: pro-drugs** | | | | | | |
| Benazepril* | carboxyl | benazeprilat | 21–22 | 5–80 mg 1–2 doses* | 2 mg | 5–20 mg 1× |
| Cilazepril | carboxyl | cilazeprilat | 8–24 | 2.5–5 mg 1× | — | — |
| Enalapril* | carboxyl | enalaprilat | 11 | 5–20 mg 1–2 doses* | 2.5 mg | Up to 10 mg 2×* |
| Fosinopril* | phosphoryl | fosinoprilat | 12 | 10–40 mg 1×* | — | — |
| Perindopril | carboxyl | perindoprilat | 27–60 | 4–8 mg 1×* | 2 mg | 2–8 mg 1× |
| Quinapril* | carboxyl | quinaprilat | 1.8 | 10–40 mg 1–2 doses* | 5 mg | 5–40 mg 1–2 doses* |
| Ramipril* | carboxyl | ramiprilat | 34–113 | 2.5–10 mg 1×* | 1.25 mg | 2.5–5 mg 1 or 2× |
| Trandolapril | carboxyl | trandolaprilat | 16–24 | 0.5–2 mg 1× | — | — |
| **Class III: water-soluble** | | | | | | |
| Lisinopril* | carboxyl | lisinoprilat | 7 or more | 10–40 mg 1×* | 2.5 mg | 2.5–40 mg 1×* |

*licensed for use by FDA

Elim T½ = elimination (terminal) half-life

Adapted from Opie L.H. Angiotensin-Converting Enzyme Inhibitors. Scientific Basis for Clinical Use, 2nd edition, 1994, with permission of Wiley-Liss/Authors' Publishing House, New York.

NEUROHUMORAL ACTIVATION IN CHF

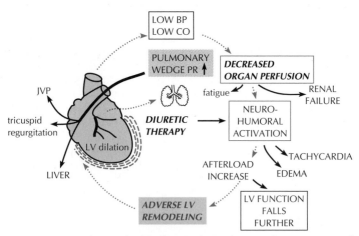

**FIGURE 5–5.** Neurohumoral adaptation in CHF. The crucial consequence of LV failure is the inability to maintain a normal blood pressure and normal organ perfusion. As a result of reflex neurohumoral activation, peripheral vasoconstriction increases to exaggerate the degree of left ventricular failure. Furthermore, increased beta-adrenergic stimulation leads to more release of renin with further formation of vasoconstrictive angiotensin-II and eventual release of aldosterone. Increasing LV wall tension and progressive neurohumoral activation lead to adverse LV remodeling. CO = cardiac output. Fig. copyright L.H. Opie and modified from Reference 1.

not metabolized, without tissue penetration, and excreted unchanged by the kidneys (Class III). Despite the lipid-solubility and tissue penetration of some of the active forms of the pro-drugs, there is no firm evidence that they perform any better than lisinopril without tissue penetration. Probably the major site of ACE inhibition is in the vascular endothelium, accessible to all ACE inhibitors, whether lipid-soluble or not.

# ACE Inhibitors in Congestive Heart Failure

## Neurohumoral Effects of Overt Heart Failure

A crucial problem in CHF is the inability of the left ventricle in severe failure to maintain a normal blood pressure and organ perfusion.[10] Enhanced activity of the renin-angiotensin system (Fig. 5–5) follows from: (1) hypotension, which evokes baroreflexes to increase sympathetic adrenergic discharge, thereby stimulating the beta$_1$ renal receptors involved in renin release; and (2) decreased renal perfusion, resulting in renal ischemia which enhances renin release. However, even in severe CHF, plasma renin may not be elevated.[25,106] Rather, to achieve consistent stimulation of the renin-angiotensin system requires simultaneous diuretic therapy.[32] Angiotensin-II promotes secretion of aldosterone, and also the release of vasopressin, to contribute to abnormal fluid retention and volume regulation in severe CHF.

The greatly increased peripheral vascular resistance, against which the failing heart must work, is explained by (1) increased formation of angiotensin-II, (2) reflex release of norepinephrine, and (3) release of vasoconstrictor **endothelin** from the dysfunctional vascular endothelium. Systemic vasoconstriction reduces renal plasma flow which detrimentally affects salt excretion and further promotes renin formation.

Vasodilator hormones of cardiac origin, such as atrial and brain natriuretic peptides, and prostaglandins of vascular origin, are also activated, but fail to dilate for complex reasons including receptor downgrading. Thus the overall peripheral vascular resistance is increased.

INCREASED LOAD ON MYOCARDIUM.   Especially during exertion, the systolic wall stress becomes too high for the depressed contractility of the failing myocardium. The inability of the left ventricle to empty itself during systole increases the preload. The combination of increased pre- and afterload, so common in CHF, leads to progressive ventricular dilation with wall remodeling (myocyte hypertrophy and slippage with matrix changes), so that the ejection fraction progressively declines with time. Load reduction and in particular angiotensin-II inhibition may retard this detrimental process.

LAPLACE LAW.   According to this law, the stress on the wall of a thin-walled sphere is proportional to the product of the intraluminal pressure and the radius, and inversely related to the wall thickness:

$$\text{Wall stress} = \frac{\text{pressure} \times \text{radius}}{2 \times \text{wall thickness}}$$

Wall stress is one of the major determinants of myocardial oxygen uptake. Afterload and preload reduction, by decreasing the radius of the left ventricle, decreases the myocardial oxygen demand. ACE inhibition, by reducing afterload and thus enhancing ventricular emptying, improves the myocardial oxygen balance.

### ACE Inhibitors for Asymptomatic or Mildly Symptomatic LV Dysfunction (Without Overt CHF)

ACE inhibitors have been used at all stages of heart failure. Two studies, the SAVE study and the SOLVD prevention study with captopril and enalapril respectively, have shown that in patients with a depressed LV ejection fraction (of about 30%) but without overt CHF, these agents can delay deterioration (Table 5–4). The SAVE study[111] was conducted specifically in postinfarct patients, while in the SOLVD study[116] 80% had a prior myocardial infarction. A minority of these patients (17% in SOLVD, 35% in SAVE) were diuretic-treated. Possibly the ACE inhibitor was limiting adverse LV remodeling,[74] and there was a claimed but controversial[59A] additional effect in a 25% reduction of reinfarction in the SAVE study.

### ACE Inhibitors as Possible Monotherapy in Early Symptomatic Heart Failure

Patients can present with significant exertional dyspnea (NYHA Classes II and III) yet without signs of sodium and water retention. Some of these will have predominant diastolic dysfunction on the basis of left ventricular hypertrophy that should respond to ACE inhibitor therapy.[63] In others, there will be predominant systolic dysfunction. Can ACE inhibitors be used as monotherapy? There have been only two small studies. Riegger[109] gave quinapril as monotherapy to 26 such patients. The increase of exercise time in those receiving quinapril was greater than in those receiving placebo. The second study showed that patients requiring diuretics could deteriorate if diuretics were replaced by an ACE inhibitor.[18] Nonetheless, the SAVE and SOLVD studies have shown that ACE inhibitors can help prevent the transition from asymptomatic to overt CHF, so that it is logical to use ACE inhibitors in early heart failure not requiring diuretics for relief of symptoms.

### ACE Inhibitors as Combination Therapy with Diuretics for Mild to Moderate CHF

Diuretic therapy is universally accepted as first-step and first-line therapy in LV failure with congestive symptoms. This section concerns studies in which patients already so treated were given additionally an ACE inhibitor or digoxin.

**TABLE 5—4**

| MAJOR TRIALS FAVORING USE OF ACE INHIBITORS AT EACH STAGE OF HEART FAILURE | | | |
|---|---|---|---|
| STAGE OF HEART FAILURE | DRUGS (S) | TRIAL (PATIENTS TREATED) | OUTCOME |
| NYHA I, 67% II, 33% | enalapril diuretic 27% digoxin 18% | SOLVD prevention (2,111) | Reduced overt CHF; death reduced 8% (NS) |
| NYHA I, 11% II, 57% III, 30% | enalapril diuretic 86% digoxin 66% | SOLVD treatment (1,285) | Reduced death 16%; reduced hospital-ization 22% |
| NYHA II, 50% III, 44% | enalapril diuretic 100% digoxin 100% | V-HeFT II (403) | Reduced death 28% vs. hydralazine-nitrate |
| NYHA IV, 100% | enalapril furosemide 77% digoxin 72% | CONSENSUS (127) | Reduced death 27% |
| Early post-infarct (3–16 days) LV dys-function* | captopril diuretic 35% digoxin 25% | SAVE (1,115) | Reduced death 19%; 37% less cardiovascular deaths |
| Early post-infarct (3–10 days) clinical CHF | ramipril diuretic 58% digoxin 12% | AIRE (1,986) | Reduced death 27% |

*ejection fraction 40% or less; mean value 31%

**ACE INHIBITION VERSUS DIGOXIN VERSUS COMBINATION IN EARLY LV FAILURE.** Kromer et al.[75] studied 19 patients with mild CHF and NYHA Class II symptoms, all treated with hydrochlorothiazide 25 mg daily. Patients were crossed over after 6 weeks of treatment with either digoxin or the ACE inhibitor, quinapril, then to the other agent, all followed by combination therapy. ACE inhibitor therapy was markedly more effective than digoxin as it increased exercise tolerance, decreased heart size, and decreased circulating norepinephrine and aldosterone levels—none of which were changed by digoxin. Combination therapy was symptomatically similar to ACE inhibition with added hemodynamic improvement.

**CAPTOPRIL-DIGOXIN MULTICENTER STUDY.** Three hundred patients with mild to moderate heart failure (NYHA Class II-III) were allocated randomly in a double-blind manner to captopril, digoxin, or placebo. Most were maintained on furosemide.[4] Effort tolerance improved with captopril and mechanical performance with digoxin. These data cannot be extrapolated to longer periods, yet support the widespread clinical impression that ACE inhibitor therapy combined with a mild diuretic is highly effective in early heart failure.

## ACE Inhibitors as Part of Triple Therapy of CHF in Combination with Diuretics and Digoxin

The first CONSENSUS study[5] showed how the addition of enala-pril to prior treatment with diuretics and digoxin reduced mortality

**TABLE 5–5      MAJOR OUTCOME TRIALS OF ACE INHIBITORS IN HEART FAILURE**

| ACRONYM AND DRUG | CONDITION | NO. OF PATIENTS | MEAN DURATION OF TRIAL | MAJOR RESULT |
|---|---|---|---|---|
| CONSENSUS enalapril | Severe heart failure | 127 | 6 months | 40% mortality reduction at 6 months, 31% at 1 year |
| SOLVD (treatment) enalapril | Mild to moderate heart failure | 1,285 | 41 months | 18% mortality reduction |
| SOLVD (prevention) enalapril | Asymptomatic LV dysfunction | 2,111 | 37 months | 37% reduction in risk of CHF |
| V-HeFT-II enalapril | Chronic heart failure | 403 | 24 months | 36% reduction in sudden death vs. nitrate-hydralazine |
| SAVE captopril | Late postinfarct LV dysfunction | 1,115 | 42 months | 37% reduction in risk of CHF |
| AIRE ramipril | Early postinfarct clinical heart failure | 1,986 | 15 months | 27% mortality reduction |

CONSENSUS = Cooperative North Scandinavian Enalapril Survival Study
SOLVD = Studies of Left Ventricular Dysfunction
V-HeFT-II = VA Cooperative Vasodilator Heart Failure Trial
SAVE = Survival and Ventricular Enlargement
AIRE = Acute Infarction Ramipril Efficacy
LV dysfunction = low ventricular ejection fraction
Adapted from Opie.[129]

in patients with severe heart failure (Table 5–5). The fundamental logic for such triple therapy (diuretic plus ACE inhibitor plus inotropic agent) lies in the self-evident difference in mode of action between these three types of agents.[114] From the hemodynamic point of view, the combination ACE inhibitor plus an inotropic agent gives better results than either type of therapy alone both in mild heart failure[75] and in severe heart failure.[9] Withdrawal of digoxin from triple therapy results in clinical deterioration, but withdrawal studies are open to criticism (Chapter 6).[104]

ACE INHIBITION VERSUS NONSPECIFIC VASODILATION. A question only recently answered is whether ACE inhibition confers any specific advantages over nonspecific vasodilators in advanced heart failure. First, captopril inhibited the release of norepinephrine from the failing heart compared with hydralazine-nitrate.[43] Second, retrospective analysis of the CONSENSUS Study gave evidence that enalapril was most effective in patients with neuroendocrine and renin-angiotensin activation.[117] Third, the Veterans Administration Heart Failure Trial (V-HeFT-II) showed the expected advantage for ACE inhibition over hydralazine-nitrate therapy.[37] Yet, in black patients, there is suggestive evidence that hydralazine-nitrate therapy is superior to ACE inhibition.[35]

NEUROHUMORAL EFFECTS OF ACE INHIBITORS ADDED TO DIGOXIN AND DIURETICS. As reviewed elsewhere,[129] in seven studies on 250 patients, the use of ACE inhibitors consistently led to an increased plasma renin (by virtue of the inhibition of the converting enzyme), and decreased angiotensin-II (also the consequence of ACE inhibition). There was also a decrease in aldosterone (formation of which is stimulated by angiotensin-II), and a fall in norepinephrine and vasopressin, the elevation of which are among consequences of severe CHF. From these data and from the CONSENSUS trial,[117] it can be concluded that chronic ACE inhibition ameliorates the adverse neurohumoral changes found in CHF.

## ACE Inhibition as Part of Quadruple Therapy of Severe CHF Including Diuretics, Digoxin, and Conventional Vasodilators

Logically, there should be scope for added vasodilator therapy to the now-standard triple therapy in CHF, the latter consisting of diuretics-digoxin-ACE inhibition. Thus, the acute administration of **isosorbide dinitrate** 40 mg every 6 hours for 24 hours relieved pulmonary hypertension and improved LV filling in 10 of 14 patients with chronic heart failure already treated with captopril, diuretic and digoxin.[87]

An indirect argument for concomitant vasodilator therapy is that in the well-known CONSENSUS study,[5] 47% of patients were already receiving nitrates, while in the treatment arm of SOLVD study,[115] 40% were on nitrates. In the Hy-C trial,[59] 84% of the patients were on nitrate therapy. Thus, in nitrate-treated patients, also receiving diuretics and digoxin, ACE inhibition can produce further clinical benefit.

In these trials, very few patients were receiving hydralazine. There is a specific disadvantage of hydralazine in that active arteriolar dilation increases reflex sympathetic output from the failing human myocardium.[43] Furthermore, when either captopril or hydralazine was added to the therapy of patients mostly already receiving digitalis, furosemide, and nitrates, mortality was worse in the hydralazine group.[59]

Therefore, when it is desired to control dyspnea persisting despite standard triple therapy, there are better arguments for adding nitrates than for adding hydralazine.

## How to Start an ACE Inhibitor in CHF

First the patient must be fully assessed clinically, including measurements of serum creatinine and urea, and electrolytes (Fig. 5–6). It is important to avoid hypotension and thereby to lessen the risk of temporary renal failure.[81] Patients at high **risk of hypotension** include those with serum sodium < 130 mmol/L, serum creatinine 150 to 300 μmol/L or 1.5 to 3.0 mg/dL, and those with hyperkalemia or treatment with potassium-retaining diuretics. Patients with creatinine values exceeding 3.0 mg/dL should be considered separately (p 117). Other groups at high risk include those on multiple diuretics or high-dose furosemide (exceeding 80 mg daily), those with pre-existing hypotension and a systolic blood pressure < 90 mmHg, and those aged 70 years or more (UK package insert, enalapril). All these patients need to have diuretic therapy stopped for 1 to 2 days and are then given a test dose under close supervision, often in hospital.

After a low test dose, and if there is no symptomatic hypotension, the chosen drug is continued, renal function monitored, and the dose increased after 3 to 4 days.[5]

If the patient is fluid-overloaded with an elevated jugular venous pressure, then the test dose of the ACE inhibitor can be given without

## CHECKS: ACE INHIBITORS IN HEART FAILURE

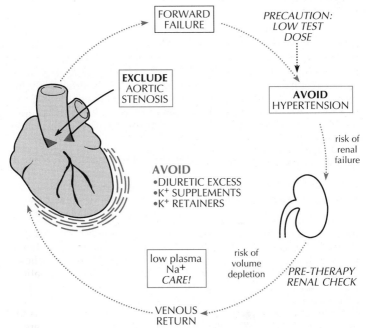

FIGURE 5-6. Potential side-effects of ACE inhibitors.

first having to stop diuretic therapy. The addition of the ACE inhibitor may call forth a diuresis, in which case the diuretic dose is decreased to avoid hypotension.

Although these procedures are often best undertaken in hospital, it is feasible in selected patients to undertake outpatient monitoring of the test dose of captopril[86] or to use perindopril[84] or a very low dose of enalapril (1.25 mg[101]). The absence of first-dose hypotension suggests that the subsequent course will be smooth.

PRE-EXISTING RENAL FAILURE. In general, the serum creatinine can be expected to rise modestly and then to stabilize. In severe CHF where renal function is already limited by poor renal blood flow and with a serum creatinine exceeding 3.0 mg/dL or 300 μmol/L, it may be a difficult decision to know whether or not to introduce ACE inhibitor therapy. The danger of exaggeration of heart failure must be balanced against the possible benefit from an improved cardiac output and decreased renal afferent arteriolar vasoconstriction resulting from ACE inhibitor therapy. Problems can be expected especially when the glomerular filtration rate (GFR) is low and the renin-angiotensin axis highly stimulated.[81] The best policy may be to improve the hemodynamic status as far as possible by the combined use of diuretics, digoxin, and conventional diuretics. Then the diuretic dose could be reduced or stopped, and a very low dose of an ACE inhibitor introduced. In the case of mild to moderate hypertension with renal failure, ACE inhibition as monotherapy does not further depress renal function, provided that renal artery stenosis is excluded and the dose adjusted downwards.[90]

HYPOTENSIVE RESPONSE TO ACE INHIBITION. Temporary renal failure is most likely to develop in patients with excess diuretic therapy and volume depletion, in whom there is a greater hypotensive response to ACE inhibitor therapy.[95] Thus it is logical to start ACE inhibitors with low initial doses, such as captopril 6.25 mg or enalapril 2.5 mg or even 1.25 mg. In elderly patients, a low initial dose of perindopril (2 mg) is less likely to cause initial hypotension than a low first dose of either enalapril (2.5 mg) or captopril (6.25 mg), for reasons that are unknown.[84] Special caution is required in diabetics in whom renal failure is a particular hazard[96] doubtlessly because diabetes predisposes one to renal disease.

HYPONATREMIA.    Patients with severe hyponatremia are 30 times more likely to develop hypotension in response to ACE inhibitor therapy and require special care. The cause of the hyponatremia is at least in part due to the release of vasopressin (antidiuretic hormone), as can result from renin-angiotensin activation[52] following intense diuretic therapy. Although the combination of furosemide and ACE inhibitor may work safely,[51] it is essential to avoid excess diuresis and volume depletion. Small-dose captopril (about 1 mg) would be a logical first choice.[91]

SALT AND WATER RESTRICTION.    Modest, tolerable salt restriction is standard practice. Patients already on strict low-sodium diets are at increased risk of first-dose hypotension. In patients who are not volume-depleted, restriction of water intake is required because delayed water diuresis may contribute to hyponatremia in severe CHF.

## Outstanding Clinical Problems

DRUG DOSE.    Whereas in hypertension the dose-response curve is flat, in CHF there is evidence with quinapril for a dose-related increase in exercise time.[100] Furthermore, in severe chronic CHF, increasing intravenous ACE inhibition progressively lessens the peripheral vascular resistance at high plasma levels exceeding those found during conventional oral doses.[103]

DIASTOLIC DYSFUNCTION.    Most studies have concentrated on the role of ACE inhibition in systolic heart failure and the indices of improvement in systolic function. Currently, however, the emphasis is shifting to diastolic heart failure, thought to be an early event particularly in left ventricular hypertrophy and in the elderly. Among the relatively few studies concerning ACE inhibitor therapy is one that shows that enalapril benefits diastolic heart failure in hypertension.[63]

VALVULAR HEART DISEASE.    ACE inhibitors have not been well studied. In chronic aortic regurgitation, acute administration of 25 mg of captopril reduced the regurgitant fraction in the absence of any fall in the blood pressure.[107] The mechanism of this benefit is speculative and may include (1) effects of the ACE inhibitor on aortic compliance, and (2) reduction of the preload and thereby an improvement of myocardial wall stress. Further studies with much longer follow-up are required.

SKELETAL MUSCLE METABOLISM IN HEART FAILURE.    Poor blood flow to working skeletal muscle may be one cause of fatigue and exercise intolerance in CHF. Captopril added to digitalis and diuretics achieved no acute benefit on leg muscle metabolism, even though peripheral vascular resistance fell.[126] With time and exercise training, muscle blood flow increases to permit increased performance.[45] Further studies over a longer period are required.

## ACE Inhibitors for Hypertension

In hypertension, increased activity of the renin-angiotensin-aldosterone system is most obvious in cases of unilateral renal artery stenosis when the decreased perfusion pressure in the renal arteries stimulates the release of renin from the juxtaglomerular apparatus. However, the renin-angiotensin system also helps to maintain blood pressure both in normal people and in essential hypertension, especially when sodium intake is restricted. Therefore, although ACE inhibition leads to the most dramatic falls of blood pressure in the presence of an underlying renal mechanism, ACE inhibition may also be an effective antihypertensive therapy in mild to moderate hypertension, possibly acting in part by indirect adrenergic modulation. In general, ACE inhibitors might be more effective in younger white patients who would also respond to beta-blockers.[85] Efficacy in other groups (black patients, the elderly) can be achieved by addition of low-dose diuretics. As ACE inhibitors do not alter glucose tolerance, blood uric acid or cholesterol levels,[17] and as these agents seldom cause subjective side-effects apart from cough, their use in hypertension is rapidly increasing.

MECHANISM OF BLOOD PRESSURE REDUCTION. ACE inhibitors appear to lower blood pressure by six mechanisms. First, by definition they inhibit the normal conversion of circulating angiotensin-I to the powerful vasoconstrictor angiotensin-II. Second, they reduce the secretion of aldosterone to induce a natriuresis. Third, specific renal vasodilation may enhance natriuresis. Fourth, the inactivation of vasodilatory bradykinins is reduced. Fifth, they inhibit local formation of angiotensin-II in vascular tissue and in myocardium.[22] Sixth, they may improve insulin resistance.

INSULIN RESISTANCE. This condition is common in obese hypertensives but also found in the nonobese and in relatives of hypertensives. It appears to contribute to the genesis of essential hypertension and to an associated metabolic syndrome including glucose intolerance and blood lipid abnormalities. ACE inhibitors act to retain body potassium by inhibiting the formation of aldosterone. Hence, they lessen the hypokalemic effects of postprandial peaks of insulin, and thereby help to maintain glucose uptake by muscle.[110] ACE inhibitors also improve insulin sensitivity.[98] Furthermore, in insulin-resistant hypertensives, a change of therapy from beta-blockade to captopril may improve glucose disposal.[28]

QUALITY OF LIFE IN HYPERTENSION. Although it is claimed that ACE inhibitors produce a good "quality of life," the classic study[6] used as comparison not placebo but two agents already known to have central and sexual side-effects, namely methyldopa and propranolol. When ACE inhibition is compared with a cardioselective beta-blocker, such as atenolol, differences in the quality of life become trivial, except for a very mild memory impairment with atenolol.[13] The reputed differences between captopril and enalapril[118] can, in practice, mostly be ignored. The quality of life with ACE inhibitors does not differ much from that with the calcium antagonist agents although the irritating side-effects may differ. For example, with ACE inhibitor therapy, cough may cause discontinuation, whereas in the case of calcium antagonists, ankle edema or headache may do likewise.

LEFT VENTRICULAR HYPERTROPHY (LVH). On the basis of the role of angiotensin-II as growth factor (Fig. 5–4), a specific role of ACE inhibition has been sought in achieving regression of LVH. Two meta-analyses of retrospective data[39,41] have supported this proposed role. Yet in only one of three prospective comparative studies has the ACE inhibitor been able to achieve better regression of LVH than other classes of antihypertensives.[40,64,120] This problem is further discussed in Chapter 7 (p 196).

ETHNIC DIFFERENCES IN ANTIHYPERTENSIVE EFFECTS OF ACE INHIBITORS. ACE inhibitors are relatively ineffective as monotherapy in blacks.[85] The proposed explanations focus on differences in the renin-angiotensin-aldosterone axis. Black patients, as a group, have a lower renin status and an impaired aldosterone response to sodium deprivation.[57] The further proposal is that a sodium load is accompanied by a tendency to intracellular sodium retention. Several studies have shown that concurrent therapy with a diuretic sensitizes black patients to an ACE inhibitor.[123]

## ACE Inhibitors for AMI or Postinfarct CHF or LV Dysfunction

Since the last edition of this book in 1991, substantial studies have revealed a place for ACE inhibitors both in the treatment and

TABLE 5–6    TRIALS OF ACE INHIBITORS GIVEN AT INITIATION OF
             TREATMENT OF ACUTE MYOCARDIAL INFARCTION

| | CONSENSUS-II | ISIS-4 | GISSI-3 |
|---|---|---|---|
| Total number treated | 3,044 | 27,442 | 9,435 |
| Drug and daily dose | Enalaprilat IV 1 mg over 2 h, then up to 20 mg 2× daily | Captopril 6.25 mg initially, increased to 50 mg 2× daily | Lisinopril 2.5–5 mg initially, increased to 10 mg 1× daily |
| Duration | 41 to 180 days | 28 days | 42 days |
| Patient population | AMI within 24 h of onset | AMI within 24 h of onset | AMI within 24 h of onset |
| Mean delay time | 15 h | 60% > 6 h | 65% > 6 h |
| Age, years | 66 mean | 72% below 70 | 63 mean |
| Gender male (%) | 73 | 74 | 78 |
| BP exclusion levels | 100/60 | 100 systolic | 100 systolic |
| Hypotension as side-effect (%) | 25 (control 10) | 21 (control 10) | 9 (control 4)[†] |
| Mortality change, absolute % | 0.8 increase | 0.46 decrease* | 0.8 decrease |
| Mortality change as risk reduction | 10% increase | 9% decrease* (p = 0.04) | 11% decrease (p = 0.03); 17% decrease with nitroglycerin (p = 0.003) |

* 35 days.

† persistent hypotension, systolic blood pressure below 90 mmHg for more than 1 hour.

Modified from Opie.[94]

prevention of postinfarct heart failure. In acute phase AMI, approximately 40,000 patients have been studied (Table 5–6).

ACUTE PHASE AMI.   Because ACE inhibitors have an indirect anti-adrenergic effect, it is logical that they have been tested in acute phase AMI, a state of excess adrenergic activation. Intravenous enalaprilat, in a fixed dose, did not work in CONSENSUS-II. In two megatrials, ISIS-IV[70] and GISSI-3,[61] ACE inhibition by captopril and lisinopril respectively achieved a 6% to 11% reduction in mortality beyond the benefit of thrombolysis and current standard therapy. Furthermore, when lisinopril was combined with intravenous nitrates, an impressive 17% reduction in mortality was found, in the same order of magnitude as in the SAVE study.[111] Possibly ACE inhibition protected from nitrate tolerance.[88] In the PRACTICAL study,[101] ACE inhibitors started within 24 hours of symptoms improved LV ejection fraction and prevented LV dilation. In this small study, enalapril but not captopril improved mortality at 12 months. The answer might lie in the greater initial hypotension in the captopril group, whose first dose (captopril 6.25 mg) was relatively higher than that of enalapril (only 1.25 mg; for effects of 2.5 mg, see Mac-

Fadyen et al.[84]). While a general recommendation cannot be made, these data support the use of oral ACE inhibitors in patients with early phase AMI and any degree of suspected heart failure (provided that first-dose hypotension is avoided).

CLINICALLY EVIDENT EARLY POSTINFARCT FAILURE.   In the AIRE study,[23] ramipril was the ACE inhibitor chosen. From the third to the tenth day postinfarct, starting from the onset of symptoms, in patients with clinically evident heart failure the addition of ramipril to other types of therapy resulted in mortality reduction of 27% over 15 months. This major benefit is not surprising, because such patients have activation of the renin-angiotensin system with levels of angiotensin-II increasing eightfold beyond those found in patients with AMI—but without clinical heart failure.[44]

POSTINFARCT LV DYSFUNCTION.   In the SAVE study,[111] captopril was given to patients with reduced ejection fractions (40% or lower), starting as early as 3 days postinfarct and continued for a mean of 42 months. The benefits included a 19% reduction in mortality from all causes, 22% reduction in development of overt CHF, and 22% reduction of first hospitalization for heart failure. In the still-unpublished TRACE study, ACE inhibition by trandolapril (not available in the USA) was given to all postinfarct patients with ejection fraction values of 35% or less, starting 3 to 7 days postinfarct and continuing for 2 to 4 years. Patients with clinically evident ischemia or heart failure (categories excluded from the SAVE study) were included. Mortality was reduced by 22%. The proposed mechanism is a lessening of the adverse **postinfarct remodeling,** whereby the left ventricle progressively enlarges with increasing mechanical dysfunction and correspondingly more renin-angiotensin activation.[113] ACE inhibition may also act by mechanically unloading the left ventricle following peripheral vasodilation and/or by inhibition of myocyte hypertrophy induced by angiotensin-II. Endothelial protection via formation of bradykinin may also help.

PREVENTION OF REINFARCTION AND CORONARY ISCHEMIC EVENTS.   An unexplained result in the SAVE study[111] was that captopril reduced reinfarction. This proposed benefit was not accepted by the FDA because the definition of MI was not clear.[59A] In the UK (but again not the USA), enalapril is licensed for the reduction of myocardial infarction and hospitalization for unstable angina pectoris, on the basis of data from the SOLVD studies.[128] One mechanism involved in these benefits may be related to the protective effects of bradykinin on the vascular endothelium, as already discussed. Additionally, angiotensin-II inhibits fibrinolysis,[108] whereas ACE inhibition promotes endogenous fibrinolysis.[126A] It must be emphasized that ACE inhibitors are not antianginal agents in the strict sense of the term, only having an indirect antianginal effect by lessening the afterload on the myocardial oxygen demand and by decreasing adrenergic activation.[27] Postinfarct, an important point is that the reduction of all-cause mortality achieved by ACE inhibition (19%) is about equal to that of beta-blockade (20% to 25%), yet there is a combined effect (33%). Whereas the benefit of beta-blockade appears to start within the first year, that of ACE inhibition becomes more evident in the second and third years.

# ACE Inhibitors for Diabetic and/or Hypertensive Renal Disease

## Diabetic Nephropathy

In diabetic nephropathy, aggressive antihypertensive treatment reduces the rate of progression toward renal failure.[99] ACE inhibitors may outperform other agents.[72] Direct proof of the efficacy of captopril in Type I diabetic nephropathy has been presented by Lewis et al.[79] in a study in which there was reduction of hard end-points, such as death, dialysis, and transplantation. The effects were found independently of the added blood pressure fall, so that the mechanism extends beyond the antihypertensive benefit. Hence, captopril is now licensed in the USA for the treatment of diabetic nephropathy (proteinuria > 500 mg per day) with retinopathy. There is no reason to suppose that other ACE inhibitors would not work equally well. Nor is there reason to doubt that the principle can be extended to Type II (noninsulin-dependent) diabetics with nephropathy.

## Diabetic Microproteinuria

In diabetics with microalbuminuria but without hypertension, enalapril reduced protein leakage, whereas hydrochlorothiazide in equivalent antihypertensive doses did not.[68] In such patients with insulin-dependent diabetes, intensive antidiabetic therapy is known to delay the onset of overt nephropathy and is basic therapy.[46] The principle of the benefits of tight diabetic control is likely to extend to noninsulin-dependent diabetes.[77] In addition, vigorous control of hypertension with blood pressure values below 140/90 mmHg is required. Experimentally, salt restriction plays a role in promoting the renoprotective effects of an ACE inhibitor.[54] In the UK, captopril is licensed for use in Type I diabetes with microproteinuria greater than 30 mg per day.

## Hypertensive Diabetics (Type II Diabetes)

In noninsulin-dependent diabetics, ACE inhibition should offer metabolic advantages over conventional therapy by thiazides and beta-blockers. ACE inhibitors, and also low-dose thiazides, calcium antagonists, and alpha-blockers (but not beta-blockers) are all recommended as first-line therapy in hypertensive diabetics.[92] If ACE inhibitors help to limit insulin resistance, they should also limit metabolic damage in diabetics. Yet, over a period of 36 months, captopril-treated patients fared no better than others treated by a variety of agents, as judged by fasting blood sugar, blood lipids, and glycosylated hemoglobin levels, although microalbuminuria was consistently reduced.[76] In a shorter study on hypertensive diabetics, over 9 months, equal control of blood pressure was achieved by verapamil or enalapril, and there were no changes in a variety of metabolic parameters.[55] Microalbuminuria again fell with the ACE inhibitor. When compared with nifedipine, enalapril was equally antihypertensive, yet both micro- and macroalbuminuria fell more in the enalapril-treated patients.[36] The crucial issue is whether ACE inhibitor therapy not only lessens microalbuminuria in hypertensive diabetics but prevents the ultimate development of hard end-points. To answer this question would require many years of follow-up study.

## Hypertensive Microalbuminuria

In nondiabetic hypertensives, as in diabetic hypertensives, ACE inhibitors have consistently reduced microalbuminuria. But are they better than other agents? Two studies say yes. In one study, enalapril was compared with nitrendipine, atenolol, and chlorthalidone[30] and in the other with nicardipine.[31] Hypothetically, the unique effect of ACE inhibitors as dilators of the efferent renal arterioles tends to relieve the intraglomerular hypertension, with a fall in the high filtration pressure that is thought to promote renal protein leakage. The opposing point of view is simple: it is the blood pressure reduction and not the type of agent that matters.[53] The latter study was, however, only for 3 months, whereas the one favoring ACE inhibitors lasted for 2 years,[31] hence being more impressive.

TABLE 5–7      **ACE** INHIBITORS: SIDE-EFFECTS AND CONTRAINDICATIONS

1. **Side-effects, Class**
   Cough—common
   Hypotension—variable (renal artery stenosis; severe heart failure)
   Deterioration of renal function (related to hypotension)
   Angioedema (rare; but potentially fatal)
   Renal failure (rare, bilateral renal artery stenosis)
   Hyperkalemia (in renal failure, or with K-retaining diuretics)
   Skin reactions
2. **Side-effects first described for high-dose captopril**
   Neutropenia especially with collagen vascular renal disease
   Proteinuria
   Loss of taste
   Oral lesions; scalded-mouth syndrome (rare)
3. **Contraindications**
   Renal—bilateral renal artery stenosis or equivalent lesions
   Pre-existing hypotension
   Severe aortic stenosis or obstructive cardiomyopathy
   Pregnancy (NB: recent FDA warning)

## Chronic Renal Failure with Hypertension

In such patients with a serum creatinine of 200 to 400 $\mu$mol/L (2.0 to 4.0 mg/dL), enalapril more effectively delayed end-stage renal failure than did a beta-blocker.[68A] Other agents (furosemide, a calcium antagonist or a central agent) were added as needed to achieve equal blood pressure control in the two groups.

# Side-effects of ACE Inhibitors

## Class Side-effects of ACE Inhibitors

COUGH.  Of the various side-effects (Fig. 5–6; Table 5–2), some serious and some not, cough has emerged as one of the most troublesome and common. This side-effect took a long time to be discovered. Patients with heart failure cough in any case, and in patients with hypertension such side-effects are generally only discovered if volunteered. Cough was not known and ignored in the well-known "quality of life" study in hypertensives.[6] In some centers, the incidence of cough is thought to be as high as 10% to 15%, whereas others report a much lower incidence. The cough is due to an increased sensitivity of the cough reflex resulting in a dry, irritating, nonproductive cough, quite different from bronchospasm. Increased formation of bradykinin and prostaglandins may play a role (Table 5–2). Several studies suggest relief of the cough by added nonsteroidal antiinflammatory drugs[14,58] with the downside of diminished antihypertensive effects.[15] As an alternative, the combination of low-dose ACE inhibitor and the calcium antagonist nifedipine lessens the cough through unknown mechanisms.[58] Another possible solution to the problem of cough is just to wait for about 4 months: it may go.[105] Logically, a change to an angiotensin-II receptor inhibitor (**losartan**) should consistently benefit.

HYPOTENSION.  Particularly in CHF, orthostatic symptoms due to excess hypotension are common and may necessitate dose reduction or even cessation of ACE inhibitor therapy. In general, so long as orthostatic symptoms do not occur, the absolute blood pressure is not crucial and many patients do well with systolic pressures of 80 to 90 mmHg.

RENAL SIDE-EFFECTS. Hypotension can in turn precipitate reversible renal failure. Predisposing factors are severe CHF or underlying renal disease including renal artery stenosis. Rarely, irreversible renal failure has occurred in patients with bilateral renal artery stenosis, which is therefore a contraindication to ACE inhibitors. In unilateral renal artery disease, with high circulating renin values, ACE inhibitors may also cause excessive hypotensive responses with oliguria and/or azotemia. To obviate and minimize such problems, a low first test dose is required with blood pressure checks. A slight stable increase in serum creatinine does not limit use.

ANGIOEDEMA. Although rare (about 0.1%), this condition is life-threatening. There is no known method of prediction. The mechanism may be by formation of bradykinin. The treatment is by prompt subcutaneous epinephrine.

HYPERKALEMIA. When given with potassium-sparing diuretics or in the presence of renal failure, the mild potassium retention induced by ACE inhibition may precipitate hyperkalemia. Thus potassium supplements or retainers should be stopped when ACE inhibition is initiated.

PREGNANCY RISKS. All ACE inhibitors are embryopathic and contraindicated in pregnancy, with the greatest risk in the second and third trimesters. The FDA requires a boxed warning in the package insert.

### Captopril-specific Side-effects

Whether the SH-groups in the captopril molecule really are the specific cause of neutropenia and/or agranulocytosis is still not clear. The association with high-dose captopril, usually occurring in patients with renal failure and especially those with a collagen vascular disorder, is undoubted. In the case of all other ACE inhibitors, there is suspicion without proof, so that the American package inserts all warn that available data for noncaptopril ACE inhibitors (i.e., all the rest) are not sufficient to exclude agranulocytosis at similar rates to those found with captopril.

## ACE Inhibitors: Drug Combinations and Interactions

ACE INHIBITORS PLUS DIURETICS. There are excellent theoretical and practical arguments for the combination of ACE inhibitors and low-dose diuretics. In **hypertension,** these agents are able to remedy the defects of each other: the diuretics invoke a sodium diuresis that sensitizes to the hypotensive effect of ACE inhibitors, whereas ACE inhibitors oppose the unwanted vasoconstriction resulting from diuretic-induced renin release. Numerous studies show the added hypotensive effects of diuretics and that low doses work well (p 189). In black patients, the combination restores their sensitivity to ACE inhibitors.[123] Diuretics should not, except in special circumstances, be potassium-retaining (**Dyazide, Moduretic, Maxzide** and spironolactone) because there is a **risk of hyperkalemia** especially in the presence of renal impairment.[1]

In **CHF,** additive effects of ACE inhibitors on the preload may lead to syncope or hypotension so that the diuretic dose is usually halved before starting ACE inhibitors. The result may be a true diuretic-sparing effect in about half of patients with mild CHF upon addition of the ACE inhibitor, while in others the full diuretic dose must be reinstituted.[16] Low-dose captopril (up to a mean of 57 mg daily) can be cautiously added to patients already treated by furosemide and spironolactone, if those reacting to the spironolactone by hyperkalemia are excluded.[42]

*Small doses of captopril* may be added to furosemide. In a fascinating report,[91] the addition of only 1 mg captopril was able to facilitate a diuresis when added to furosemide (median dose 80 mg/day). In contrast, 25 mg captopril decreased blood pressure and hence the glomerular filtration rate, and limited the diuretic response to furosemide.

ACE Inhibitors Plus Digoxin for CHF.   In CHF, ACE inhibitors are frequently combined with diuretics and digoxin. Digoxin decreases heart size and rate, whereas ACE inhibitors decrease the load, so that the combination should be better hemodynamically than either agent alone.[9]

ACE Inhibitors Plus Beta-blockade.   This combination has been widely used in hypertension, although theoretically it is not ideal because both agents have in common an ultimate antirenin effect. Incomplete data suggest that there could be an additive effect.[2] Post-infarct, the protective effects of these two types of agents are additive.[111]

ACE Inhibitors Plus Calcium Antagonists.   This combination, now increasingly used in the therapy of hypertension, is logical. There are two different modalities of attack, first on the renin-angiotensin system and second on the increased peripheral vascular resistance found especially in moderate and severe hypertension. Furthermore, both agents should be free of CNS side-effects and are metabolically neutral. Nifedipine may unexpectedly diminish the cough induced by an ACE inhibitor.[58] Of interest, in subtotally nephrectomized rats, an ACE inhibitor decreases intraglomerular pressure, whereas a calcium antagonist inhibits glomerular growth,[50] with added renoprotection from the combination. Such experimental data are supported by studies in diabetic microalbuminuria in which verapamil and enalapril together decrease protein leakage more than either agent singly.[56]

ACE Inhibitors Plus Other Vasodilators.   As different vasodilators have different supplementary qualities, each patient has to be considered on a pragmatic basis. Combination of ACE inhibitors with other vasodilators such as nitrates, calcium antagonists, or hydralazine should be undertaken with care because of the added risk of hypotension. The combination of high-dose hydralazine plus captopril may have an added risk of altered immune function, so that careful monitoring of neutrophils is advisable.

ACE Inhibitors and Nonsteroidal Anti-inflammatories (NSAIDs).   Formation of bradykinin and thereby prostaglandins may play an important role in peripheral vasodilation. Hence, nonsteroidal anti-inflammatories and especially indomethacin and naproxen lessen the effectiveness of ACE inhibitors in CHF and in hypertension.[58] Aspirin may also interfere with ACE inhibitor hemodynamic effects,[67] although lower doses (aspirin 236 mg daily) interfere less.[122]

## Specific ACE Inhibitors

### Captopril

Captopril (**Capoten; Lopril** in France; **Lopirin** in Germany; **Captopril** in Japan), the first widely available ACE inhibitor, was originally seen to be an agent with significant and serious side-effects such as loss of taste, renal impairment, and neutropenia. Now it is recognized that these are rather rare side-effects that can be avoided largely by reducing the daily dose and by appropriate monitoring. Captopril is licensed in the USA for hypertension, heart failure, postinfarct LV dysfunction, and diabetic nephropathy. It has the widest range of approved indications. In the UK, it is also licensed for prevention of reinfarction and for diabetic microproteinuria.

PHARMACOKINETICS.   After absorption from the stomach, captopril is metabolized by the liver and kidney with an elimination half-life of approximately 4 to 6 hours (Table 5–3). A dose of 20 mg given orally to normal volunteers blocks the pressor response to exogenous angiotensin-I within 15 minutes and for over 2 hours.[1] In hypertension, its biological half-life is long enough to allow twice-daily dosage.

DOSE AND INDICATIONS. In **hypertension,** captopril has an average daily dose of 25 to 50 mg orally given twice daily (instead of much higher three-times-daily doses previously prescribed). For maximum bioavailability, captopril should be taken on an empty stomach, yet food has little influence on the overall antihypertensive effect.[1] Although twice-daily doses are conventional, a single daily dose of 50 to 100 mg may be used with dietary salt restriction.[1] The risk of excess hypotension is highest in patients with high renin states (renal artery stenosis, pre-existing vigorous diuretic therapy, or severe sodium restriction) when the initial dose should be low (6.25 to 12.5 mg). Whether captopril can improve hard end-points in hypertension is the subject of the current CAPPP study.[34] For **severe hypertension,** sublingual captopril (25 mg chewed) reduces the blood pressure,[1] but renal contraindications must first be excluded.

In **CHF,** the usual maintenance dose is 37.5 to 150 mg daily in three divided doses; twice-daily therapy is logical.[8] Captopril may cause excessive hypotension especially in vigorously diuresed patients so that a **test dose** of 6.25 mg is required (if given sublingually the safety can be assessed within 1 hour) followed by 12.5 mg three times daily, and working up to 50 mg three times daily if tolerated. The diuretic should be stopped for 24 to 48 hours prior to captopril to avoid an excess renin state.

In **renal disease,** when captopril is not contraindicated (next section), the dose is reduced.

In **diabetic nephropathy,** captopril improves proteinuria and decreases hard end-points, such as death, transplantation, or dialysis.[79]

In **postinfarct patients with LV dysfunction** (ejection fraction 40% or lower), captopril is licensed to prevent overt heart failure and, in the UK, to reduce recurrent myocardial infarction and coronary revascularization procedures.

In **rheumatoid arthritis,** captopril appears to exert a modest antiarthritic effect by virtue of the sulfhydryl (SH) group.[1]

In **nitrate tolerance,** some data suggest amelioration of tolerance by captopril,[11] possibly by virtue of the protective SH-groups in captopril.[88] Furthermore, captopril can potentiate the antianginal effects of a single dose of isosorbide dinitrate.[89]

CONTRAINDICATIONS. These include bilateral renal artery stenosis; renal artery stenosis in a single kidney; immune-based renal disease, especially collagen vascular disease; severe renal failure (serum creatinine > 3 mg/dL or > 300 umol/L, see p 117); pre-existing neutropenia; systemic hypotension; and pregnancy. *Relative contraindications* include coadministration of other drugs likely to alter immune function such as procainamide, hydralazine and probenecid.

SIDE-EFFECTS. In general, the side-effects are seldom serious provided that the total daily dose is 150 mg daily or less.[1] Cough is the most common and frequently troublesome side-effect. Other class side-effects include renal failure, angioedema, and hyperkalemia. Immune-based side-effects are probably specific to captopril, such as taste disturbances, certain immune-based skin rashes, and (in a subgroup of patients) neutropenia.

**Neutropenia** ($< 1,000/mm^3$) may occur with captopril, extremely rarely in hypertensive patients with normal renal function (1/8,600 according to the package insert), more commonly (1/500) with pre-existing impaired renal function with a serum creatinine of 1.6 mg/dL or more, and as a grave risk (1/25) in patients with both collagen vascular disease and renal impairment. When captopril is discontinued, recovery from neutropenia is usual except when there is associated serious disease, such as severe renal or heart failure or collagen vascular disease.

**Proteinuria** occurs in about 1% of patients receiving captopril, especially in the presence of pre-existing renal disease or with high doses of captopril (> 150 mg/day[1]). There is a double mechanism for renal damage induced by captopril: first, an altered immune response, and second, excess hypotension, as shared with enalapril.[1] Paradoxically, captopril is used in the therapy of diabetic nephropathy with proteinuria.[79]

**Other side-effects** include hypotension (frequent in the treatment of CHF), impaired taste (2% to 7%), skin rashes (4% to 10%) sometimes with eosinophilia, and (rarely) serious angioedema (1/100 to 1/1,000). Hepatic damage is also very rare. Renal failure in patients with CHF may be exacerbated by captopril.

PRETREATMENT PRECAUTIONS. Bilateral renal artery stenosis must be excluded as far as possible. Patients with renal impairment caused by collagen disease, or patients receiving immunosuppressives or immune system modifiers such as steroids and hydralazine, should be excluded, as should patients with a history of hematological disease or pretreatment depression of neutrophils or platelets. Pretreatment hypotension excludes therapy.

PRECAUTIONS DURING TREATMENT. Regular monitoring of neutrophil counts is required in patients with pre-existing serious renal impairment, especially on the basis of collagen vascular disease (pretreatment count, then 2 weekly counts for 3 months). The risk of renal damage from captopril may be reduced by keeping total daily doses below 150 mg/day.[1]

## Enalapril

Enalapril (**Vasotec** in the USA; **Innovace** in the UK; **Xanef, Renitec** or **Pres** in Europe; **Renivace** in Japan) is the standard pro-drug. It has been extensively tested in heart failure (Tables 5–4 and 5–5). The chief differences from captopril are: (1) a longer half-life; (2) a slower onset of effect because of the requirement of hydrolysis of the pro-drug to the active form, enalaprilat, in the liver so that the therapeutic effect depends on hepatic metabolism (Class II pattern of pharmacokinetics, Table 5–3); and (3) the absence of the SH-group from the structure, thus theoretically lessening or removing the risk of immune-based side-effects. Enalapril is approved for hypertension, heart failure, and to decrease the development of overt heart failure in symptomatic patients with LV dysfunction (ejection fraction equal to or less than 35%). In the latter group of patients, enalapril is also licensed in the UK to prevent coronary ischemic events.

PHARMACOKINETICS. About 60% of the oral dose is absorbed[1] with no influence of meals. Enalapril is de-esterified in the liver and kidney to the active form, enalaprilat. Time to peak serum concentration is about 2 hours for enalapril, and about 5 hours for enalaprilat,[1] with some delay in CHF. Excretion is 95% renal as enalapril or enalaprilat (hence the lower doses in renal failure). The elimination half-life of enalaprilat is about 4 to 5 hours in hypertension and 7 to 8 hours in CHF.[1] Following multiple doses, the effective elimination half-life of enalaprilat is 11 hours (package insert). One oral 10 mg dose of enalapril yields sufficient enalaprilat to cause significant ACE inhibition for 19 hours.[1] In hypertension and in CHF, the peak hypotensive response to enalapril occurs about 4 to 6 hours after the oral dose, and may account for the marked depression of renal function which may occur at that time.[1] Peak effects on cardiac index and other hemodynamic parameters occur earlier, after about 1 to 2 hours, and are sustained for at least 12 hours.[1] In severe liver disease, the dose may have to be increased (impaired conversion of enalapril to enalaprilat).

DOSE. In **hypertension,** the dose is 2.5 to 20 mg as 1 or 2 daily doses. Doses higher than 10 to 20 mg daily give little added benefit.[20,21] A low initial dose (2.5 mg) is a wise precaution, especially when enalapril is added to a diuretic or the patient is salt-depleted,[1] in the elderly, or when high-renin hypertension is suspected. In **asymptomatic LV dysfunction** and in **CHF,** in the SOLVD trials,[115,116] enalapril was started with an initial dose of 2.5 mg twice daily and worked up to 10 mg twice daily (mean daily dose 17 mg). Yet when added to digoxin and diuretics, a low dose of only 5 mg daily achieved good short-term hemodynamic results.[3] Logically, the dose could be keyed to the severity of CHF. In **renal failure** (glomerular filtration rate below 30 ml/min), the dose of enalapril must be reduced. In **early phase AMI,** within 24 hours of symptoms, an initial dose of only 1.25 mg at 2-hourly intervals for 3 doses was followed by 5 mg three times daily[101] with long-term benefits.

INTRAVENOUS DOSE. **Enalaprilat** is now available for intravenous use, the indication being hypertension when oral use is contraindicated. Concurrent furosemide has an approximately additive effect on the blood pressure. The dose of enalaprilat is 1.25 mg every 6 hours given intravenously over 5 minutes; a response in the blood pressure can be expected within 15 minutes. The dose is halved for patients receiving prior diuretic therapy or with renal impairment or those thought for any other reason to be at risk of excess hypotension. In early AMI, the CONSENSUS-II study[38] showed that the use of fixed-dose enalaprilat (1 mg infused over 2 hours, then oral enalapril 2.5 mg up to 5 mg twice daily, then 20 mg daily) led to excess hypotension and the trial was stopped.

SIDE-EFFECTS. Cough is most common, as for all ACE inhibitors. In animals, very high doses of enalapril may cause renal tubular damage, probably the result of excess prolonged hypotension. Rarely neutropenia has been reported, and the relationship to enalapril has not been proven. Taste disturbances are not listed in the package insert. Enalapril may be safer when captopril has induced a skin rash.[1] As for all ACE inhibitors, angioedema is a rare risk highlighted in the package insert.

PRECAUTIONS. As in the case of captopril, (1) the major risk is excess hypotension (use low initial dose); and (2) pretreatment evaluation of renal function and of drug cotherapy is essential. It is presumed that enalapril, without the SH-group found in captopril, does not produce the same immune-based toxic effects, and regular monitoring of the neutrophil count or proteinuria is not essential. Nonetheless, the package insert points out that available data are insufficient to show that enalapril does not cause neutropenia, so that monitoring of the white cell count is still advisable, especially in those with collagen vascular disease and renal failure.

CONTRAINDICATIONS. In hypertensives, bilateral renal artery stenosis or stenosis in a single kidney must be excluded. Pregnancy (see captopril).

## Other Pro-drugs

FOSINOPRIL. (**Monopril** in the USA, **Staril** in the UK). Chemically, this compound differs from other ACE inhibitors in that it uses phosphinic acid as the zinc ligand. Although it is a pro-drug belonging to Class II (Table 5–3), it has unique pharmacokinetic features in that there are dual routes of excretion, hepatic and renal. The result is that in chronic renal failure the active fosinoprilat form accumulates less in the blood than would enalaprilat or lisinopril.[112] In a large clinical trial with concurrent placebo controls, 40 to 80 mg fosinopril once daily was antihypertensive.[26] A dose of 10 mg was less effective but 20 mg was not tested. Addition of a diuretic was required in about half the patients. In the elderly, the major reason for decreasing doses of other ACE inhibitors is renal impairment. In the case of fosinopril, no dosage adjustment is required.

QUINAPRIL. (**Accupril** in the USA; **Accupro** in the UK). This agent has only a short plasma half-life, but appears to be tightly bound to the angiotensin-converting enzyme, so that in practice it can be given once or twice daily. In the UK, it is licensed for once-daily therapy for hypertension (5 to 40 mg daily) and twice-daily therapy for CHF (2.5 mg upwards). In the USA, quinapril (10 to 40 mg given once or twice daily) is currently licensed for hypertension only, but it works in CHF.[100,109] It is the drug being used in the QUIET study,[102] an outcome study on 1,740 patients with previous angioplasty or atherectomy randomized to placebo or quinapril. Quinapril has a high magnesium content and may interfere with the absorption of tetracycline.

RAMIPRIL (**Altace** in the USA; **Ramace, Tritace** elsewhere). This agent is a long-acting antihypertensive in a 2.5 to 10 mg dose once daily. It is proposed as a tissue-specific ACE inhibitor without that claim being translated into any definite clinical differences from others. In the AIRE study[23] ramipril 2.5 mg twice daily and then 5 mg twice daily, as tolerated, was used to show a major fall (27%) in mortality of patients with early postinfarct heart failure diagnosed clinically (Table 5–4).

SOME OTHER PRO-DRUGS. **Benazepril** (**Lotensin** in the USA) has an optimal dose of 10 mg twice daily in hypertension. **Cilazapril** (**Vasace** in the UK) has similar kinetics to enalapril. The half-life of the active form appears to be 8 to 24 hours. **Perindopril** (**Coversyl** in the UK, 4 to 16 mg once daily for hypertension) is long-acting and well studied in relation to a beneficial effect on the vascular structure in hypertension. In CHF, the effect of a first dose of 2 mg is well studied and appears to cause little or no hypotension, in contrast to low-dose enalapril or captopril.[84] This interesting property warrants further study.

### Lisinopril: A Kinetic Class of Its Own

This ACE inhibitor (**Zestril, Prinivil**), approved for hypertension and CHF in the USA, differs from all the others in its unusual pharmacokinetic properties (Table 5–4). It is not a pro-drug, it is not metabolized by the liver, it is water-soluble, and it is excreted unchanged by the kidneys (reminiscent of the kinetic patterns of water-soluble beta-blockers). Therefore, it can be given a class of its own, Class III (Table 5–3). The half-life is sufficiently long to give a duration of action exceeding 24 hours. Once-daily dosing for **CHF** is licensed in the USA. The initial dose is 2.5 to 5 mg in heart failure, and the maintenance dose 5 to 20 mg per day. In **hypertension,** the initial dose is 10 mg once daily and the usual dose range is 20 to 40 mg per day. In **diuretic-treated patients,** the manufacturers recommend an initial dose of 5 mg while the patient is being supervised for 2 hours. In **renal impairment** and in the **elderly,** the dose should also be reduced.

Lisinopril was the drug used in the GISSI-3 megastudy in acute phase AMI (Table 5–5) and is the agent used in the ATLAS study (Assessment of Treatment with Lisinopril and Survival). The latter study in CHF aims to test whether even higher doses of lisinopril than currently used might give additional benefits.[100]

### Choice of ACE Inhibitor

*In general, we see little advantage for any one agent compared with others.* They all work in hypertension, heart failure (Table 5–5), and (probably) in postinfarct protection and in diabetic renal disease. However, some drugs are much better tested for each of these situations than others. **Captopril,** the first agent available, has the widest range of approved indications. Furthermore, captopril is very well tested for its quality of life in hypertension, and is the only ACE inhibitor licensed for diabetic nephropathy, yet it must be given twice or three times daily. There are certain borderline indications where the SH-group may possibly be an advantage, such as associated rheumatoid arthritis, the treatment of nitrate tolerance, and, hypothetically, reperfusion damage. Captopril is often chosen for a test dose. Not being a pro-drug it has a rapid onset of action. On the other hand, captopril in high doses may incur the risk of certain side-effects specific to the SH-group, including ageusia and neutropenia. **Enalapril** is very well tested for all stages of heart failure in several landmark studies including the CONSENSUS study,[5] V-HeFT-II[125] and the more recent SOLVD studies (prevention and treatment arms).[115,116] It is the drug with the best data on reduction of mortality in CHF. Yet it is not clearly a once-a-day drug and was used twice daily in all these studies. In early phase AMI, enalapril in a very low initial dose of 1.25 mg and then worked up to 5 mg three times daily exerted long-term benefits over 12 months.[101] Yet the trial was very small. **Ramipril** is well tested in early postinfarct clinical heart failure, where it reduced mortality substantially. Although long-acting, it was given twice daily. A practical advantage is that it is cheaper than some others. **Lisinopril** is clearly a once-a-day preparation with simple metabolism, being water-soluble, with no liver transformation and renal excretion, making it an easy drug to use and understand. It has advantages when SH-groups should be avoided or when several other agents are being administered because there is no risk of hepatic pharmacokinetic interactions.

## Angiotensin-II Receptor Antagonists

Because ACE inhibitors have their major effects by inhibiting the formation of angiotensin-II, it follows that direct antagonism of these receptors should duplicate many or most of the effects of ACE inhibition. The angiotensin-II receptors ($AT_1$) concerned are blocked by **losartan,** a new orally active agent well into preregistration clinical trials, and registered for use in hypertension in Scandinavia. The possible indications are hypertension and heart failure. In volunteers, losartan 100 mg daily decreased the blood pressure and increased circulating renin and angiotensin-II levels.[62] In patients with CHF, acute administration of losartan 25 mg reduced systemic vascular resistance and increased plasma renin and angiotensin-II levels.[65] The ELITE study (Evaluation of Losartan In The Elderly) will compare **losartan** and captopril in CHF in those over 70 years with mortality as end-point. The theoretical advantage of losartan over ACE inhibitors is the total absence of cough, the latter hypothetically being induced by bradykinin and prostaglandins. Also, losartan is claimed to reduce blood cholesterol levels. Losartan might, theoretically, be able to avoid the hormonal escape (hyperreninemia and increase in angiotensin-II) found during prolonged administration of ACE inhibitors.[119] A potential disadvantage of losartan is the absence of those beneficial effects of ACE inhibitors ascribed to the formation of bradykinin, such as renal vasodilation[66] and endothelial protection. This consideration might be of special importance in the treatment of heart failure.

## Conventional Vasodilators Used Either in Heart Failure or in Hypertension

Vasodilation, once a specialized procedure, is now commonplace in the therapy of CHF and hypertension, as the peripheral circulation has become one of the prime sites of cardiac drug action. Vasodilators may be classified according to the site of action in the circulation.

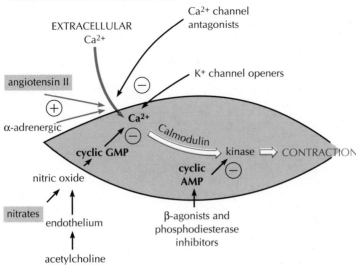

**FIGURE 5–7.** Cellular mechanisms of actions of vasodilators. Kinase, myosin light chain kinase. Fig. copyright L.H. Opie.

Preload reducers (predominantly venodilators) may be separated from those reducing primarily the afterload (predominantly arteriolar dilators), while mixed agents act on both pre- and afterload and are combined veno-arteriolar dilators. The cellular sites of action of these agents are shown in Fig. 5–7. ACE inhibitors can be regarded as specialized vasodilators. Whereas other vasodilators, especially the arteriolar dilators, reflexively activate the renin-angiotensin axis, ACE inhibitors both vasodilate and inhibit this system.

**PRELOAD REDUCTION.** Normally as the preload (the LV filling pressure) increases so also does the peak LV systolic pressure, and the cardiac output rises (ascending limb of the Frank-Starling curve, Fig. 5–8). In diseased hearts the increase in cardiac output is much less than normal, and the output fails to rise and may even fall as the filling pressure rises (the apparent descending limb of Frank-Starling curve). However, the optimal filling pressure for the diseased heart is very variable, not always being higher than normal. Reduction of the preload is generally but not always useful. Clinically, the major drugs reducing the preload in CHF are (1) furosemide by its diuretic effect and (2) the nitrates that dilate the systemic veins to reduce the venous return and thus the filling pressure in both the right and left heart chambers.

**AFTERLOAD REDUCTION.** The therapeutic aim is reduction of the peripheral vascular resistance to lessen the load on the heart, improved renal function, and better skeletal muscle perfusion (Fig. 5–9). Reduction of the systemic vascular resistance is not the same as blood pressure reduction, because in CHF a compensatory increase in the cardiac output tends to maintain the arterial pressure during afterload reduction.

Specific afterload reducers are few and limited in practice to two. First, hydralazine is a nonspecific agent whose cellular mode of action is still undecided, although it may well act as a potassium channel opener. Second, the calcium antagonists are also afterload reducers and widely used in hypertension. They often have a negative inotropic effect, thereby restricting their use in CHF. Nonetheless, felodipine and amlodipine are undergoing formal testing in CHF, mostly in patients already treated by diuretics, ACE inhibition and digitalis.

**COMBINED PRE- AND AFTERLOAD REDUCTION.** Sodium nitroprusside,

## HEMODYNAMICS OF VASODILATORS IN CHF

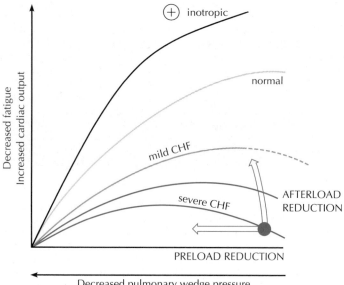

**FIGURE 5–8.** Theoretical Frank-Starling curves in CHF. Note effects of preload reduction on dyspnea and pulmonary wedge pressure, and afterload reduction on cardiac output and muscle fatigue. Nitrates reduce the preload, hydralazine the afterload, and angiotensin-converting enzyme inhibitors and sodium nitroprusside reduce both preload and afterload. Inotropic agents, such as digoxin, put the heart onto a higher Frank-Starling curve. Fig. copyright, L.H. Opie.

## ARTERIOLAR vs. VENOUS VASODILATORS

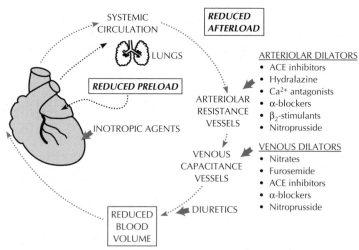

**FIGURE 5–9.** Comparatives sites of action of agents reducing afterload, reducing preload, inotropic agents and diuretics. Fig. copyright, L.H. Opie.

used for very severe hypertension or CHF, must be given intravenously under close supervision and careful monitoring. The **alpha-adrenergic blockers** give combined pre- and afterload reduction, the latter explaining their antihypertensive effect. Theoretically, they should also work in CHF. Yet prazosin evokes tolerance and is no better than placebo during chronic testing in heart failure. On the other hand, the longer-acting **doxazosin** has shown promising results in a study over 17 weeks in that exercise tolerance was increased and there were fewer morbid and mortal cardiac events when compared with placebo.[47] Clearly these results need confirmation and extension of the test period. Nonetheless, it is possible to hypothesize that the shorter-acting prazosin caused intermittent vasodilation with intermittent reflex neuroendocrine activation, whereas the longer-acting doxazosin did not (by analogy with short- and long-acting calcium antagonists). Two combined alpha-beta-blockers, **labetalol**[78] and **carvedilol**[60] both appear to improve heart failure. The beta-blocking component of these drugs should be able to inhibit beta-mediated myocardial toxicity resulting from neuroadrenergic activation, and the alpha-blocking component to reduce peripheral vasoconstriction. Nonetheless, the overall status of alpha-receptor or alpha-beta-receptor blockade in the long-term therapy of heart failure still remains an open question. At present, data for carvedilol look best.

## Nitroprusside

Intravenous nitroprusside (**Nipride, Nitropress**) remains the reference vasodilator for severe low-output left-sided heart failure provided that the arterial pressure is reasonable, because it acts rapidly and has a balanced effect, dilating both arterioles and veins (Fig. 5–9). Nitroprusside seems particularly useful for increasing LV stroke work in severe refractory heart failure caused by mitral or aortic incompetence. Hemodynamic and clinical improvement also are observed in patients with severe pump failure complicating AMI, in heart failure after cardiac surgery, and in patients with acute exacerbation of chronic heart failure. Because of the increased stroke volume there may be considerable hemodynamic improvement without much hypotension; but in general, some hypotension accompanies and may limit the therapeutic effect of nitroprusside. Because of the need for careful continuous monitoring and its light sensitivity, nitroprusside is being replaced in severe CHF by nitrates or by the inotropic dilators such as milrinone, and in hypertensive crises by intravenous nicardipine or enalaprilat.

Pharmacokinetics. With infusion of nitroprusside, the hemodynamic response (direct vasodilation) starts within minutes and stops equally quickly. Nitroprusside given intravenously is converted to cyanmethemoglobin and free cyanide in the red cells; the free cyanide is then converted to thiocyanate in the liver and is cleared by the kidneys (half-life 7 days).

Dose. An initial infusion of 10 $\mu$g/min is increased by 10 $\mu$g/min every 10 minutes up to 40 to 75 $\mu$g/min with a top dose of 300 $\mu$g/min.

Precautions. The infusion rate needs careful titration against the blood pressure, which must be continously monitored to avoid excess hypotension. Nitroprusside must not be abruptly withdrawn because of the danger of rebound hypertension. Extravasation must be avoided. The solution in normal saline (avoid alkaline solutions) must be freshly made and then shielded from light during infusion; it should be discarded when 4 hours old, or before if discolored. Cyanide may accumulate with prolonged high doses of nitroprusside to produce a lactic acidosis. Toxicity can be avoided by monitoring blood lactate and blood thiocyanate (toxic level 100 $\mu$g/mL). But in lactic acidosis due to poor tissue perfusion nitroprusside may be beneficial.

Indications. These include the following situations: (1) for hemodynamic improvement in selected patients with myocardial infarction and LV failure; (2) severe CHF with regurgitant valve disease; (3) in hypertensive crises associated with LV failure; (4) in dissecting aneurysm; and (5) after coronary bypass surgery, when patients frequently have reactive hypertension as they are removed from hypothermia, so that nitroprussides or nitrates are routinely given by most cardiovascular surgical units for 24 hours provided that hypotension is no problem.

CONTRAINDICATIONS. Pre-existing hypotension (systolic < 90 mmHg, diastolic < 60 mmHg). All vasodilators are contraindicated in severe obstructive valvular heart disease (aortic or mitral or pulmonic stenosis, or obstructive cardiomyopathy). AMI is not a contraindication, provided that excess hypotension is avoided.

SIDE-EFFECTS. Overvigorous treatment may cause an excessive drop in LV end-diastolic pressure, severe hypotension, and myocardial ischemia. Fatigue, nausea, vomiting, and disorientation tend to arise especially when treatment continues for more than 48 hours. In patients with renal failure, thiocyanate accumulates with high-dose infusions and may produce hypothyroidism after prolonged therapy. Hypoxia may result from increased ventilation-perfusion mismatch with pulmonary vasodilation.

COMBINATION WITH OTHER AGENTS. Nitroprusside may be combined with inotropic agents such as dopamine, dobutamine or digitalis to optimize the hemodynamic benefit. Maintaining an adequate ventricular filling pressure is essential with these combined therapies and invasive monitoring is required.

### Nitrates

Nitrates are now used in the therapy of both acute and chronic heart failure (p 42). Their major effect is venous rather than arteriolar dilation, thus being most suited to patients with raised pulmonary wedge pressure and clinical features of pulmonary congestion. Nitrates produce a "pharmacologic phlebotomy." Intravenous nitrates are usually chosen above nitroprusside for acute pulmonary edema of myocardial infarction, because of the extensive experience with nitrates in recent large trials.

### Hydralazine

Hydralazine is predominantly an arteriolar dilator and may have some indirect positive inotropic effect. It causes a marked increase in cardiac output with little or no decrease in pulmonary wedge or right atrial pressures. Hydralazine is particularly effective in patients with mitral regurgitation. It increases forward stroke volume and decreases regurgitant volume. In the VeHeFT-I and II trials,[124,125] the dose of hydralazine, combined with isosorbide dinitrate, was 150 to 300 mg in 4 divided daily doses.

PHARMACOKINETICS. Hydralazine is rapidly absorbed from the gut (peak concentration 1 to 2 hours). It is metabolized via acetylation in the liver with subsequent excretion in the urine. The plasma half-life is 2 to 8 hours, but the hypotensive effect is longer lasting, possibly because hydralazine is avidly taken up by the arterial wall. In severe renal failure, the dosage should be reduced. Patients with fast acetylation rates need a dose about 25% higher than those with slow rates. Lupus syndrome is more likely to develop in slow acetylators.

DOSE AND INDICATIONS. In **chronic LV failure,** in the Ve-HeFT trials,[124,125] the dose of hydralazine combined with isosorbide dinitrate was 150 to 300 mg daily in four divided doses. The role of hydralazine alone in patients already treated by diuretics, ACE inhibitors, and digoxin is not clear.

In **mild to moderate hypertension,** the usual dose is 50 to 75 mg every 6 to 8 hours, but two divided doses a day are equally effective. In **myocardial hypertrophy of hypertension,** hydralazine can bring down the pressure without causing regression of the hypertrophy, presumably because of the partial inotropic effect or reflex adrenergic stimulation. For IV use, see p 199.

In **sinus bradycardia,** hydralazine is one of the options to increase the heart rate.[12]

In **heart failure following cardiac surgery,** hydralazine (test dose 2.5 to 5.0 mg IV, up to 7.5 mg every 4 to 6 hours) generally gives improvement within 8 hours.[1]

SIDE-EFFECTS. Side-effects include fluid retention (renin release) that may necessitate diuretic therapy. In hypertension, the direct inotropic effect and the tachycardia limit the usefulness of hydralazine in patients with angina pectoris not on beta-blockade. In contrast, in CHF, reflex tachycardia is unusual, perhaps because reflex arcs are blunted. The lupus syndrome is rare with doses below 200 mg a day or with total doses below 100g. Patients on higher doses or prolonged therapy should be checked for antinuclear factors. Headache, nausea, and abdominal pain are not unusual at the start of therapy. Postural hypotension is occasionally seen in patients with CHF. Polyneuropathy (usually responsive to pyridoxine) and drug fever are rare side-effects.

# Alpha-Adrenergic Receptor Antagonists

Two types of alpha-receptors have been defined—the presynaptic alpha$_2$-receptors and the postsynaptic or vascular alpha$_1$-receptors. In addition, there are postsynaptic alpha$_2$-receptors that may facilitate vasoconstriction. No specific alpha$_2$-receptor blockers are yet available for clinical use. Presently the only approved use for alpha$_1$-blockers is against hypertension and not CHF.

## Prazosin

Prazosin (**Minipress**) is used in the therapy of hypertension, both in combination with diuretics or beta-blockade or as monotherapy. In CHF, it is no better than placebo.[124] Specific attractions are the favorable effects on the blood lipid profile and the benefit in prostatic outflow obstruction. As an antihypertensive, prazosin had no conspicuous advantages when compared with five other agents and was among the less well-tolerated.[85]

PHARMACOLOGY. Prazosin dilates both peripheral arterial and venous systems. The venous effects may account for first-dose syncope, unless a low dose is used. Arteriolar dilation should cause a reflex tachycardia, yet the heart rate usually rises little in hypertension. Besides blocking the postsynaptic alpha$_1$-receptors, prazosin may also decrease release of epinephrine by peripheral and central mechanisms.[19] It does not increase plasma renin activity.

PHARMACOKINETICS. Prazosin has to be given orally and is well absorbed. The plasma half-life is 3 to 4 hours, yet the antihypertensive effect is prolonged. Although thrice-daily doses are conventional, twice-daily doses suffice. Prazosin can be used in renal failure because renal blood flow is not altered and the drug is chiefly excreted in the feces. Substantial first-pass liver metabolism indicates the need for caution in patients with liver disease.

DOSE. The initial dose should be low and taken at night (2 mg for heart failure, 0.5 or 1 mg for hypertension) then twice daily (previously three times daily was recommended). As the dose is worked up to a maximum of 20 mg/day, it is convenient to give 1 mg then 2 mg then 5 mg tablets twice daily. There is no evidence that 30 mg daily gives a better response than 20 mg. Sharp increases in the dose may cause syncope.

SIDE-EFFECTS. **First-dose syncope** may be due to decreased preload and is especially likely when there is no LV failure or during cotherapy with nitrates or potent diuretics. Chronic postural dizziness is a less frequent side-effect. Several double-blind studies show that prazosin is not effective in the long-term therapy of CHF. Tachyphy-laxis may also occur in the therapy of hypertension[1] and may explain why upward adjustment of the dose of prazosin is so frequently needed.

**Nonspecific side-effects** include drowsiness, lack of energy,[85] nasal congestion, and depression. Tachycardia is usually not common but in some patients can precede syncope. Positive antinuclear factors may develop without clinical lupus.

## Doxazosin

This agent (**Cardura**) resembles prazosin in its receptor effects but is longer acting with a plasma half-life of 11 to 13 hours. It is used for hypertension and is under investigation for CHF.

DOSE. The major hazard is hypotension if the initial dose is too high. Treatment is started with 1 mg, no more, the first dose given only at night to minimize postural hypotension. Thereafter, the dose is titrated upward at 1- to 2-week intervals to 16 mg once daily.

SIDE-EFFECTS. Dizziness, fatigue, and malaise are double the incidence in placebo (package insert). Patients should be told that postural hypotension may occur and instructed to sit or lie down if needed. Somnolence is a side-effect in 5% and may impair driving (package insert). The incidence of postural hypotension increases with doses above 4 mg and is about 10% at 16 mg daily.

PROLONGED USE IN MILD HYPERTENSION. In the TOMH study,[120] doxazosin given over 4 years induced significant decreases in serum total and LDL-cholesterol with an increase in the ratio of HDL to total cholesterol. There was a small but significant decrease in the quality of life when compared with acebutolol.

## Terazosin

Terazosin (**Hytrin**) has similar pharmacologic properties to doxazosin. The dose is 1 to 20 mg daily starting with the low dose at night and titrating upwards. In the UK it is also approved for benign prostatic hypertrophy.

# New Vasodilators

## Dopamine-receptor Stimulators

**Fenoldopam** is a dopamine agonist ($DA_1$) able to reduce blood pressure in severe hypertension with a sodium diuresis in contrast to nitroprusside which causes sodium retention.[7]

**Ibopamine** is an orally active dopamine agonist which inhibits neurohumoral activation in mild to moderate CHF.[121] It is less effective than digoxin when added to low-dose furosemide.

## Atrial Natriuretic Peptide

This peptide, also called **atrial natriuretic factor** or ANF, is secreted by the cardiac atria in response to volume distension. It is the natural hypovolemic agent, acting on the renal vasculature to cause a powerful vasodilation and diuresis. Thereby the polyuria frequently associated with paroxysmal supraventricular tachycardia can be explained. ANP acts on vascular cells to produce vasodilatory cyclic GMP. ANP therapy is likely to be of limited benefit in CHF because levels of ANP are already high and downgrading of ANP receptors occurs. **Brain natriuretic peptide (BNP),** with similar properties to ANP, is also released from the left ventricle in heart failure.

The **endopeptidase inhibitors** act by decreasing the degradation of ANP and can improve hemodynamics and renal function in CHF; their clinical use has not yet been established.

# Summary

## ACE Inhibitors

In **congestive heart failure** (CHF), several large trials have focused attention on the important therapeutic and potential prophylactic role of the ACE inhibitors. These trials have shown that reduction of "hard" end-points, such as mortality, hospitalization, and prevention of disease progression, can be achieved in certain patient populations. In a minority of patients, ACE inhibitors fail to benefit and might harm via hypotension. The benefits of ACE inhibitors can be explained by inhibition of the activated renin-angiotensin-aldosterone system. The present trend is to start therapy with diuretics and ACE inhibition in mild to moderate symptomatic heart failure, combined with digoxin in more severe failure, or when there is atrial fibrillation.

In **hypertension,** there is no doubt that the ACE inhibitors can reduce the blood pressure by multiple mechanisms, including decreased vasoconstriction (lessening the effect of angiotensin-II). New experimental evidence, showing that angiotensin-II is an important regulator of cellular growth in vascular smooth muscle and myocardium, has led to the proposal that ACE inhibitors may also exhibit specific protective effects acting by limitation of vascular or myocardial hypertrophy. These are both undesirable complications of hypertension. Yet ACE inhibitors have not yet been proven to reduce hard hypertensive end-points such as stroke, heart failure, coronary heart disease, or nephropathy. Likewise, despite the potential mechanisms whereby insulin resistance in hypertensive patients can be diminished by these agents, there are no large trials convincingly proving any patient benefit.

In **acute myocardial infarction,** ACE inhibitors were given in the early phase of two megatrials[61,70] to show a modest, statistically significant reduction in mortality (6% to 11%). Lisinopril combined with intravenous and then transdermal nitroglycerin reduced mortality by an impressive 17%. This regime seems especially appropriate for clinically diagnosed heart failure.

In **early postinfarct heart failure,** an ACE inhibitor, ramipril, has shown a striking reduction of 27% in mortality.

In **asymptomatic left ventricular (LV) dysfunction,** whether postinfarct or otherwise, ACE inhibitors can prevent the development of overt CHF, as shown by two large trials.[111,115]

In **diabetic nephropathy,** ACE inhibition added to insulin and to other antihypertensives has achieved reduction of hard end-points, such as death, dialysis, and renal transplantation. Because these benefits were apparently achieved over and beyond any added hypotensive effect of the ACE inhibitor, a renovascular protective mechanism seems to be involved.

**Contraindications** to ACE inhibitors are few: bilateral renal artery stenosis, hypotension, or pregnancy.

Therefore, ACE inhibitors are increasingly used for a widening group of cardiac and vascular indications. Their major documented benefit on hard end-points remains in heart failure. Large-scale preventative trials still in progress may establish definitive benefits on hard end-points in hypertension and in ischemic heart disease.

## Conventional Vasodilators

Whereas vasodilators such as the alpha-adrenergic blockers and hydralazine have a confirmed place in the therapy of hypertension, there are no studies to prove that either of these types of agents alone can improve outlook in CHF. Hydralazine combined with isosorbide dinitrate gives benefit in CHF beyond that obtained by digitalis and diuretics alone, but inferior to that obtained by ACE inhibition plus diuretics plus digoxin. Therefore, the addition of hydralazine-nitrates to standard triple therapy for severe CHF (diuretics, ACE inhibition and digoxin) is generally only undertaken when the patient's problems persist, except in black patients where vasodilation may be more effective than expected. Short-acting nitrates are used to help relieve pulmonary symptoms. Occasionally, in very severely ill patients, infusions of sodium nitroprusside or inotropic dilators (p 165) may help to see the patient through. The role of long-acting alpha-blockers or combined alpha-beta-blockers in the chronic therapy of CHF is not yet clarified, but early data for doxazosin and especially carvedilol look promising.

# References

*For references from Second Edition, see Opie et al. (1991)*

1. Opie LH, Chatterjee K, Poole-Wilson PA, Sonnenblick E. Angiotensin-converting enzyme inhibitors and conventional vasodilators. In: Opie LH (ed), Drugs for the Heart, Third Edition. WB Saunders Company, Philadelphia, 1991, pp 100–128.

*References from Third Edition*

2. Belz GG, Essig J, Erb K, et al. Br J Clin Pharmacol 1989; 27:317S–322S.
3. Brilla CG, Kramer B, Hoffmeister HM, et al. Cardiovasc Drugs Ther 1989; 3:211–218.
4. Captopril Multicenter Research Group. J Am Coll Cardiol 1983; 2:755–763.
5. CONSENSUS Trial Study Group. N Engl J Med 1987; 316:1429–1435.
6. Croog SH, Levine S, Testa MA, et al. N Engl J Med 1986; 314:1657–1664.
7. Elliott WJ, Weber RR, Nelson KS, et al. Circulation 1990; 81:970–977.
8. Flapan AD, Shaw TRD, Stewart S, et al. Br Heart J 1987; 57:82–83.
9. Gheorghiade M, Hall V, Lakier JB, Goldstein S. J Am Coll Cardiol 1989; 13:134–142.
10. Harris P. Br Heart J 1987; 58:190–203.
11. Levy WS, Katz RJ, Buff L, Wasserman AG. Circulation 1989; 80 (Suppl II):II–214.
12. Lewis BS, Rozenman Y, Merdler A, et al. Am J Cardiol 1987; 59:93–96.
13. Lichter I, Richardson PJ, Wyke MA. Br J Clin Pharmacol 1986; 21:641–645.
14. McEwan JR, Choudry NB, Fuller RW. Circulation 1989; 80 (Suppl II):II–128.
15. Nishimura H, Kubo S, Ueyama M, et al. Am Heart J 1989; 117:100–105.
16. Odemuyiwa O, Gilmartin J, Kenny D, Hall RJC. Eur Heart J 1989; 10:586–590.
17. Pollare T, Lithell H, Berne C. N Engl J Med 1989; 321:868–873.
18. Richardson A, Bayliss J, Scriven et al. Lancet 1987; 2:709–711.
19. Riegger GAJ, Haeske W, Kraus C, et al. Am J Cardiol 1987; 59:906–910.
20. Salvetti A, Arzilli F. Am J Hypertens 1989; 2:352–354.
21. Sassano P, Chatellier G, Billaud E, et al. J Cardiovasc Pharmacol 1989; 13:314–319.
22. Williams GH. N Engl J Med 1988; 319:1517–1525.

*New References*

23. AIRE study—The Acute Infarction Ramipril Efficacy (AIRE) Study Investigators. Effect of ramipril on mortality and morbidity of survivors of acute myocardial infarction with clinical evidence of heart failure. Lancet 1993; 342:821–828.
24. Ajayi AA, Campbell BC, Meredith PA, et al. The effect of captopril on the reflex control heart rate: Possible mechanisms. Br J Clin Pharmacol 1985; 20:17–25.
25. Anand IS, Ferrari R, Kalra GS, et al. Edema of cardiac origin. Studies of body water and sodium, renal function, hemodynamic indexes, and plasma hormones in untreated congestive cardiac failure. Circulation 1989; 80:299–305.
26. Anderson RJ, Duchin KL, Gore RD, et al. Once-daily fosinopril in the treatment of hypertension. Hypertension 1991; 17:636–642.
27. Bartels L, Remme WJ, van der Ent M, Kruikssen D. ACE inhibitors reduce myocardial ischemia through modulation of ischemia-induced catecholamine activation. Experience with perindoprilat (abstr). J Am Coll Cardiol 1993; 23:19A.
28. Berntorp K, Lindgarde F, Mattiasson I. Long-term effects on insulin sensitivity and sodium transport in glucose-intolerant hypertensive subjects when beta-blockade is replaced by captopril treatment. J Human Hypertens 1992; 6:291–298.
29. Berridge MJ. Inositol trisphosphate and calcium signalling. Nature 1993; 361:315–325.
30. Bianchi S, Bigazzi R, Baldari G. Microalbuminuria in patients with essential hypertension: Effects of several antihypertensive drugs. Am J Med 1992; 93:525–528.
31. Bigazzi R, Bianchi S, Baldari D, et al. Long-term effects of a converting enzyme

inhibitor and a calcium channel blocker on urinary albumin excretion in patients with essential hypertension. Am J Hypertens 1992; 6:108–113.

32. Broqvist M. Dahlstrom U, Karlberg BE, et al. Neuroendocrine response in acute heart failure and the influence of treatment. Eur Heart J 1989; 10:1075–1083.

33. Campbell DJ, Kladis A, Duncan A-M. Bradykinin peptides in kidney, blood, and other tissues of the rat. Hypertension 1993; 21:155–165.

34. CAPPP group. The Captopril Prevention Project: A prospective intervention trial of angiotensin converting enzyme inhibition in the treatment of hypertension. J Hypertens 1990; 8:985–990.

35. Carson PE, Johnson GR, Singh SN, et al. for the VA Cooperative Study Group. Differences in vasodilator response by race in heart failure: VHeFT (abstr). J Am Coll Cardiol 1994; 23:382A.

36. Chan JCN, Cockram CS, Nicholls MG, et al. Comparison of enalapril and nifedipine in treating non-insulin dependent diabetes associated with hypertension: One year analysis. Br Med J 1992; 305:981–985.

37. Cohn JN, Johnson G, Ziesche S, et al. Comparison of enalapril with hydralazine-isosorbide dinitrate in the treatment of chronic congestive heart failure. N Engl J Med 1991; 325:303–310.

38. CONSENSUS II—Swedberg K, Held P, Kjekshus J, Rasmussen K, et al. On behalf of the CONSENSUS II Study Group. Effects of the early administration of enalapril on mortality in patients with acute myocardial infarction. Results of the Cooperative New Scandinavian Enalapril Survival Study II (CONSENSUS II). N Engl J Med 1992; 327:678–684.

39. Cruickshank JM, Lewis J, Moore V, Dodd C. Reversibility of left ventricular hypertrophy by differing types of antihypertensive therapy. J Human Hypertens 1992; 6:85–90.

40. Dahlof B, Hansson L. Regression of left ventricular hypertrophy in previously untreated essential hypertension: Different effects of enalapril and hydrochlorothiazide. J Hypertens 1992; 10:1513–1524.

41. Dahlof B, Pennert K, Hansson L. Reversal of left ventricular hypertrophy in hypertensive patients. A meta-analysis of 109 treatment studies. Am J Hypertens 1992; 5:95–110.

42. Dahlstrom U, Karlsson E. Captopril and spironolactone therapy for refractory congestive heart failure. Am J Cardiol 1993; 71:29A–33A.

43. Daly P, Rouleau J-L, Cousineau D, et al. Effects of captopril and a combination of hydralazine and isosorbide dinitrate on myocardial sympathetic tone in patients with severe congestive heart failure. Br Heart J 1986; 56:152–157.

44. Dargie HJ, McAlpine HM, Morton JJ. Neuroendocrine activation in acute myocardial infarction. J Cardiovasc Pharmacol 1987; 9 (Suppl 2):S21–S24.

45. Demopoulos L, LeJemtel TH. Peripheral factors in the management of congestive heart failure. Cardiovasc Drugs Ther 1994; 8:75–82.

46. Diabetes Control and Complications Trial Research Group. The effect of intensive treatment of diabetes on the development and progression of long-term complications in insulin-dependent diabetes mellitus. N Engl J Med 1993; 329:977–986.

47. DiBianco R, Parker JO, Chakko S, et al. Doxazosin for the treatment of chronic congestive heart failure: Results of a randomized double-blind and placebo-controlled study. Am Heart J 1991; 121:372–380.

48. Dostal DE, Baker KM. Evidence for a role of an intracardiac renin-angiotensin system in normal and failing hearts. Trends Cardiovasc Med 1993; 3:67–74.

49. Durante W, Schini VB, Scott-Burden T, et al. Platelet inhibition by an L-arginine-derived substance released by IL-1 beta-treated vascular smooth muscle cells. Am J Physiol 1991; 261:H2024–H2030.

50. Dworkin LD, Benstein JA, Parker M, et al. Calcium antagonists and converting enzyme inhibitors reduce renal injury by different mechanisms. Kidney Int 1993; 43:808–814.

51. Dzau VJ, Hollenberg NK. Renal response to captopril in severe heart failure: Role of furosemide in natriuresis and reversal of hyponatremia. Ann Intern Med 1984; 100:777–782.

52. Dzau VJ, Packer M, Lilly LS, et al. Prostaglandins in severe congestive heart failure. Relation to activation of the renin-angiotensin system and hyponatremia. N Engl J Med 1984; 310:347–352.

53. Erley CM, Haefele U, Heyne N, Braun N, Risler T. Microalbuminuria in essential hypertension. Reduction by different antihypertensive drugs. Hypertension 1993; 21:810–815.

54. Fabris B, Jackson B, Johnston CI. Salt blocks the renal benefits of ramipril in diabetic hypertensive rats. Hypertension 1991; 17:497–503.

55. Ferrier C, Ferrari P, Weidmann P, et al. Swiss hypertension treatment programme with verapamil and/or enalapril in diabetic patients. Drugs 1992; 44 (Suppl 1):74–84.

56. Fioretto P, Frigato F, Velussi M, et al. Effects of angiotensin converting enzyme inhibitors and calcium antagonists on atrial natriuretic peptide release and action and on albumin excretion rate in hypertensive insulin-dependent diabetic patients. Am J Hypertens 1992; 5:837–846.

57. Fisher NDL, Gleason RE, Moore TJ, et al. Regulation of aldosterone secretion in hypertensive blacks. Hypertension 1994; 23:179–184.

58. Fogari R, Zoppi A, Tettamanti F, et al. Effects of nifedipine and indomethacin

on cough induced by angiotensin-converting enzyme inhibitors: A double-blind, randomized, cross-over study. J Cardiovasc Pharmacol 1992; 19:670–673.

59. Fonarow GC, Chelimsky-Fallick C, Stevenson LW, et al. Effect of direct vasodilation with hydralazine versus angiotensin-converting enzyme inhibition with captopril on mortality in advanced heart failure: the Hy-C Trial. J Am Coll Cardiol 1992; 19:842–850.

59A. Ganley CJ, Hung HMJ, Temple R. More on the Survival And Ventricular Enlargement trial. N Engl J Med 1993; 329:1204–1205.

60. Gilbert EM, Olsen SL, Renlund DG, et al. Chronic beta-blockade with carvedilol results in sustained improvement in left ventricular function in patients with heart failure (abstr). Circulation 1993; 88:I–104.

61. GISSI-3—Gruppo Italiano per lo Studio della Sopravvivenza Nel'Infarto Miocardico. GISSI-3: effects of lisinopril and transdermal glyceryl trinitrate singly and together on 6-week mortality and ventricular function after acute myocardial infarction. Lancet 1994; 343:1115–1122.

62. Goldberg MR, Tanaka W, Barchowsky A, et al. Effects of losartan on blood pressure, plasma renin activity, and angiotensin-II in volunteers. Hypertension 1993; 21:704–713.

63. Gonzalez-Fernandez RA, Altieri PI, Diaz LM, et al. Effects of enalapril on heart failure in hypertensive patients with diastolic dysfunction. Am J Hypertens 1992; 5:480–483.

64. Gottdiener J, Reda D, Notargiacomo A, Metersen B. VA Cooperative Study Group on Antihypertensive Agents. Comparison of monotherapy effects on LV mass regression in mild-to-moderate hypertension: differences between short- and long-term therapy (abstr). J Am Coll Cardiol 1992; 19:85A.

65. Gottlieb SS, Dickstein K, Fleck E, et al. Hemodynamic and neurohormonal effects of the angiotensin-II antagonist losartan in patients with congestive heart failure. Circulation 1993; 88 (part 1):1602–1609.

66. Hajj-ali AF, Zimmerman BG. Kinin contribution to renal vasodilator effect of captopril in rabbit. Hypertension 1991; 17:504–509.

67. Hall D, Zeitler H, Rudolph W. Counteraction of the vasodilator effects of enalapril by aspirin in severe heart failure. J Am Coll Cardiol 1992; 20:1549–1555.

68. Hallab M, Gallois Y, Chatellier G, et al. Comparison of reduction in microalbuminuria by enalapril and hydrochlorothiazide in normotensive patients with insulin-dependent diabetes. Br Med J 1993; 306:175–182.

68A. Hannedouche T, Landais P, Goldfarb B, et al. Randomised controlled trial of enalapril and beta-blockers in non-diabetic chronic renal failure. Br Med J 1994; 309:833–837.

69. Hollenberg NK, Williams GH. Abnormal renal function, sodium-volume homeostasis, and renin system behavior in normal-renin essential hypertension. In: Laragh JH, Brenner BM (eds), Hypertension, Pathophysiology, Diagnosis, and Management. Raven Press, New York, 1990, pp 1349–1370.

70. ISIS-IV study (1994)(Fourth International Study of Infarct Survival)—Ferguson JJ. Meeting highlights. Circulation 1994; 89:545–547.

71. Johnston CI. Tissue angiotensin-converting enzyme in cardiac and vascular hypertrophy, repair, and remodeling. Hypertension 1994; 23:258–268.

72. Kasiske BL, Kalil RSN, Ma JZ, et al. Effect of antihypertensive therapy on the kidney in patients with diabetes: A meta-regression analysis. Ann Intern Med 1993; 118:129–138.

73. Kojima M, Shiojima I, Yamazaki T, et al. Angiotensin-II receptor antagonist TCV-116 induces regression of hypertensive left ventricular hypertrophy in vivo and inhibits the intracellular signaling pathway of stretch-mediated cardiomyocyte hypertrophy in vitro. Circulation 1994; 89:2204–2211.

74. Konstam MA, Kronenberg MW, Rousseau MF, Udelson JE, SOLVD Investigators. Effects of the angiotensin-converting enzyme inhibitor enalapril on the long-term progression of left ventricular dilatation in patients with asymptomatic systolic dysfunction. Circulation 1993; 88:2277–2283.

75. Kromer EP, Elsner D, Riegger GAJ. Digoxin, converting-enzyme inhibition (quinapril), and the combination in patients with congestive heart failure functional Class II and sinus rhythm. J Cardiovasc Pharmacol 1990; 16:9–14.

76. Lacourciere Y, Nadeau A, Poirier L, Tancrede G. Captopril or conventional therapy in hypertensive Type II diabetics. Three year analysis. Hypertension 1993; 21:786–794.

77. Lasker RD. The Diabetes Control and Complications Trial. Implications for policy and practice. N Engl J Med 1993; 329:1035–1036.

78. Leung W-H, Lau C-P, Wong C-K, et al. Improvement in exercise performance and hemodynamics by labetalol in patients with idiopathic dilated cardiomyopathy. Am Heart J 1990; 119:884–890.

79. Lewis EJ, Hunsicker LG, Bain RP, Rohde RD for the Collaborative Study Group. The effect of angiotensin-converting enzyme inhibition on diabetic nephropathy. N Engl J Med 1993; 329:1456–1462.

80. Linz W, Scholkens BA. A specific beta$_2$-bradykinin receptor antagonist HOE 140 abolishes the antihypertrophic effect of ramipril. Br J Pharmacol 1992; 105:771–772.

81. Ljungman S, Kjekshus J, Swedberg K. Renal function in severe congestive heart failure during treatment with enalapril (the Cooperative North Scandinavian Enalapril Survival Study [CONSENSUS] Trial). Am J Cardiol 1992; 70:479–487.

82. Lüscher TF. Angiotensin, ACE inhibitors and endothelial control of vasomotor tone. Basic Res Cardiol 1993; 88:Suppl 1, 15–24.

83. Lyall F, Dornan ES, McQueen J, et al. Angiotensin-II increases proto-oncogene expression and phosphoinositide turnover in vascular smooth muscle cells via the angiotensin-II $AT_1$ receptor. J Hypertens 1992; 10:1463–1469.

84. MacFadyen RJ, Lees KR, Reid JL. Differences in first dose response to ACE inhibition in congestive cardiac failure—a placebo controlled study. Br Heart J 1991; 66:206–211.

85. Materson BJ, Reda DJ, Cushman WC, et al. Single-drug therapy for hypertension in men. A comparison of six antihypertensive agents with placebo. N Engl J Med 1993; 328:914–921.

86. McLay JS, McMurray J, Bridges A, Struthers AD. Practical issues when initiating captopril therapy in chronic heart failure. Eur Heart J 1992; 13:1521–1527.

87. Mehra A, Ostrzega E, Shotan A, et al. Persistent hemodynamic improvement with short-term nitrate therapy in patients with chronic congestive heart failure already treated with captopril. Am J Cardiol 1992; 70:1310–1314.

88. Meredith IT, Alison JF, Zhang F-M, et al. Captopril potentiates the effects of nitroglycerin in the coronary vascular bed. J Am Coll Cardiol 1993; 22:581–587.

89. Metelitsa VI, Martsevich SY, Kozyreva MP, Slastnikova ID. Enhancement of the efficacy of isosorbide dinitrate by captopril in stable angina pectoris. Am J Cardiol 1992; 69:291–296.

90. Miller MA, Texter M, Gmerek A, et al. Quinapril hydrochloride effects on renal function in patients with renal dysfunction and hypertension: A drug-withdrawal study. Cardiovasc Drugs Ther 1994; 8:271–275.

91. Motwani JG, Fenwick MK, Morton JJ, Struthers AD. Furosemide-induced natriuresis is augmented by ultra low-dose captopril but not by standard doses of captopril in chronic heart failure. Circulation 1992; 86:439–445.

92. National High Blood Pressure Education Program Working Group. National high blood pressure education program working group report on hypertension in diabetes. Hypertension 1994; 23:145–158.

93. Ondetti MA, Cushman DW. Design of specific inhibitors of angiotensin-converting enzyme: New class of orally active antihypertensive agents. Science 1977; 196:441–444.

94. Opie LH. The new trials: AIRE, ISIS-4 AND GISSI-3. Is the dossier on ACE inhibitors now complete? Cardiovasc Drugs Ther, 1994; 8:469–472.

95. Packer M, Lee WH, Medina N, et al. Functional renal insufficiency during long-term therapy with captopril and enalapril in severe chronic heart failure. Ann Intern Med 1987a; 106:346–354.

96. Packer M, Lee WH, Medina N, et al. Influence of diabetes mellitus on changes in left ventricular performance and renal function produced by converting enzyme inhibition in patients with severe chronic heart failure. Am J Med 1987b; 82:1119–1126.

97. Pahor M, Gambassi G, Carbonin P. Antiarrhythmic effects of ACE inhibitors: A matter of faith or reality? Cardiovasc Res 1994; 28:173–182.

98. Paolisso G, Gambardella A, Verza M, et al. ACE inhibition improves insulin-sensitivity in aged insulin-resistant hypertensive patients. J Human Hypertens 1992; 6:175–179.

99. Parving H-H, Andersen AR, Smidt UM, Svendsen PA. Early aggressive antihypertensive treatment reduces rate of decline in kidney function in diabetic nephropathy. Lancet 1983; 1:1175–1178.

100. Pouleur H. High or low dose of angiotensin-converting enzyme inhibitor in patients with left ventricular dysfunction? Cardiovasc Drugs Ther 1993; 7:891–892.

101. PRACTICAL study—Foy SG, Crozier IG, Turner JG, et al. Comparison of enalapril versus captopril on left ventricular function and survival three months after acute myocardial infarction (the "PRACTICAL" Study). Am J Cardiol 1994; 73:1180–1186.

102. QUIET study—Texter M, Lees RS, Pitt B, et al. The QUinapril Ischemic Event Trial (QUIET) design and methods: Evaluation of chronic ACE inhibitor therapy after coronary artery intervention. Cardiovasc Drugs Ther 1993; 7:273–282.

103. Rademaker M, Shaw TRD, Williams BC, et al. Intravenous captopril treatment in patients with severe cardiac failure. Br Heart J 1986; 55:187–190.

104. RADIANCE study—Packer M, Gheorghiade M, Young JB, et al for the RADIANCE study. Withdrawal of digoxin from patients with chronic heart failure treated with angiotensin-converting enzyme inhibitors. N Engl J Med 1993; 329:1–7.

105. Reisin L, Schneeweiss A. Complete spontaneous remission of cough induced by ACE inhibitors during chronic therapy in hypertensive patients. J Human Hypertens 1992; 6:333–335.

106. Remes J, Tikkanen I, Fyhquist F, Pyorala K. Neuroendocrine activity in untreated heart failure. Br Heart J 1991; 65:249–255.

107. Reske SN, Heck I, Kropp J, et al. Captopril mediated decrease of aortic regurgitation. Br Heart J 1985; 54:415–419.

108. Ridker PM, Gaboury CL, Conlin PR, et al. Stimulation of plasminogen activator inhibitor in vivo by infusion of angiotensin-II. Evidence of a potential interaction between the renin-angiotensin system and fibrinolytic function. Circulation 1993; 87:1969–1973.

109. Riegger GAJ. Effects of quinapril on exercise tolerance in patients with mild to moderate heart failure. Eur Heart J 1991; 12:705–711.

110. Santoro D, Natali A, Palombo C, et al. Effects of chronic angiotensin-converting enzyme inhibition on glucose tolerance and insulin sensitivity in essential hypertension. Hypertension 1992; 20:181–191.

111. SAVE study—Pfeffer MA, Braunwald E, Moye LA, et al. Effect of captopril on mortality and morbidity in patients with left ventricular dysfunction after myocardial infarction. Results of the Survival and Ventricular Enlargement Trial (SAVE). N Engl J Med 1992; 327:669–677.

112. Sica DA, Cutler RE, Parmer RJ, Ford NF. Comparison of the steady-state pharmacokinetics of fosinopril, lisinopril and enalapril in patients with chronic renal insufficiency. Clin Pharmacokinet 1991; 20:420–427.

113. Sigurdsson A, Held P, Swedberg K. Short- and long-term neurohormonal activation following acute myocardial infarction. Am Heart J 1993; 126:1068–1076.

114. Smith TW, Pfeffer MA. The rationale for combined use of diuretics, digitalis and vasodilators in congestive heart failure. Cardiovasc Drugs Ther 1989; 3:13–17.

115. SOLVD study—The SOLVD Investigators. Effect of enalapril on survival in patients with reduced left ventricular ejection fractions and congestive heart failure. N Engl J Med 1991; 325:293–302.

116. SOLVD study—The SOLVD Investigators. Effect of enalapril on mortality and the development of heart failure in asymptomatic patients with reduced left ventricular fractions. N Engl J Med 1992; 327:685–691.

117. Swedberg K, Eneroth P, Kjekshus J, Wilhelmsen L, for the CONSENSUS Trial Study Group. Hormones regulating cardiovascular function in patients with severe congestive heart failure and their relation to mortality. Circulation 1990; 82:1730–1736.

118. Testa MA, Anderson RB, Nackley JF, Hollenberg NK and the Quality of Life Hypertension Study Group. Quality of life and antihypertensive therapy in men. A comparison of captopril with enalapril. N Engl J Med 1993; 328:907–913.

119. Timmermans PBMWM, Wong PC, Chiu AT, et al. Angiotensin-II receptors and angiotensin-II receptor antagonists. Pharmacol Rev 1993; 45:205–251.

120. TOMH study—Neaton JD, Grimm RH, Prineas RJ, et al. for the Treatment of Mild Hypertension (TOMH) Study Research Group. Treatment of mild hypertension study. Final results. JAMA 1993; 270:713–724.

121. van Veldhuisen DJ, Man in't Veld AJ, Dunselman PHJM, et al. Double-blind placebo-controlled study of ibopamine and digoxin in patients with mild to moderate heart failure: Results of the Dutch Ibopamine Multicenter Trial (DIMT). J Am Coll Cardiol 1993; 22:1564–1573.

122. van Wijngaarden J, Smit AJ, de Graeff PA, et al. Effects of acetylsalicylic acid on peripheral hemodynamics in patients with chronic heart failure treated with angiotensin-converting enzyme inhibitors. J Cardiovasc Pharmacol 1994; 23:240–245.

123. Veterans Administration Co-operative Study Group. Racial differences in response to low-dose captopril are abolished by the addition of hydrochlorothiazide. Br J Clin Pharmacol 1982; 14:97S–101S.

124. V-HeFT I study—Cohn JN, Archibald DG, Ziesche S, et al. for the V-HeFT I study. Effect of vasodilator therapy on mortality in chronic congestive heart failure. Results of a Veterans Administration Cooperative Study. N Engl J Med 1986; 314:1547–1552.

125. V-HeFT II study—Cohn JN, Johnson G, Ziesche S, et al. for the V-HeFT II study. A comparison of enalapril with hydralazine-isosorbide dinitrate in the treatment of chronic congestive heart failure. N Engl J Med 1991; 325:303–310.

126. Wilson JR, Ferraro N. Effect of the renin-angiotensin system on limb circulation and metabolism during exercise in patients with heart failure. J Am Coll Cardiol 1985; 6:556–563.

126A. Wright RA, Flapan AD, Alberti KGMM, et al. Effects of captopril therapy on endogenous fibrinolysis in men with recent, uncomplicated myocardial infarction. J Am Coll Cardiol 1994; 24:67–73.

127. Yoshioka T, Mitarai T, Kon V, et al. Role for angiotensin-II in an overt functional proteinuria. Kidney Int 1986; 30:538–545.

128. Yusuf S, Pepine CJ, Carces C, et al. Effect of enalapril on myocardial infarction and unstable angina in patients with low ejection fractions. Lancet 1992; 340:1173–1178.

*Book*

129. Opie LH. Angiotensin-Converting Enzyme Inhibitors. Scientific Basis for Clinical Use, 2nd edition. Wiley-Liss and Authors' Publishing House, New York, 1994.

## Notes

ACE INHIBITION FOR SYNDROME X (microvascular angina).

In these patients with effort angina and normal enalapril (10 mg daily for 2 weeks) improved exercise J Am Coll Cardiol 1994; 23:652.

The proposed mechanism sympathetic-induced coronary vasoconstriction.

## ACE Inhibitors and Early Phase Acute Myocardial Infarction

Data continue to come in supporting the early use of ACE inhibitors in acute myocardial infarction. In the still-unpublished TRACE
study (TRAndolapril Cardiac Evaluation), patients 3 to 7 days after
the onset of AMI and with echocardiographic evidence of LV dysfunction, mostly with reduced ejection fractions of 35% or below,
were given trandolapril 1 to 4 mg once daily and followed for up
to 4 years. There was a 22% reduction in overall mortality and
cardiovascular mortality and morbidity fell. These patients did not
necessarily have any clinical evidence of congestive heart failure.

In the SMILE study (New England Journal of Medicine, in press;
also see ref. 133A, Chapter 11), the ACE inhibitor zofenopril was
started within 24 hours of symptoms in patients with acute anterior
infarction but not given thrombolytic therapy. The dose was 7.5 up
to 30 mg twice daily. After 6 weeks the combined end-point (death
and congestive heart failure) was reduced by about one-third.

Taken together with the modestly positive results for captopril in
ISIS-4, and for lisinopril in GISSI-3, the case for the use of ACE inhibi-
tors within the first 24 hours of AMI or even earlier becomes stronger.
This is especially so when combined with intravenous nitrates (as in
GISSI-3), or when there is anterior myocardial infarction (as in
SMILE), or with clinical congestive heart failure (as in AIRE), or
tachycardia (as a sign of threatened CHF), or when echocardiographic
LV function is impaired. Clearly, hypotension is the Achilles heel of
ACE inhibition, as shown by CONSENSUS-II in which early intrave-
nous enalaprilat seemed deleterious. Thus, hypotension is a clear
contraindication to ACE inhibition in early phase AMI.

Because the mortality benefit for ACE inhibition in postinfarct
patients only began to emerge after one year in the SAVE study and
the curves still appeared to diverge even at the end of 4 years, the
case for continuing ACE inhibition indefinitely in patients with either
overt or threatened left ventricular failure becomes strong. It will
be recalled from the SAVE study that the effects of ACE inhibition
were still found in the presence of beta-blockade and, therefore, the
combination may be given with added effect.

## Future Studies with ACE Inhibitors

To explore the possiblity raised by SAVE and SOLVD that ACE
inhibitors prevent reinfarction or lessen the rate of progression of
coronary atheroma, or act in some other beneficial manner radically
to alter the course of coronary artery disease, two large-scale studies
have been planned. In the HOPE (Heart Outcomes Prevention Evaluation) study in Canada, patients with established coronary disease
will be treated by either an ACE inhibitor or Vitamin E or the
combination in a $2\times$ factorial design and the end-point will be
myocardial infarction and death. This study will include patients
thought to be at high risk of clinical coronary artery disease such
as those with diabetes mellitus.

In the PEACE (Prevention of Events by ACE inhibition) study,
patients with a previous myocardial infarction but with an ejection
fraction exceeding 40% will be observed for 4 to 5 years. The hypothesis under test in this NIH-sponsored study is that ACE inhibition
reduces the clinical manifestations of coronary disease.

Thus, the emphasis with ACE inhibitors has shifted from the
initial observations on the benefits in the treatment of CHF, then to
prevention of CHF, then to postinfarct prevention of remodeling,
then to use in acute myocardial infarction with overt or threatened
LV failure, and now to the possibility that the natural history of
coronary artery disease might in some way be fundamentally altered
for the better. (Dr. E. Braunwald is thanked for the information given
in this paragraph).

## Notes

# 6 Digitalis and Acute Inotropes

F.I. Marcus ♦ L.H. Opie ♦ E.H. Sonnenblick
K. Chatterjee

*"Digitalis is effective, but is it safe?"*[39]

## Chronic Versus Acute Heart Failure

Chronic heart failure differs from acute failure in the aims of therapy.

In **chronic heart failure,** there are complex aims including relief of symptoms, improvement of the hemodynamic status, prevention of deterioration and frequent hospitalizations, and, above all, a decrease in the mortality rate. Successive trials first with vasodilators and then with ACE inhibitors have now established the disabling nature of conventionally treated congestive heart failure (CHF) if left to run its natural course. Nonetheless, CHF is not a uniform condition. It stretches all the way from mild exertional dyspnea through to disabling symptoms at rest (NYHA Classes I to IV). In mild to moderate heart failure (Classes I and II), digoxin is no longer compulsory therapy. Rather, ACE inhibitors and diuretics are now often combined in mild early heart failure, primarily because of evidence (summarized in Chapter 5) that ACE inhibitors can lessen the rate of progression toward overt CHF, evidence not available for digoxin. In more severe heart failure, triple therapy with diuretics, ACE inhibitors and digoxin has become standard practice. Although digoxin is only a weak inotropic drug, it does have a unique profile of properties. Besides its inotropic effect, it slows the ventricular rate, especially in atrial fibrillation, which allows better ventricular filling. Digoxin also decreases the sympathetic drive generated by the failing circulation. The optimal use of digoxin, the major topic of this chapter, requires a thorough knowledge of the multiple factors governing its efficacy and toxicity, including numerous drug interactions.

In **acute heart failure,** urgent reduction of pulmonary capillary pressure and right atrial filling pressure is sought along with an increased cardiac output if the latter is reduced. These aims can be achieved by a variety of intravenous inotropes, including dopamine, dobutamine, amrinone (or milrinone) and others. Some of these, such as high-dose dopamine and also norepinephrine, cause peripheral vasoconstriction, which may aid in increasing the blood pressure in shocklike states. Another group, such as amrinone, milrinone, and low-dose dopamine, have a prominent vasodilator component to their action that is desired if the blood pressure is relatively well maintained. Such inotropic-dilator therapy should be combined with diuretics. Added preload reduction by nitrates is often useful. Because the effects of digoxin in the acutely ill patient with hypoxia and electrolyte disturbances are often difficult to predict, digoxin is usually best delayed until the acute phase has successfully been managed.

INOTROPIC, VAGAL & SYMPATHOLYTIC EFFECTS OF DIGITALIS

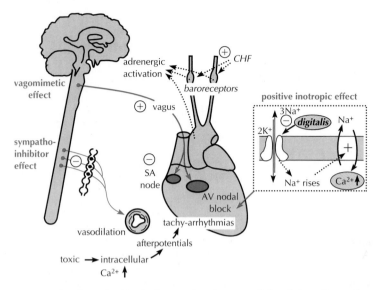

**FIGURE 6–1.** Digitalis has both neural and myocardial cellular effects. The inotropic effect of digitalis is due to inhibition of the sodium pump in myocardial cells. Slowing of the heart rate and inhibition of the atrioventricular node by vagal stimulation and the decreased sympathetic nerve discharge are important therapeutic benefits. Toxic arrhythmias are less well understood, but may be caused by calcium-dependent afterpotentials. Fig. copyright L.H. Opie. Modified from Fig. 18–7, L.H. Opie, The Heart: Physiology, Metabolism, Pharmacology and Therapy, Grune and Stratton, Orlando, 1984.

# Digitalis Compounds

*The combined inotropic-bradycardic action of digitalis is unique when compared to the many sympathomimetic inotropes that all tend to cause tachycardia.* Furthermore, no other inotropes are currently approved for oral use in the USA. Therefore digitalis, whatever its defects, remains the basic inotrope, despite the narrow therapeutic-toxic margin and the "intensifying myriad of interactions."[1]

## Pharmacologic Properties of Digitalis

All cardiac glycosides share an aglycone ring wherein the pharmacologic activity resides, usually combined with one to four molecules of sugar that modify the pharmacokinetic properties. Digoxin is a polar compound with an OH group binding to the steroid nucleus, whereas digitoxin is nonpolar with lesser central nervous system penetration.

**Sodium pump inhibition** explains the myocardial cellular effect of digitalis. As the sodium pump (Na/K-ATPase) is inhibited, there is a transient increase in intracellular sodium close to the sarcolemma, which in turn promotes calcium influx by the sodium-calcium exchange mechanism.[1] The end result is an increased cytosolic calcium ion concentration with enhanced myocardial contractility (Fig. 6–1).

**Parasympathetic activation** results in sinus slowing and atrioventricular (AV) nodal inhibition. The extent of the inhibitory effect on the AV node depends partly on the degree of vagal tone, which varies from person to person.[1] An ill-understood direct depression of nodal tissue may account for those effects of digitalis still found after vagal blockade.[1] Part of the toxic symptoms of digitalis may be explained by parasympathomimetic effects, such as nausea, vomiting, and anorexia.

**TABLE 6–1     DIGOXIN PHARMACOKINETICS**

1. 75% of oral dose rapidly absorbed; rest inactivated in lower gut to digoxin reduction products by bacteria.
2. Circulates in blood, unbound to plasma proteins; "therapeutic level" 1–2 ng/mL; blood half-life about 36 hr.
3. Binds to tissue receptors in heart and skeletal muscle.
4. Lipid-soluble; brain penetration.
5. Most of absorbed digoxin excreted unchanged in urine (tubular excretion and glomerular filtration). About 30% undergoes nonrenal clearance, more in renal failure.
6. In chronic renal failure, reduced volume of distribution.
7. With small lean body mass, reduced total binding to skeletal muscle.

**Sympathetic inhibition** may play an important role in the effects of digitalis in CHF.[24] Digitalis inhibits sympathetic nerve discharge, an effect which occurs before any observed hemodynamic changes. A similar action could not be achieved by dobutamine infusion.[5]

**Renin release** from the kidney is inhibited because digoxin decreases the activity of the renal sodium pump[48] with a natriuretic effect. Less renin release should lead to vasodilation to help offset the direct vasoconstrictor mechanism of digoxin (next paragraph).

The **hemodynamic effects** of intravenous digoxin were first described in a classic paper by McMichael and Sharpey-Schafer[9] who showed that acute digitalization improved cardiac output and heart failure. The fall in the venous pressure they found is probably best explained by a decreased sympathetic drive. The direct effect of digoxin on peripheral veins and arteries is mild vasoconstriction, because intracellular calcium increases. Likewise there is coronary constriction.[30] The action of digoxin on AV conduction which it slows, and on the AV refractory period, which it prolongs, is primarily dependent on vagal tone and only to a minor extent on the direct effect of digoxin.[1] The inhibitory effect on the AV node is usually preceded by the inotropic effect; the two effects differ in their mechanisms.

PHARMACOKINETICS OF DIGOXIN   (Table 6–1). The serum half-life is 1.5 days. The major portion is ultimately excreted by the kidneys unchanged. About 30% is excreted by nonrenal routes (stools, hepatic metabolism) in those with normal renal function.[29] In digitalized subjects, about half of the digoxin is bound to skeletal muscle receptors accounting (with blood) for most of the volume of distribution. The "fit" between digitalis and the receptor is much less "tight" for skeletal muscle than for the myocardium, which remains the major site of action.[52] In approximately 10% of patients, **intestinal flora** convert digoxin to an inactive reduction product, dihydrodigoxin; in such patients the blood level stays low unless the gut flora are inhibited by antibiotics such as erythromycin or tetracycline.[7] Multiple pharmacokinetic factors influence the blood level obtained with a given dose of digoxin (Tables 6–2 and 6–3). If **renal function** is subnormal, excretion is impaired and the maintenance dose is lower. The loading dose may also be lower (next section).

DOSE OF DIGOXIN.   Various nomograms have been designed for calculation of the dose, taking into account lean body mass and renal function,[1] but none appears to be more effective than the experienced physician's intuitive estimation of the correct digoxin dosage.[1]

A **loading dose** may be required for urgent indications because a certain amount of digoxin is required to saturate the skeletal muscle receptors throughout the body and for tissue penetration until equilibrium is reached. Thus the loading dose is governed by the lean body weight (reduced in old age and severe renal insufficiency).

TABLE 6–2    CAUSES OF LOW SERUM DIGOXIN LEVEL

**Dose too low or not taken.**
**Poor absorption**
   Malabsorption, high bran diet
   Drug interference: cholestyramine, sulfasalazine, neomycin, PAS,
     kaolin-pectin, rifampin (= rifampicin)
   Hyperthyroidism (additional mechanisms possible)
   Enhanced intestinal conversion to inactive metabolites
**Enhanced renal secretion**
   Improved GFR as vasodilator therapy enhances renal blood flow

  PAS = paraaminosalicylic acid
  GFR = glomerular filtration rate

The calculated effects of an oral loading dose of 0.75 mg followed by 6-hourly oral doses each of 0.25 mg on peak blood levels are shown in Fig. 6–2. The inotropic effect is near its maximum at 6 hours and not much less than that achieved by doubling the digoxin dose.

**Digitalization** is now commonly started with multiple doses over a longer period (0.5 mg twice daily for 2 days or 0.5 mg three times daily for 1 day followed by 0.25 mg daily) to allow for variable gastrointestinal (GI) absorption, variable cardiac responses, and possible drug interactions. When no loading dose is given, steady-state plasma and tissue concentrations are achieved in 5 to 7 days. **Rapid digitalization** can be achieved by a combination of intravenous digoxin (0.5 mg IV) and oral digoxin (0.25 mg, one or two doses) to a total of 0.75 to 1.0 mg.

The **maintenance dose** is usually 0.25 mg daily. The optimal dose required varies from 0.1 to 0.75 mg daily and renal function is the most important determinant (for impaired renal function, see p 151). In the RADIANCE study,[47] the mean dose of digoxin was 0.3 mg to achieve blood levels of 0.9 to 2.0 ng/ml. A **single evening dose** to allow a steady-state situation for blood digoxin assays in the morning is advised; timing in relation to meals is not important. Each patient's dose must be individually adjusted. To aim for "the highest possible dose tolerated" is no longer acceptable practice; rather the dose is adjusted according to the blood digoxin level.

## Digitalis Indications: Changes in Practice

CHF WITH ATRIAL FIBRILLATION.    The most solid indication for digitalis is still the **combination of chronic CHF with atrial fibrillation.** It

TABLE 6–3    DRUG INTERACTIONS AND OTHER CAUSES OF HIGH SERUM
               DIGOXIN LEVELS

**Excess initial dose for body mass** (small lean body mass)
**Decreased renal excretion**
   Severe hypokalemia (< 3 mEq/L)
   Concurrent cardiac drugs (quinidine, verapamil, amiodarone)
   Depressed renal blood flow (congestive heart failure, beta-blockers)
   Depressed GFR (elderly patients, renal disease)
**Decreased nonrenal clearance**
   Antiarrhythmic drugs (quinidine, verapamil, amiodarone, propafenone)
   Calcium antagonists (verapamil and possibly others)
**Decreased conversion in gut to digoxin reduction products**
   In unusual patients, antibiotics can inhibit bacteria converting digoxin
     to inactive reduction products (erythromycin, tetracycline)

## Digoxin Loading Doses

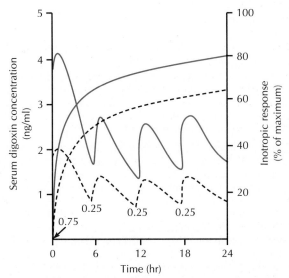

**FIGURE 6–2.**   Despite much lower digoxin levels after a low oral loading dose regime (dashed lines) than with a high oral dose regime (solid lines), the effects on contractile activity are not too different. The high loading dose regime consisted of 1.5 mg digoxin orally, then 0.5 mg every 6 hours, whereas the low loading dose had half of the above regime. Digoxin levels of only 0.9 to 1.2 ng/ml may be therapeutically as effective as higher values according to a clinical analysis.[60] Modified from Kelly and Smith[31] with permission.

is also used for atrial fibrillation from other causes and sometimes for the treatment of acute supraventricular tachycardias. In such arrhythmias, it may be used alone or in combination with verapamil, diltiazem or beta-blocking drugs. It is preferred to these other drugs if there is heart failure. However, toxicity must be excluded prior to electrical cardioversion.

**CHF WITH SINUS RHYTHM.**   In the approach to the management of **low-output heart failure** with sinus rhythm, digitalis has gone through three phases.[8] First, it was regarded with the diuretics as essential first-line therapy. Thereafter reports on ineffectiveness or development of tolerance came in, so that its use declined, especially in the UK. More recently, the benefits of digitalis have been re-established as a result of several well-controlled blinded studies[38] and the two major withdrawal studies.[46,47] In patients with NYHA Classes II and III symptoms, digoxin lessens effort intolerance and reduces morbidity.[32,39] The more advanced the heart failure, the more effective is digoxin.[27]

### Other Possible Indications

In **paroxysmal atrial fibrillation,** digoxin often neither controls the ventricular rate nor terminates a paroxysm,[23] although there are small benefits.[42] Drug control of paroxysmal atrial fibrillation has shifted from digoxin to specific antiarrhythmics such as flecainide, sotalol, and amiodarone (Chapter 8).

In **chronic atrial fibrillation without CHF,** digoxin is much less effective than propranolol or verapamil in controlling the heart rate during exercise.[41] Thus, in practice, small doses of beta-blockers or verapamil are often added to digoxin for better control of the exercise heart rate (note verapamil-digoxin interaction, p 154).

In **mitral stenosis with sinus rhythm,** prophylactic digoxin is not ideal (p 329). Rather, anticoagulants and antiarrhythmics are important, especially if there is intermittent atrial fibrillation.

**Acute left ventricular (LV) failure** is generally treated by more potent inotropic drugs such as dopamine, dobutamine, amrinone, milrinone, or intravenous diuretics before digitalis is considered.

In **valvular heart disease** with failure, digitalization is conventionally used early, but is probably best combined with ACE inhibition in regurgitation. The general rule is to replace the damaged valve whenever possible.

In **children,** digitalis is preferred to diuretic therapy as first-line treatment of heart failure even in high-output states with left or right shunts.[1] Nevertheless, its efficacy is not without dispute.[33]

## Digitalis Contraindications

These are many: (1) **Hypertrophic obstructive cardiomyopathy** (hypertrophic subaortic stenosis, asymmetrical septal hypertrophy) is a contraindication (unless there is atrial fibrillation and severe myocardial failure), because the inotropic effect can worsen outflow obstruction. (2) The possibility of **digitalis toxicity** is a frequent contraindication, pending a full history of digitalis dosage, renal function tests and measurement of serum digoxin. (3) In some cases of **Wolff-Parkinson-White (WPW) syndrome,** digitalization may accelerate antegrade conduction over the bypass tract to precipitate ventricular tachycardia or ventricular fibrillation.[1] (4) Significant **AV nodal heart block.** Intermittent complete heart block or second degree AV block may be worsened by digitalis, especially if there is a history of Stokes-Adams attacks or when conduction is likely to be unstable as in acute myocardial infarction (AMI) or acute myocarditis. (5) **Diastolic dysfunction,** seen most notably with concentric ventricular hypertrophy as in hypertension or aortic stenosis, and associated with the paradox of a normal or high ejection fraction, probably does not respond to digitalis.

RELATIVE CONTRAINDICATIONS. Relative contraindications occur (1) if a poor response can be expected, as when low-output states are caused by valvular stenosis or chronic pericarditis; (2) in high-output states[1] including chronic cor pulmonale and thyrotoxicosis; (3) when atrial fibrillation occurs without heart failure or when atrial fibrillation is caused by thyrotoxicosis; (4) in all conditions increasing digitalis sensitivity to apparently therapeutic levels such as hypokalemia, chronic pulmonary disease, myxedema, acute hypoxemia; (5) in early AMI and postinfarct because of the risk of increased arrhythmias; (6) in renal failure—a lower dose, monitoring of plasma potassium, and a watch for digitalis toxicity are needed; (7) in sinus bradycardia or sick sinus syndrome—occasional patients will show a marked fall in sinus rate or sinus pauses, especially during cotherapy with other drugs inhibiting the sinus node, such as beta-blockers, diltiazem, verapamil, reserpine, methyldopa, and clonidine; (8) in cotherapy with other drugs inhibiting AV conduction (verapamil, diltiazem, beta-blockers, amiodarone); here intravenous digoxin may be hazardous; (9) in cotherapy with drugs altering digoxin levels, especially quinidine which may precipitate arrhythmias more easily; (10) in heart failure accompanying acute glomerulonephritis because renal excretion of digoxin is impaired; (11) in severe myocarditis, which may predispose to digoxin-induced arrhythmias and decreased digoxin effect; (12) in cardioversion—the digoxin level should be in the therapeutic range to avoid postconversion ventricular arrhythmias. If digoxin toxicity is suspected, elective cardioversion should be delayed. If urgent cardioversion is required, the energy level used should be minimal at first and carefully increased.

## Clinical States Altering Digitalis Activity

DIGOXIN IN THE ELDERLY. In the elderly, the etiology of CHF is often complex and multifactorial[49] requiring astute clinical diagnostic skills to detect any reversible cause. As in younger patients, digoxin is indicated especially for chronic atrial fibrillation combined with CHF

**TABLE 6–4**     FACTORS ALTERING SENSITIVITY TO DIGOXIN AT APPARENTLY
THERAPEUTIC LEVELS

**Physiologic effects**
  Enhanced vagal tone (increased digoxin effect on SA and AV nodes)
  Enhanced sympathetic tone (opposite to vagal effect)
**Systemic factors or disorders**
  Renal failure (reduced volume of distribution and excretion)
  Low lean body mass (reduced binding to skeletal muscle)
  Chronic pulmonary disease (hypoxia, acid-base changes)
  Myxedema (? prolonged half-life)
  Acute hypoxemia (sensitizes to digitalis arrhythmias)
**Electrolyte disorders**
  Hypokalemia (most common; sensitizes to toxic effects)
  Hyperkalemia (protects from digitalis arrhythmias)
  Hypomagnesemia (caused by chronic diuretics; sensitizes to toxic
    effects)
  Hypercalcemia (increases sensitivity to digitalis)
  Hypocalcemia (decreases sensitivity)
**Cardiac disorders**
  Acute myocardial infarction (may cause increased sensitivity)
  Acute rheumatic or viral carditis (danger of conduction block)
  Thyrotoxic heart disease (decreased sensitivity)
**Concomitant drug therapy**
  Diuretics with $K^+$ loss (increased sensitivity via hypokalemia)
  Drugs with added effects on SA or AV nodes (verapamil, diltiazem,
    beta-blockers, clonidine, methyldopa, or amiodarone)

and, secondly, for significant systolic failure. The place for digoxin
in mild to moderate CHF in sinus rhythm is not yet settled.[49]

The **pharmacokinetics** of digitalis in the elderly have been well
studied.[1] Digoxin absorption is delayed but not decreased. A decreased skeletal muscle and lean body mass cause increased digoxin
levels (Table 6–4). The latter are also promoted by a decreasing
glomerular filtration rate (GFR), especially after the fifth and sixth
decades. Creatinine clearance may be substantially reduced before
a rise in serum creatinine alerts the clinician. Digoxin half-life may
be prolonged up to 73 hours in the elderly, depending on the decrease
in renal function. There is no solid evidence of any alteration in
myocardial sensitivity or in the response to digoxin in older individuals.

The traditional **dose** of digoxin in the elderly is 0.125 mg daily.
Logically, however, dose reduction below 0.25 mg daily should only
be in response to impaired renal function, so that a dose of 0.25 mg
is usually better.[59] At this higher dose, there is a small increased risk
of excessive bradycardia.

DIGOXIN AND RENAL FUNCTION.  *The most important determinant of the
daily digoxin dosage in all age groups is renal function* (creatinine clearance or GFR). The clinician usually relies upon measurement of
the blood urea nitrogen or serum creatinine. These parameters are
influenced by factors other than glomerular filtration. For example,
serum creatinine may be normal in an elderly patient with a GFR
that is half normal if there is a marked decrease in muscle mass,
because the amount of creatinine released daily is diminished. Even
the GFR provides only a rough estimate of the renal excretion of
digoxin, since it is excreted both by the glomerulus and by the
tubules. In **severe renal insufficiency,** there is a decrease in the
volume of distribution of digoxin, so that it is not exact to use a
nomogram to estimate the maintenance dose based on creatinine
clearance.[1] One practical policy is to start with a maintenance dose

of 0.125 mg/day in patients with severe renal insufficiency and rely on serum digoxin levels for dose adjustment.

In less severe renal insufficiency, a "guestimate" of the digoxin dose can be made as follows: the creatinine clearance can be estimated from age, sex, body weight and serum creatinine if direct measurement is impractical. In elderly patients with renal impairment, the following approximations hold:[1]

| Creatinine clearance | Approximate digoxin dose |
|---|---|
| 10–25 mL/min | 0.125 mg/day |
| 26–49 mL/min | 0.1875 mg/day |
| 50–79 mL/min | 0.25 mg/day |

As an example, for a 70 kg male aged 70, the "guestimated" digoxin dose is 0.25 mg for serum creatinine up to about 1.5 mg/dL (140 μmole/L) and 0.125 mg when the creatinine exceeds about 3.0 mg/dL (275 μmole/L). These values are only approximations, stressing the important role of renal function in determining digoxin dosage. In this situation, nothing can improve on regular monitoring of blood digoxin levels. In severe renal failure, more digoxin is eliminated by metabolism.

DIGOXIN AND PULMONARY HEART DISEASE.   Not only is digoxin not beneficial in patients with right heart failure due to cor pulmonale, but it may be especially hazardous since such patients may exhibit a sensitivity to digoxin intoxication because of hypoxia, electrolyte disturbances, and sympathetic discharge.[1] By contrast, when right ventricular failure is the result of LV failure, digoxin is indicated.[1]

DIGOXIN AND EARLY MYOCARDIAL INFARCTION.   Acute intravenous digoxin is now seldom given in early phase AMI, especially since it constricts epicardial coronary arteries[30] and experimentally increases infarct size.[37] When **atrial fibrillation** develops with a rapid ventricular response, esmolol or verapamil or diltiazem more quickly reduce the ventricular rate.

When **mild to moderate postinfarct CHF** persists for several days, digoxin exerts a modest but detectable positive inotropic effect. This benefit may be achieved without decreasing myocardial perfusion or any apparent increase in infarct size.[1] However, a better-tested combination for this situation is the addition of ACE inhibitors to diuretics, which can lessen mortality (AIRE study, table 5–5).

CHRONIC ISCHEMIC HEART DISEASE AND BETA-BLOCKADE.   In anginal patients with cardiomegaly, digitalization may avert the precipitation of cardiac failure by beta-blockade.[1] In the large dilated hearts of chronic ischemic cardiomyopathy, the response to digoxin is variable.

POSTINFARCT DIGOXIN.   Substantial doubts remain about the safety of digoxin in postinfarct patients.[38] Several studies suggest that postinfarct digoxin may increase mortality,[11] presumably acting by induction of arrhythmias or by increasing the myocardial oxygen demand. In the absence of a randomized, controlled trial, finality cannot be reached. It is prudent to use digoxin in postinfarct patients only when strictly required and with frequent checks of serum digoxin levels and potassium. A suitable patient would be one with dilated ventricles and systolic dysfunction, and a third heart sound despite therapy by diuretics, ACE inhibitors, and beta-blockers.

It should be recalled that beta-blockers reduce postinfarct mortality by about one-quarter. Thus, although not well documented, a logical combination for postinfarct CHF is beta-blockade (initial low dose) plus diuretic therapy plus ACE inhibition and then, if needed, the further combination with digoxin.

Regarding prevention of postinfarct CHF, the reduction of ejection fraction that follows an acute myocardial infarction is directly related to the size of the infarction. Following a large infarct, the diastolic size of the heart tends to increase slowly but progressively over

## K⁺ AND TOXIC DIGOXIN LEVELS

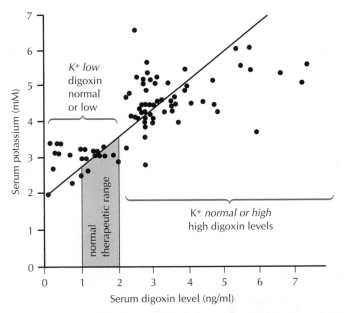

FIGURE 6–3. As the serum potassium falls the heart is sensitized to the arrhythmias of digitalis toxicity. Conversely, as the serum potassium rises a higher serum digoxin level is tolerated. Modified from Shapiro W. Am J Cardiol 1978; 41:852–859, with permission.

months (adverse **remodeling**). Prevention of this dilation may help prevent late heart failure. ACE inhibitors are useful in this regard (Chapter 5); any additional role for diuretics or digoxin requires further study.

### Ideal Serum Digoxin Levels

The major problem with digoxin remains the narrow therapeutic-to-toxic ratio. Serum digoxin levels can help, to some extent, in the assessment of the therapeutic effect and, at the very least, can prove that the patient is taking the drug and that it is being absorbed from the gut. *The major error with digoxin levels is taking the blood too soon after the last dose.* The usual therapeutic level ranges between 1 and 2 ng/mL (= 1.3 to 2.6 nmole/L).[1] Although values above that range may indicate digitalis toxicity and below may indicate underdigitalization, there are numerous problems in relating digoxin levels to digoxin efficacy. The sensitivity to digoxin at apparently therapeutic levels may be altered by a host of factors, the chief of which is the enhancing effect of hypokalemia (Table 6–4). In practice, digoxin levels of 0.9 to 1.2 ng/mL give as good a therapeutic response in CHF as higher values.[60]

In the presence of **hypokalemia,** digoxin-induced arrhythmias can arise even when the serum levels are within the therapeutic range (Fig. 6–3).

The *pharmacokinetics of digoxin also influence interpretation of serum levels.* The blood for sampling should not be taken less than 4 hours after an intravenous dose, 6 to 8 hours after an oral dose, or 10 to 12 hours after an intramuscular dose. The multiplicity of factors altering the effects of any given digoxin level (Table 6–4) needs to be taken into account in deciding whether the serum level is inappropriately high or low for that particular patient.

Clinical judgement may override digoxin levels. Thus, when a patient in sinus rhythm appears to suffer from toxicity, such as early arrhythmias, the dose should be reduced even if the digoxin level is in the therapeutic range.

| TABLE 6–5 | ANTIARRHYTHMIC DRUGS WHICH HAVE NO PHARMACOKINETIC INTERACTIONS WITH DIGOXIN |
|---|---|
| Class IA agents: | procainamide, disopyramide |
| Class IB agents: | lidocaine, phenytoin, tocainide, mexiletine |
| Class IC agents: | moricizine |
| Class II agents: | beta-blockade, unless renal blood flow critical |
| Class III agent: | sotalol (but not amiodarone) |
| Class IV agent: | diltiazem (modest elevation compared with verapamil) |

## Drug Interactions with Digoxin

The number of drug interactions is still increasing (Table 6–3). Although there are no rules to guide the clinician, it is of interest that several of the offending drugs are either antiarrhythmics or calcium antagonists.

The **quinidine-digoxin** interaction is best known. The concomitant administration of quinidine causes the blood digoxin level approximately to double, probably by reducing both renal and extrarenal clearance. **Quinine,** an agent sometimes used in the therapy of muscle cramps, acts likewise. The **verapamil-digoxin** interaction is equally important. However, verapamil does not alter the volume of distribution of digoxin so that the loading dose of digoxin is unaltered.[1] **Amiodarone** and **propafenone** (Chapter 8) also elevate serum digoxin levels. Other antiarrhythmics, including procainamide, have no interaction with digoxin (Table 6–5).

**Diuretics** may induce hypokalemia which (1) sensitizes the heart to digoxin toxicity and (2) shuts off the tubular secretion of digoxin when the plasma potassium falls to below 2 to 3 mEq/L.

**ACE inhibitors,** frequently combined with digoxin in the therapy of CHF, occasionally precipitate renal failure to decrease the renal excretion of digoxin and to increase its blood levels.[3]

## Digitalis Toxicity

The typical patient with digitalis toxicity (Table 6–6) is elderly with advanced heart disease and atrial fibrillation with abnormal renal function. Hypokalemia is common (Fig. 6–3). Digitalis toxicity should, however, be considered in any patient receiving digoxin or other digitalis compounds who presents with a new GI, ocular, or central nervous system complaint, or in whom a new arrhythmia or AV conduction disturbance develops. Symptoms do not necessarily precede serious cardiac arrhythmias. The *cellular mechanism* of digitalis toxicity resides in part in (1) intracellular calcium overload that predisposes to calcium-dependent delayed afterdepolarizations which may develop into ventricular automaticity; (2) excess vagal stimulation, predisposing to sinus bradycardia and AV block; and (3) an added "direct" depressive effect of digoxin on nodal tissue.

| TABLE 6–6 | FEATURES OF DIGITALIS TOXICITY | |
|---|---|---|
| **SYSTEM** | **SYMPTOMS AND SIGNS** | |
| Gastrointestinal | Anorexia, nausea, vomiting, diarrhea | |
| Neurologic | Malaise, fatigue, confusion, facial pain, insomnia, depression, vertigo, colored vision (green or yellow halos around lights) | |
| Cardiologic | Palpitations, arrhythmias, syncope | |
| Blood | High digoxin level; may be normal level with low potassium; check magnesium, urea, creatinine. | |

## DIGITALIS TOXICITY: Ca$^{2+}$ OVERLOAD

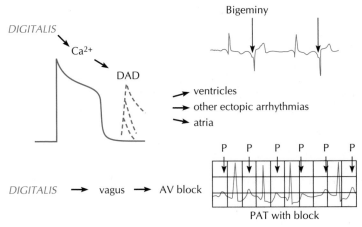

**FIGURE 6–4.** The cellular basis of the arrhythmias of digitalis toxicity lies in calcium overload, as a result of excess inhibition of the sodium pump (see Fig. 6–1). The result is the formation of delayed afterdepolarizations (DADs) and risk of ventricular ectopy, typically bigeminy, or atrial arrhythmias such as paroxysmal atrial tachycardia (PAT). Added excess vagal stimulation (Fig. 6–1) causes the typical ECG of PAT with block, as shown above. Fig. copyright L.H. Opie.

Digoxin may precipitate ischemic arrhythmias, some of which have calcium overload as their basis (Fig. 6–4).

TYPICAL DIGITALIS ARRHYTHMIAS. These are largely explained by increased vagal tone and include AV block, unexplained sinus bradycardia, and atrial fibrillation with a ventricular response of less than 50/min.[40] Digoxin toxicity also increases the automaticity of junctional and His-Purkinje tissue. Thus, accelerated atrial, junctional or ventricular arrhythmias may result and when combined with AV nodal block are highly suggestive of digitalis toxicity (Fig. 6–4). Classically, increased ventricular ectopic beats give the pattern of bigeminy.

When cotherapy elevates digoxin levels, the features of toxicity may depend on the agent added. With quinidine, tachyarrhythmias become more likely; amiodarone and verapamil seem to repress the ventricular arrhythmias of digoxin toxicity, so that bradycardia and AV block are more likely.[1]

The **diagnosis** of digoxin toxicity is confirmed if the arrhythmias resolve when the drug is discontinued; and/or if the digoxin blood level is inappropriately high for the patient in the presence of suspicious clinical features. Provided that hypokalemia is excluded (Fig. 6–3), an inappropriately low plasma digoxin level strongly suggests that an arrhythmia or conduction disturbance is not due to digoxin toxicity. Occasionally, intravenous digoxin antibodies are given for diagnosis of suspected digoxin toxicity when blood levels are not diagnostic or the clinical problem is too complex to solve otherwise.

TREATMENT OF DIGOXIN TOXICITY. Much depends on the clinical severity. With only suggestive symptoms, **withdrawal of digoxin** is sufficient while awaiting confirmation by elevated plasma levels. With dangerous arrhythmias and a low plasma potassium, potassium chloride may be infused intravenously very cautiously as 30 to 40 mEq in 20 to 50 ml of saline at 0.5 to 1 mEq/min into a large vein through a plastic catheter (infiltration of potassium solution can cause tissue necrosis and infusion into small veins causes local irritation and pain). **Oral potassium** (4 to 6 g potassium chloride, 50 to 80 mEq) may be given orally in divided doses when arrhythmias are not urgent (eg., PVCs). Potassium is contraindicated if AV conduction block or hyperkalemia are present, because potassium further increases AV block.[1]

**Lidocaine** is usually chosen for ventricular ectopy since it does not impair the AV conduction frequently present. **Phenytoin,** in addition, reverses the high-degree AV block, possibly acting by a central mechanism.[1] The dose is 100 mg intravenously every 5 minutes to a total of 1,000 mg or until side-effects appear.[40] Quinidine must be avoided because it displaces digoxin from binding sites to increase blood digoxin levels. Disopyramide can have a marked negative inotropic effect. Beta-blockers should be avoided because of added nodal depression.

**Interacting drugs** need attention. Any drugs elevating the blood digoxin level should be stopped (verapamil, quinidine), as also should beta-blockade (added AV or sinus nodal inhibition). On the other hand, because of its very long half-life, there is little point in stopping amiodarone.

Temporary transvenous **ventricular pacing** may be required for marked sinus bradycardia or advanced heart block not responsive to atropine.

**Digoxin-specific antibodies (Digibind)**, can be strikingly effective therapy for life-threatening digoxin intoxication, especially when there is severe ventricular tachycardia or significant hyperkalemia ($> 5.5$ mEq/L). In the latter case the digoxin level is likely to be very high (Fig. 6–3). The reversal of toxicity is rapid and not accompanied by adverse effects except that hypokalemia may develop as the sodium pump activity is regained and potassium is transferred from blood to muscle.[40] Anaphylactic shock is possible but extremely rare. Digoxin assays become unreliable unless a protein-free ultrafiltrate of the serum is used.

In patients with **renal failure,** the elimination half-life of antigen-binding fragments increases from the usual 15 hours to over 300 hours. The danger is dissociation of the antigen-antibody combination with renewed digoxin toxicity. *Plasmapheresis* is required.

**Activated charcoal** (50 to 100 g) is used to enhance GI clearance of digoxin. **Cholestyramine** (p 295) has a similar but less powerful effect.

## Digitoxin

Its pharmacokinetics include virtually complete absorption, so that the oral and intravenous digitalizing doses are the same. Because it is chiefly metabolized or excreted in the gut, *blood levels are not much altered by poor renal function.* The loading dose ranges from 0.8 to 1.2 mg in 24 hours given in four divided doses 6 hours apart. The maintenance dose is usually 0.1 to 0.15 mg of digitoxin daily. The great disadvantage is the long half-life (6 to 7 days compared with 36 hours for digoxin), which complicates the treatment of toxicity, as does the lack of a widely available assay.

The management of digitalis toxicity changes in patients given digitoxin because of (1) the much longer half-life than that of digoxin, (2) the enterohepatic circulation with recycling of 25% so that cholestyramine or activated charcoal must be given to promote excretion of digitoxin by the gut.[1]

## Other Oral Inotropes

A number of drugs used for CHF have had an apparent benefit at lower doses with adverse or lesser effects at higher doses. These include digoxin itself, xamoterol (beta-blocker with a high level of ISA), pimobendan, flosequinan (an inotropic dilator, withdrawn), and vesnarinone. Possibly the excess inotropic stimulation could have predominantly adverse effects, for example by calcium overload or by increasing the myocardial oxygen demand. Experimental inotropic agents that have not been approved by the FDA include **vesnarinone,** and the calcium-sensitizer **pimobendan.**

### Current Position of Digoxin in the Therapy of CHF

The separate and combined hemodynamic effects of digoxin and captopril have been studied.[6] To achieve marked improvements in hemodynamics at rest and during exercise in patients with CHF already receiving diuretics, both digoxin and an ACE inhibitor are needed. When compared with enalapril in patients receiving diuretics, digoxin was at least as effective as the ACE inhibitor and had a lower adverse reaction profile.[2] Also arguing for early digoxin use is an unexpected result in patients with NYHA Classes II–III apparently initially off all therapy and then randomized to digoxin.[22] According to the preliminary report, patients randomized to digoxin had a better quality of life with fewer side-effects than those treated by captopril or placebo. Decisive will be the outcome of a large prospective NIH-sponsored study (DIG; Digitalis Investigators Group) which will specifically test the effects of digoxin versus placebo on hard end-points in 7,500 patients with CHF in sinus rhythm. Currently, the ACE inhibitor-diuretic combination is especially advocated for mild to moderate heart failure (NYHA Classes I and II) and added digoxin for Classes II and III.[20,32]

Favoring the use of digoxin in CHF are two recent well-conducted withdrawal studies. The PROVED study[46] and the RADIANCE study[47] showed clinical worsening of heart failure on digoxin withdrawal. Such deterioration occurred especially in those patients with more severe symptoms and signs.[27] Yet withdrawal studies have a serious inherent limitation.[55]

It is often debated whether to use diuretics and ACE inhibitors or diuretics and digoxin or all three agents for mild to moderate CHF. Nonetheless, it must be acknowledged that the long-term effects of digoxin are not as well studied as those of ACE inhibitors, nor is there any evidence that digoxin prevents the development of overt heart failure as in the case of ACE inhibitors (SAVE and SOLVD studies, p 113). Hence diuretics are now often combined with ACE inhibitors rather than with digoxin as standard therapy for mild to moderate heart failure.

# Predominant Diastolic Dysfunction

Strategies for LV failure in the presence of relatively well-maintained systolic but impaired diastolic function are not well defined. Hypothetically, cytosolic calcium overload is to blame. Dyspnea, often prominent, leads to the use of diuretics, yet overdiuresis will reduce LV filling pressure which is critically important in this situation. Digoxin is contraindicated because increased cytosolic calcium levels could worsen diastolic dysfunction.[14] Logically, beta-stimulants such as dobutamine should accelerate diastolic filling because they enhance the uptake of calcium into the sarcoplasmic reticulum.[61] Conversely, beta-blockers should increase diastolic dysfunction. Calcium antagonists might help to lessen cytosolic calcium. In one of the few studies reported, verapamil was strikingly successful in patients with diastolic dysfunction mainly caused by hypertension.[54] Unexpectedly, verapamil seemed to benefit patients with diastolic dysfunction even in the presence of pulmonary congestive symptoms, yet there is no large prospective study.

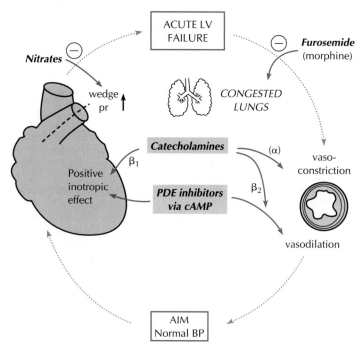

**FIGURE 6–5.** Some principles of therapy for acute LV failure. Note opposing effects of (i) vasoconstriction resulting from alpha-effect (norepinephrine, high doses of epinephrine or dopamine) and (ii) vasodilation resulting from vascular cyclic AMP elevation from beta$_2$-effects or PDE inhibition. Fig. copyright L.H. Opie.

## Acute Sympathomimetic Inotropes and Vasodilators

Physiologically, the basis of the acute inotropic response to an increased adrenergic drive is the rapid increase in the tissue levels of the second messenger, cyclic AMP. Pharmacologically, acute inotropic support uses the same principles, either by administration of exogenous catecholamines which stimulate the beta-receptor, or by inhibition of the breakdown of cyclic AMP by PDE inhibitors (Fig. 6–5). To give acute support to the failing circulation may require temporary peripheral vasoconstriction by alpha-adrenergic stimulation. Hence there are a variety of catecholamine-like agents used for acute heart failure, depending on the combination of acute inotropic stimulation, acute vasodilation and acute vasoconstriction that may be required. In addition, in acute heart failure, pulmonary congestion is countered by intravenous furosemide and nitrates.

### Adrenergic Receptors and Inotropic Effects

**Norepinephrine** is the endogenous catecholamine that is synthesized and stored in granules in adrenergic nerve endings in the myocardium. When sympathetic nerves to the heart are activated, norepinephrine is released from its stores and stimulates specific **beta$_1$-adrenergic receptors** (Fig. 1–1). Stimulation of these beta$_1$-receptors increases the rate of discharge of the sinoatrial node, thereby increasing heart rate, AV conduction, and the force and speed of contraction of atrial and ventricular myocardium. Beta$_1$-stimulation also enhances the rate of relaxation of the myocardium (**lusitropic effect**). Most of the released norepinephrine is subsequently taken

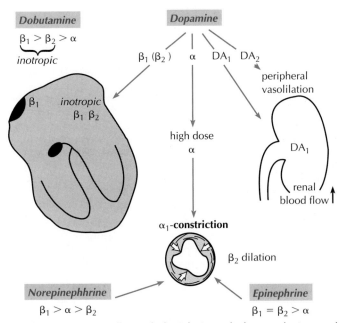

**FIGURE 6–6.** Receptor effects of physiologic and pharmacologic catechol-amines. For concepts regarding adrenergic receptor stimulation by dobutamine, see Ruffolo.[50] For norepinephrine, see Bristow.[15] Fig. copyright L.H. Opie.

up by the same adrenergic nerve endings and stored for renewed release. Smaller amounts are metabolized. Norepinephrine also has vasoconstrictive effects that result from stimulation of the vascular alpha-receptors, so that the blood pressure rises. Hence the positive inotropic effect of norepinephrine (Fig. 6–6) is accompanied by an elevation of systolic and diastolic blood pressure.

**Alpha-adrenergic myocardial stimulation** may also contribute a limited calcium-mediated inotropic effect. The most prominent consequence of alpha-receptor stimulation is, however, arteriolar vasoconstriction.

**Beta$_2$-adrenergic receptors** convey another type of beta-mediated sympathomimetic effect, namely that causing dilation of the smooth muscles of the blood vessels, bronchi, and uterus. A subpopulation of **beta$_2$-receptors** is also found in the heart with effects similar to those of the beta$_1$-receptors; these beta$_2$-receptors mediate more stimulation of adenylate cyclase, i.e., the coupling is tighter. In severe CHF, as beta$_1$-receptors downgrade, beta$_2$-receptors relatively increase to about 40% but become mildly uncoupled.[15]

**Epinephrine**, released from the adrenal glands, is a mixed beta$_1$- and beta$_2$-stimulant with high-dose alpha effects.

### Cardiovascular Therapeutic Effects of Adrenergic Agents

ADRENERGIC EFFECTS ON BLOOD PRESSURE. In the case of norepinephrine, the net effect is blood pressure elevation (dominant peripheral alpha-effects), whereas in the case of epinephrine at physiological doses, the vasodilatory effects of beta$_2$-stimulation seem to offset the blood pressure elevating effects of alpha-stimulation. The net effect of epinephrine is an elevation only of systolic blood pressure (increased stroke volume) with a fall of diastolic blood pressure (beta$_2$-peripheral dilation). Only at high pharmacological doses of epinephrine does alpha-constriction elevate diastolic blood pressure.

THE FAILING HEART. Sympathomimetic agents could thus benefit the failing heart: beta$_1$-stimulation by an inotropic effect, beta$_2$-stimulation by afterload reduction (peripheral arterial vasodilation), and alpha-stimulation by restoring pressure in hypotensive states. Experimental work unfortunately shows that catecholamine stimulation as exemplified by norepinephrine infusion should be used with caution in the low-output state of AMI. Beta$_1$-effects may precipitate arrhythmias and tachycardia, which can potentially increase ischemia, while excessive alpha-effects increase the afterload as the blood pressure rises beyond what is required for adequate perfusion. Although beta$_2$-stimulation achieves beneficial vasodilation and also mediates some inotropic effect, such stimulation also causes hypokalemia with enhanced risk of arrhythmias. A further and serious problem is that prolonged or vigorous beta$_1$-stimulation may lead to or increase receptor downgrading with a diminished inotropic response (Chapter 1, Fig. 1–1). Consequently, there is an ongoing search for new catecholamine-like agents, including PDE inhibitors, that lack the undesirable effects.

### Measures for Acute Heart Failure

CHOICE OF INOTROPIC STIMULANT. A crucial feature is whether it is desired to increase the blood pressure solely by inotropic support or by a combination of inotropic and peripheral vasoconstrictory effects, or only by peripheral vasoconstriction. Although the latter aim can be achieved by pure **alpha-stimulants,** such as **phenylephrine** (5 to 20 mg in 500 mL slow infusion) or **methoximine** (5 to 10 mg at 1 mg/min), this option is not logical, because heart failure automatically invokes reflex adrenergic vasoconstriction. Both these alpha-stimulants may be useful in anesthetic hypotension. Occasionally phenylephrine is still used in primary vasodilatory conditions, such as **septic shock.** The real therapeutic aim in the latter condition is inhibition of formation of excess vasodilatory nitric oxide.

Generally a mixture of inotropic and vasoconstrictory effects are required, as may for example be achieved by high-dose dopamine. Furthermore, bearing in mind that there are often defects in the rate of formation of cyclic AMP in chronically myopathic hearts, when there is acute-on-chronic heart failure, then a logical combination becomes dopamine plus a PDE inhibitor such as milrinone. If only inotropic stimulation is required, dobutamine is the agent of choice. If inotropic stimulation plus peripheral vasodilation is required, then low-dose dopamine or milrinone is appropriate. Drugs acting in this way are termed **inotropic-vasodilators** or **inodilators** (Fig. 6–7; Table 6–7).

PRELOAD REDUCTION. Acute venodilation is often of benefit to the patient with severe pulmonary congestion. Either sublingual or intravenous nitrates give most rapid relief.

COMBINED AFTERLOAD AND PRELOAD REDUCTION. When these qualities are required without any direct inotropic effect, sodium nitroprusside is still used (table 7–4).

AFTERLOAD REDUCTION. In severe CHF, inotropic dilators may lose some of their inotropic effect to become chiefly arteriolar dilators. Specific afterload reduction can also be achieved by hydralazine (table 7–4).

ACUTE DIURESIS. Furosemide is given intravenously for its acute diuretic and vasodilatory effects.

## Mixed Adrenergic Intravenous Inotropes (Beta > Alpha-adrenergic Stimulation)

These agents have as their common property the stimulation of both beta and alpha-adrenergic receptors to a varying degree. Alpha-adrenergic stimulation also results in some positive inotropic response in the human heart,[16] of greater importance when alpha-receptors are relatively upgraded as in severe CHF. Included in

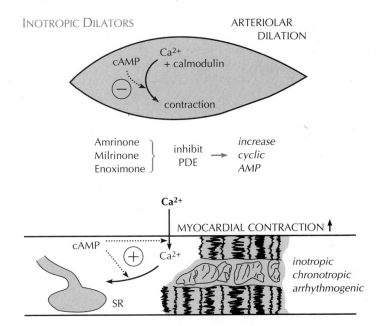

FIGURE 6–7.   Inotropic vasodilators (inodilators) have as their mechanism of action an increase of cyclic AMP in vascular smooth muscle (top) and in myocardium (bottom). For cellular mode of action of cyclic AMP in vascular smooth muscle, see Fig. 5–2. PDE, phosphodiesterase. Fig. copyright L.H. Opie and modified from Reference 1.

this group of mixed adrenergic agents is dobutamine, previously considered as highly selective for beta$_1$-receptors, but now thought also to stimulate beta$_2$- and alpha-receptors.

## Dobutamine

Dobutamine (**Dobutrex**), a synthetic analog of dopamine, is a beta-adrenergic stimulating agent. Its major characteristic is that it exerts a potent inotropic effect with only limited undesirable side-effects on heart rate and blood pressure. "The relative lack of positive chronotropic effect is not well understood."[35] One proposal is that the inotropic response is jointly mediated by beta$_1$- and alpha-receptors, the latter causing an inotropic component that is independent of any chronotropic effect. The proposed explanation for the relative lack of effect on the blood pressure is that the vasoconstrictive alpha$_1$-mediated effect is offset by beta$_2$-mediated vasodilation.[50] Dobutamine does not directly release norepinephrine as does dopamine, nor does it affect the dopamine receptors (Fig. 6–6). Dobutamine can be used cautiously as an inotropic agent in heart failure to increase cardiac output while reducing ventricular filling pressures. It may also be used in selected cases of evolving myocardial infarction with heart failure and low output, without great risk of increasing infarct size or inducing arrhythmias.[1]

PHARMACOKINETICS.   An infusion is rapidly cleared (half-life 2.4 minutes).

DOSE.   The standard intravenous dose is 2.5 to 10 µg/kg/min, occasionally up to 40 µg/kg/min.[1] The drug can be infused for up to 72 hours with monitoring. There is no oral preparation.

INDICATIONS.   Refractory heart failure; severe acute myocardial failure (AMI, after cardiac surgery); cardiogenic shock; excess beta-blockade; peri-operative spasm of internal thoracic artery.[43]

**TABLE 6-7  OVERALL PROPERTIES OF BETA-STIMULANTS, INOTROPIC VASODILATORS AND ADRENERGIC RECEPTOR BLOCKADE**

| | MIXED $\beta_1$-$\beta_2$-$\alpha$ | DOPAMINERGIC | MIXED $\beta_1$-$\alpha$ | MIXED $\beta_1$-$\beta_2$ (HIGH DOSE $\alpha$) | PURE $\beta$ | $\beta_2 > \beta_1$ | PDE INHIBITORS | MIXED $\beta$-$\alpha$ BLOCKADE |
|---|---|---|---|---|---|---|---|---|
| Drug examples | Dobutamine | Dopamine | NE | Epinephrine | Isoproterenol | Terbutaline[1] Albuterol | Amrinone Milrinone | Carvedilol* |
| Inotropic effect | ++ | ++ | + | ++ | +++ | + | + | 0 |
| Arteriolar vasodilation | + | ++ | 0 | + | + | ++ | ++ | + |
| Vasoconstriction | + | +(HD) | ++ | +(HD) | 0 | 0 | 0 | 0 |
| Chronotropic effect | + | 0/+ | + | ++ | +++ | + | 0 | 0 |
| Effect on BP | + | 0/+(HD) | + | 0/+ | +SBP | 0/– | 0/– | – |
| Direct diuretic effect | 0 | ++ | + | 0 | 0 | 0 | 0 | 0 |
| Arrhythmia risk | +/++ | 0/+(HD) | + | +++ | +++ | +/0 | +/++ | 0 |
| Effects in CHF | 0,+ | ++ | + | 0 | 0 | + | ++ | + |
| Effects in resuscitation and acute CHF | ++ | ++ | + | ++ | +/0 | 0 | 0 | 0 |

* investigational; + = increase; 0 = no effect; – = negative effect; NE = norepinephrine; CHF = congestive heart failure; PDE = phosphodiesterase; SBP = systolic blood pressure; HD = high-dose dopamine or epinephrine

1. See Schafers et al.[51]

SIDE-EFFECTS.   In severe CHF, dobutamine can cause tachycardia,[1] but there is a dose-related increase in cardiac output.[1] Although there may be less tachycardia and arrhythmias than with dopamine or isoproterenol, all inotropic agents have risk of enhanced arrhythmias. Tolerance to the inotropic effect may develop after prolonged infusion.[57]

PRECAUTIONS.   Dilute in sterile water or dextrose or saline, not in alkaline solutions. Use within 24 hours. Hemodynamic monitoring of patient required. Check blood potassium to minimize arrhythmias.

CLINICAL USE.   The ideal candidate for dobutamine therapy is the patient who has severely depressed LV function with a low cardiac index and elevated LV filling pressure, but in whom extreme hypotension is not present (mean arterial BP not < 70 mmHg).[1] The potential disadvantages of dobutamine are (1) that in severe CHF the beta-receptors may be downgraded so that dobutamine may not be as effective as anticipated, and (2) prolonged therapy with dobutamine itself could cause receptor downgrading, especially after 72 hours.[58] Relief of CHF may improve peripheral blood flow and enhance renal function indirectly. A logical combination is that of dobutamine with a vasodilator, acting through a different mechanism such as low-dose dopamine, or with a PDE inhibitor.

## Dopamine

Dopamine (**Intropin**) is a catecholamine-like agent used for therapy of severe heart failure and cardiogenic shock. Physiologically it is both the precursor of norepinephrine and releases norepinephrine from the stores in the nerve-endings in the heart (Fig. 6–6). However, in the periphery this effect is overridden by the activity of the prejunctional dopaminergic $DA_2$-receptors, inhibiting norepinephrine release and thereby helping to vasodilate.[1] Therefore, overall dopamine stimulates the heart by both beta- and alpha-adrenergic responses and causes vasodilation through dopamine receptors. Theoretically, dopamine has the valuable property in severe CHF or shock of specifically increasing blood flow to the renal,[1] mesenteric, coronary, and cerebral beds by activating the specific postjunctional dopamine $DA_1$-receptors. At high doses, however, dopamine causes alpha-receptor stimulation with peripheral vasoconstriction; the peripheral resistance increases and renal blood flow falls.[1] The dose should therefore be kept as low as possible to achieve the desired ends; a combination of dopamine and vasodilator therapy or dopamine and dobutamine would be better than increasing the dose of dopamine into the vasoconstrictor range.[1]

PHARMACOLOGY.   Dopamine, a "flexible molecule," also fits into many receptors to cause direct $beta_1$- and $beta_2$-receptor stimulation, as well as alpha-stimulation. The latter explains why in high doses dopamine causes significant vasoconstriction. By increasing renal blood flow, dopamine may induce diuresis or it may potentiate the effects of furosemide.

PHARMACOKINETICS.   Dopamine is inactive orally. Intravenous dopamine is metabolized within minutes by dopamine beta-hydroxylase and monoamine oxidase.

DOSE AND INDICATIONS.   In **refractory cardiac failure,** dopamine can only be given intravenously, which restricts its use to short-term treatment.[1] The dose starts at 0.5 to 1 µg/kg/min and is raised until an acceptable urinary flow, blood pressure or heart rate is achieved; vasoconstriction begins at about 10 µg/kg/min and becomes marked at higher doses, then calling for an added alpha-blocking agent or sodium nitroprusside. In a few patients vasoconstriction can begin at doses as low as 5 µg/kg/min. In **cardiogenic shock** or **AMI,** 5 µg/kg/min of dopamine is enough to give a maximum increase in stroke volume, while renal flow reaches a peak at 7.5

$\mu g/kg/min$, and arrhythmias may appear at 10 $\mu g/kg/min$.[1] In **septic shock,** dopamine has an inotropic effect and increases urine volume.[1] Dopamine is widely used for **myocardial failure** after cardiac surgery.[1] It is sometimes given in **acute renal failure** for diuresis.

PRECAUTIONS. Dopamine must not be diluted in alkaline solutions. Blood pressure, electrocardiogram, and urinary flow are monitored constantly with intermittent measurements of cardiac output and pulmonary wedge pressure if possible. For oliguria, first correct hypovolemia; try furosemide.

SIDE-EFFECTS AND INTERACTIONS. Dopamine is contraindicated in ventricular arrhythmias, and in pheochromocytoma. Use with care in aortic stenosis. Extravasation can cause sloughing, prevented by infusing the drug into a large vein through a plastic catheter, and treated by local infiltration with phentolamine. If the patient has recently taken a monoamine-oxidase inhibitor, the rate of dopamine metabolism by the tissue will fall and *the dose should be cut to one-tenth* of the usual.

COMPARISON OF DOPAMINE AND DOBUTAMINE. After cardiac surgery dobutamine may be best for the patient with depressed cardiac output with modest hypotension, particularly when the patient has sinus tachycardia or ventricular arrhythmias. Dopamine, on the other hand, is preferred in the patient who requires both a pressor effect (high-dose alpha-effect) and increase in cardiac output, and who does not have marked tachycardia or ventricular irritability.[1] *Dopamine may be especially beneficial when renal blood flow is impaired in severe CHF.*[1] In cardiogenic shock, infusion of equal concentrations of dopamine and dobutamine may afford more advantages than either drug singly.[1]

## Epinephrine (Adrenaline)

Epinephrine gives mixed $beta_1$-$beta_2$-stimulation with some added alpha-mediated effects at a high dose. A low physiologic infusion rate ($< 0.01$ $\mu g/kg/min$) decreases blood pressure (vasodilator effect), whereas $> 0.2$ $\mu g/kg/min$ increases peripheral resistance and blood pressure (combined inotropic and vasoconstrictor effects). It is used chiefly when combined inotropic/chronotropic stimulation is urgently desired as in cardiac arrest. Then the added alpha-stimulatory effect of high-dose epinephrine helps to maintain the blood pressure and overcomes the peripheral vasodilation achieved by $beta_2$-receptor stimulation. The acute *dose* is 0.5 mg subcutaneously or intramuscularly (0.5 ml of 1 in 1,000), or 0.5 to 1.0 mg into the central veins, or 0.1 to 0.2 mg intracardiac. The *terminal half-life* is 2 minutes. *Side-effects* include tachycardia, arrhythmias, anxiety, headaches, cold extremities, cerebral hemorrhage and pulmonary edema. *Contraindications* include late pregnancy because of risk of inducing uterine contractions.

### Norepinephrine (Noradrenaline)

Norepinephrine is given in an *intravenous dose* of 8 to 12 $\mu g/min$ with a terminal half-life of 3 minutes. This catecholamine has prominent $beta_1$- and alpha-effects with less $beta_2$-stimulation.[15] Norepinephrine chiefly stimulates alpha-receptors in the periphery (with more marked alpha-effects than epinephrine) and beta-receptors in the heart. Logically, norepinephrine should be of most use when a shock-like state is accompanied by peripheral vasodilation (*"warm shock"*). In the future, drugs inhibiting the formation of vasodilatory nitric oxide will probably be of greater use in such patients. *Side-effects* of norepinephrine include headache, tachycardia, bradycardia and hypertension. Note the risk of necrosis with extravasation. *Combination therapy* with PDE inhibitors helps to avoid their hypotensive effects. *Contraindications* include late pregnancy (see epinephrine) and pre-existing excess vasoconstriction.

## Isoproterenol (Isoprenaline)

This relatively pure beta-stimulant (beta$_1$ > beta$_2$) is still sometimes used. Its cardiovascular effects closely resemble those of exercise including a positive inotropic and vasodilatory effect.[34] Theoretically, it is most suited to situations where the myocardium is poorly contractile and the heart rate slow, yet the peripheral resistance high as, for example, after cardiac surgery in patients with prior beta-blockade. Another ideal use is in beta-blocker overdose. The intravenous dose is 0.5 to 10 μg/min, the plasma half-life is about 2 minutes, and the major problem lies in the risk of tachycardia and arrhythmias. Furthermore, it may drop the diastolic blood pressure by its beta$_2$-vasodilator stimulation. Other side-effects are headache, tremor and sweating. Contraindications include myocardial ischemia, which can be worsened, and arrhythmias.

## Beta$_2$-agonists

In healthy volunteers, beta$_2$-receptors mediate chronotropic, inotropic, and vasodilator responses.[51] Although not well tested in CHF where there is known to be cardiac beta$_2$-receptor uncoupling, yet some evidence suggests clinical benefit in patients already treated by diuretics and digoxin.[1] The drugs used are basically bronchodilators (terbutaline; albuterol = salbutamol) and should therefore be ideal for the combination of chronic obstructive airways disease and CHF. By inducing hypokalemia and prolonging the QT-interval, beta$_2$-agonists may increase the risk of arrhythmias.

## Ibopamine

This orally active agent, not available in the USA or UK, acts by release in the blood of epinine, with properties similar to dopamine. In mild to moderate CHF treated by furosemide, it had only modest effects when compared with digoxin.[21] In severe CHF, it may be able to increase renal plasma flow and the GFR.[28]

# Mixed Inotropic-Vasodilator Agents ("Inodilators")

Although "inodilation" is a term relatively recently coined,[10] the rationale goes back at least to 1978 when Stemple et al.[12] combined the advantages of the vasodilator effects of nitroprusside with the inotropic effect of dopamine. Recognition of the sympatholytic properties of digoxin[5] strictly speaking leads to its inclusion in the group of inodilators. Nonetheless, it is the PDE inhibitors that are the prototypical agents.

## Phosphodiesterase-III Inhibitors

These agents, epitomized by amrinone and milrinone, inhibit the breakdown of cyclic AMP in cardiac and peripheral vascular smooth muscle, resulting in augmented myocardial contractility and peripheral arterial and venous vasodilation (Fig. 6–7). For ill-understood reasons, these effects occur with relatively little change in heart rate or blood pressure.[1] The added dilator component may explain relative conservation of the myocardial oxygen consumption.[1] Nonetheless, the increased levels of myocardial cyclic AMP may predispose to ventricular arrhythmias,[36] which could explain the findings in the Milrinone-Digoxin trial in which milrinone was no better than digoxin and led to an increase in ventricular arrhythmias.[4]

## Amrinone

Amrinone (**Inocor Lactate**) is a phosphodiesterase-III inhibitor with both inotropic and vasodilating properties. The intravenous preparation has been approved by the FDA for patients with severe CHF, who are not adequately responsive to digoxin, diuretics and/or vasodilators. In patients with severe CHF, the vasodilator effect dominates with a variable direct positive inotropic effect contribution.[1] Although orally active, a multicenter investigation[1] showed no sustained improvement in cardiac function beyond that provided by standard treatment.

PHARMACOKINETICS. Intravenous amrinone is rapidly distributed in the circulation with an elimination half-life of 4 hours (prolonged in CHF). About 20 to 40% is plasma bound and the therapeutic plasma level is about 3 μg/mL. Most is excreted unchanged in the urine, some is metabolized, and some is excreted in the feces.

DOSE. Intravenously, therapy is initiated with 0.75 mg/kg bolus over 2 to 3 minutes followed by an infusion of 5 to 10 μg/kg/min. An added bolus dose may be given 30 minutes later. Higher infusion doses have also been used (10 to 20 μg/kg/min).[1]

PRECAUTIONS. Amrinone ampules should be protected from the light, and amrinone should not be mixed with glucose (dextrose) for infusion. Predrug and repeated platelet counts are required (decrease drug or discontinue if platelets fall below 150,000/mm³). Monitor fluid balance and blood potassium (risk of added hypokalemia). Monitor liver and renal function.

INDICATIONS. Severe CHF resistant to conventional therapy; acute LV failure; AMI with cardiogenic shock when dopamine or dobutamine are ineffective. For the same increase in cardiac output, amrinone is more potent than these other agents in reducing both right and left filling pressures.

CONTRAINDICATIONS. AMI (risk of arrhythmias); aortic or pulmonic stenosis (as for all vasodilators); hypertrophic cardiomyopathy (may aggravate obstruction).

SIDE-EFFECTS. Serious side-effects, which are rare during intravenous use, include thrombocytopenia, ventricular arrhythmias, hepatotoxicity, hypotension, and possibly hypersensitivity reactions. The hypotension may be due to excessive reduction in filling pressure and/or excessive vasodilation.

COMBINATION THERAPY. The effects of amrinone and dobutamine are additive in augmenting cardiac output and reducing filling pressure.[1] Amrinone has been combined with digoxin (check blood digoxin and $K^+$ levels for risk of arrhythmias), diuretics (monitor blood $K^+$), ACE inhibitors, and vasodilators such as hydralazine and nitrates (watch for additive hypotension). The combined inotropic-vasodilator effects of amrinone are additive to the effects of dobutamine (different mechanisms of stimulating formation of cyclic AMP), dopamine (different mechanisms of vasodilation) and hydralazine.[1]

## Milrinone

Milrinone (**Primacor**) is approved for intravenous use in the USA and UK. Its pharmacologic mechanisms of action resemble those of amrinone. It is 20× more potent than amrinone, with a similar mechanism of action, also with a prominent vasodilatory component.[1] When given acutely, its inotropic and vasodilator effects occur with only a modest change in heart rate or blood pressure,[1] although tachycardia can be a side-effect.

INTRAVENOUS DOSE. A slow intravenous injection (over 10 minutes, diluted before use, 50 μg/kg) is followed by an intravenous infusion at a rate of 375 to 750 nanograms/kg/min, usually for up to 12 hours following surgery or for 48 to 72 hours in congestive heart failure; maximum daily dose is 1.13 mg/kg. Reduce dose in renal failure.

COMBINATION THERAPY. Milrinone also gives added hemodynamic

benefit to patients already receiving ACE inhibitors, with however a high risk of vasodilatory side-effects.[19] Milrinone may also be combined with modest doses of dobutamine, enhancing the inotropic effects while lowering filling pressures. When the blood pressure is low, milrinone could logically be combined with high-dose dopamine.

CHRONIC ORAL ADMINISTRATION. The PROMISE Research Study Group[45] found increased mortality particularly in Class IV heart failure, a result which led to suspension of further trials with the oral preparation in the USA. Chronic oral milrinone has also been compared with digoxin in patients with moderately severe heart failure.[4] Overall there was a marked superiority of digoxin and an adverse effect of milrinone on heart rhythm.

### Enoximone

This investigational agent, also acting by enhancement of cyclic AMP levels, is being widely evaluated and is now available as **Perfan** for intravenous use in the UK (90 µg/kg/min over 10 to 30 minutes) against acute heart failure or in bridging situations such as for patients awaiting transplantation. In a double-blind placebo-controlled multicenter study, enoximone only transiently improved the patients, and 48% of enoximone-treated patients dropped out of the study.[13] Furthermore, in this rather small trial, more patients in the enoximone group died. Thus, it seems that enoximone has not overcome the general problem of PDE inhibitors, namely the risk of serious arrhythmias.

## Logic for Combined Inotropic Support

There are several reasons for combining agents with different inotropic mechanisms. First, the beta-stimulants such as dobutamine may become progressively ineffective over many hours, probably due to increasing beta-receptor downregulation. Hence the addition of a PDE inhibitor which bypasses the beta-receptor to increase cyclic AMP is logical. Second, pre-existing beta-receptor desensitization in severe CHF may limit even the early response to beta-stimulating agents.[18] Third, acute heart failure is a complex situation requiring multiple drugs acting at various sites (Fig. 6–5). Hence, once early intravenous management of acute heart failure by combined inotropic therapy has stabilized the patient, rapid oral digitalization is often considered. Heart failure is accompanied by abnormalities of baroreflex control which may be reverted by digoxin.[53] Furthermore, ACE inhibitors are likely to be introduced soon after the acute phase is over.

Another logical combination is that of a PDE inhibitor with a beta-blocker, the latter to counteract excess tachycardia induced by the former.[26]

## Acute Versus Chronic Effects of Sympathomimetics and Vasodilators

In **acute LV failure,** sympathomimetic inotropes and inotropic dilators may achieve dramatic short-term benefits to remedy the added deterioration that usually accompanies and promotes the condition. Together with loop diuretics and nitrates, the positive inotropes or inotropic vasodilators frequently save the patient from drowning in his own secretions. In contrast, in **chronic severe heart failure,** the major limitation is the underlying state of the myocardium, which is usually damaged beyond repair, so that all therapy has inherent limitations.[1] Therapy is now aimed at improving the

MAXIMAL THERAPY FOR SEVERE CHF

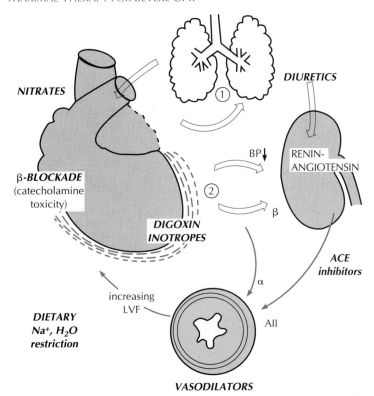

**FIGURE 6–8.** Principles of maximum therapy for CHF. Diuretics are given for back pressure into the lungs with edema (1) yet stimulate the renin-angiotensin system. Poor LV function also activates this system (2) by a low blood pressure with decreased renal perfusion and/or by reflex β-adrenergic (β) baroreceptor activation. Vasoconstriction results from formation of angiotensin-II (AII) and/or from alpha-adrenergic activity. Fig. copyright L.H. Opie.

peripheral circulation[1] and the neurohumoral status by ACE inhibition, digoxin (acting as a sympathoinhibitory agent), and judicious supplementary beta-blockade while achieving optimal diuresis (Fig. 6–8). In a third and intermediate situation, **chronic mild to moderate CHF,** the myocardium is still theoretically capable of at least some response to inotropic stimulation, and may also be better able to withstand possible side-effects of inotropic agents such as arrhythmias and aggravation of ischemia. In this setting, prevention of further cardiac dilation and resultant functional mitral regurgitation may help to prevent or delay ventricular deterioration. It is in this category that there is most potential for the benefits of new oral inotropic agents, for example the calcium sensitizers. At present such patients are best treated by diuretics and ACE inhibition with, sometimes, the addition of digoxin.

## Maximum Therapy of Congestive Heart Failure

Although the myocardium might be largely destroyed, symptomatic improvement is still possible using a judicious mixture of diuretics, ACE inhibition, digoxin, vasodilation, and beta-adrenergic blockade (Fig. 6–8).

**Diuretic doses** must be carefully adjusted to steer the course between optimal relief of edema and excess diuresis with ionic disturbances and prerenal azotemia. Following the principle of sequential nephron blockade (Fig. 4–1), combination diuretic therapy will often be used. In those unusual patients who have severe heart failure with major restriction of the GFR (below 15 to 20 ml/min), high doses of furosemide alone or combined with metolazone are used. In diuretic-resistant patients, first check for interacting drugs especially NSAIDs (Fig. 4–2). Intermittent dopamine infusions could help to improve renal blood flow and to induce diuresis.

**ACE inhibitors** should be used in a dose which is as high as possible (p 118), yet avoiding excess hypotension. When an ACE inhibitor is introduced for the first time to a patient already receiving high-dose diuretics (and therefore with intense renin-angiotensin activation), the diuretic dose must first be dropped and care be taken to minimize or avoid first-dose hypotension.

**Digoxin** is now re-established for CHF in sinus rhythm, and appears to be more effective in patients with severe symptoms and signs.[27] Blood potassium should be normal. Dose reduction is required in patients with renal impairment. Watch for interacting drugs and factors altering the sensitivity to digoxin (Table 6–4).

**Vasodilators** have the inherent problem of the development of tolerance. Nonetheless, nitrates have a specific role in reducing the preload and relieving dyspnea. They can be given intermittently (to avoid tolerance) in anticipation of exertional dyspnea or at bedtime to avoid nocturnal dyspnea. Hydralazine-nitrate may be preferred to ACE inhibition in black patients,[17] or if ACE inhibitor therapy induces excess hypotension.

**Beta-blockers,** although not yet approved for use in CHF, have increasing support from trials mostly in idiopathic cardiomyopathy. Recently, their benefit has also been confirmed for ischemic cardiomyopathy.[25] It is essential to start with a very low dose of the beta-blocker, to set aside those patients reacting adversely, and then to work up to a standard dose.

**Antiarrhythmics** may be required. Ventricular tachyarrhythmias may be fatal in CHF. Nonetheless, there are no established principles to deal with such arrhythmias in heart failure, except to avoid predisposing factors such as hypokalemia, digoxin excess, or chronic use of PDE inhibitors. Judging by the recent GESICA study,[44] long-term **amiodarone** may be considered in a low dose. Over 2 years total mortality in a prospective open study was reduced by 28%. In contrast, a double-blind study gave no mortality benefit for amiodarone (p 241).

**Short-term inotropic support** by amrinone or milrinone or the sympathomimetics may give dramatic relief. This is essentially a rescue operation.

**General measures for CHF** include salt restriction and, in the presence of poor renal perfusion, water restriction. Although periodic bed rest may be required to achieve optimal diuresis (the patient returning to bed for 1 to 2 hours of supine rest after taking the diuretic), in principle physical activity should be maintained and, if possible, an exercise rehabilitation program undertaken.

**Cardiac transplantation** remains as the last option for the patient remaining severely symptomatic. Nonetheless, it should be considered that the prognosis in such patients, given modern medical management, may be more favorable than previously anticipated.[56]

## Summary

**Digoxin,** by its unique combination of a positive inotropic effect and vagally-induced bradycardia with inhibition of AV nodal conduction and its sympatholytic effects, remains the oral inotrope of choice. A thorough understanding of its pharmacokinetics, numerous interactions with other drugs, and correct use in various clinical situations is mandatory. Chronic digoxin therapy should be undertaken only for clearly defined indications, in the absence of which the benefit will be limited yet involve the risk of digoxin toxicity.

The strongest indications for digoxin remain (1) the combination of atrial fibrillation and congestive heart failure, and (2) severe heart failure albeit in sinus rhythm.

**Beta-receptor stimulatory inotropes** are often used in the acute therapy of severe heart failure. The problem of beta-receptor down-regulation may require added PDE inhibition. Although dobutamine provides dominant beta-receptor stimulation, the full pattern of receptor stimulation is still not well understood. Dopamine has added effects on dopaminergic renal vascular receptors to increase renal blood flow and, sometimes, to induce a diuresis especially in patients with pre-existing severe CHF. High-dose dopamine is accompanied by alpha-receptor stimulation which increases the blood pressure. Predominant beta$_2$-stimulation can be achieved by oral terbutaline or by albuterol (salbutamol). Such therapy is logical for patients with both bronchospasm and CHF, although not well tested.

Although **PDE inhibitors** are no longer used in oral form, the intravenous preparations with their inotropic and vasodilator effects should be especially useful in patients with beta-receptor downgrading, as in severe CHF or during prolonged therapy with dobutamine or other beta$_1$-stimulants, or after chronic beta-blockade. Thus amrinone and milrinone have a place in the management of short-term therapy of heart failure.

**The major new approach** to the management of CHF is inhibition of the beta-adrenergic response by beta-blockers initially given in very low doses.

# References

*For references from Second Edition, see Marcus et al. (1991)*

1. Marcus FI, Opie LH, Sonnenblick EH. Digitalis and other inotropes. In: Opie LH (ed), Drugs for the Heart, Third Edition. WB Saunders Company, Philadelphia, 1991, pp 129–154.

### *References from Third Edition*

2. Beaune J, for the Enalapril vs Digoxin French Multicenter Study Group. Am J Cardiol 1989; 63:22D–25D.
3. Cleland JGF, Dargie HJ, Pettigrew A, et al. Am Heart J 1986; 112:130–135.
4. DiBianco R, Shabetai R, Kostuk W, et al. N Engl J Med 1989; 320:677–683.
5. Ferguson DW, Berg WJ, Sanders JS, et al. Circulation 1989; 80:65–77.
6. Gheorghiade M, Hall V, Lakier JB, Goldstein S. J Am Coll Cardiol 1989; 13:134–142.
7. Lindenbaum J, Rund DG, Butler VP, et al. N Engl J Med 1981; 305:789–794.
8. Marcus FI. Cardiovasc Drugs Ther 1989; 3:473–476.
9. McMichael J, Sharpey-Schafer EP. Qtly J Med 1944; 13:123–135.
10. Opie LH. Cardiovasc Drugs Ther 1989; 3:1041–1054.
11. Poole-Wilson PA, Robinson K. Cardiovasc Drugs Ther 1989; 2:733–741.
12. Stemple DR, Kleiman JH, Harrison DC. Am J Cardiol 1978; 42:267–275.
13. Uretsky BF, Jessup M, Konstam MA, et al. Circulation 1989; 80 (Suppl II):II–175.

### *New References*

14. Bolognesi R, Cucchini F, Iavernaro A, et al. Effects of acute strophantidin administration on left ventricular relaxation and filling phase in coronary artery disease. Am J Cardiol 1992; 69:169–172.
15. Bristow MR. Changes in myocardial and vascular receptors in heart failure. J Am Coll Cardiol 1993; 22 (Suppl A):61A–71A.
16. Bristow MR, Minobe W, Rasmussen R, et al. Alpha-1 adrenergic receptors in the nonfailing and failing human heart. J Pharmacol Exp Ther 1988; 247:1039–1045.
17. Carson PE, Johnson GR, Singh SN, et al, for the VA Cooperative Study Group. Differences in vasodilator response by race in heart failure: VHeFT (abstr). J Am Coll Cardiol 1994; 23:382A.
18. Colucci WS, Ribeiro JP, Rocco MB, et al. Impaired chronotropic response to exercise in patient with congestive heart failure. Role of postsynaptic beta-adrenergic desensitization. Circulation 1989; 80:314–323.
19. Colucci WS, Sonnenblick EH, Adams KF, et al. Efficacy of phosphodiesterase inhibition with milrinone in combination with converting enzyme inhibitors in patients with heart failure. J Am Coll Cardiol 1993: 22 (Suppl A):113A–118A.

20. Crozier I, Ikram H. Angiotensin-converting enzyme inhibitors versus digoxin for the treatment of congestive heart failure. Drugs 1992; 43:637–650.

21. DIMT trial—van Veldhuizen DJ, Man in 't Veld AJ, Dunselman PHJM, et al. Double-blind placebo-controlled study of ibopamine and digoxin in patients with mild to moderate heart failure: Results of the Dutch Ibopamine Multicenter Trial (DIMT). J Am Coll Cardiol 1993; 22:1564–1573.

22. Drexler H, Schumacher M, Siegrist J, Just H, for the CADS Multicenter Study Group. Effect of captopril and digoxin on quality of life and clinical symptoms in patients with coronary artery disease and mild heart failure (abstr). J Am Coll Cardiol 1992; 19:260A.

23. Falk RH, Leavitt JI. Digoxin for atrial fibrillation: A drug whose time has gone? Ann Intern Med 1991; 114:573–575.

24. Ferguson DW. Digitalis and neurohumoral abnormalities in heart failure and implications for therapy. Am J Cardiol 1992; 69:24G–33G.

25. Fisher ML, Gottlieb SS, Plotnick GD, et al. Beneficial effects of metoprolol in heart failure associated with coronary artery disease: A randomized trial. J Am Coll Cardiol 1994; 23:943–950.

26. Galie N, Branzi A, Magnani G, et al. Effect of enoximone alone and in combination with metoprolol on myocardial function and energetics in severe congestive heart failure: Improvement in hemodynamic and metabolic profile. Cardiovasc Drugs Ther 1993; 7:337–347.

27. Gheorghiade M, Young JB, Uretsky B, et al, on behalf of the PROVED and RADI-ANCE Investigators. Predicting clinical deterioration after digoxin withdrawal in heart failure (abstr). Circulation 1993; 88:I–604.

28. Girbes ARJ, Kalisvaart CJ, Van Veldhuisen DJ, et al. Effects of ibopamine on renal haemodynamics in patients with severe congestive heart failure. Eur Heart J 1993; 14:279–283.

29. Hinderling PH, Hartmann D. Pharmacokinetics of digoxin and main metabolites/derivatives in healthy humans. Therapeutic Drug Monitoring 1991; 13:381–400.

30. Indolfi C, Piscione F, Russolillo E, et al. Digoxin-induced vasoconstriction of normal and atherosclerotic epicardial coronary arteries. Am J Cardiol 1991; 68:1274–1278.

31. Kelly RA, Smith TW. Use and misuse of digitalis blood levels. Heart Disease and Stroke 1992: 1:117–122.

32. Kelly RA, Smith TW. Digoxin in heart failure: Implications of recent trials. J Am Coll Cardiol 1993; 22 (Suppl A):107A–112A.

33. Kimball TR, Daniels SR, Meyer RA, et al. Effect of digoxin on contractility and symptoms in infants with a large ventricular septal defect. Am J Cardiol 1991; 68:1377–1382.

34. Krasnow N, Rolett EL, Yurchak PM, et al. Isoproterenol and cardiovascular performance. Am J Med 1964; 37:514–523.

35. Le Jemtel TH, Sonnenblick E. Nonglycosidic cardioactive agents. In: Schlant RC, Alexander RW (eds). The Heart, Eighth Edition. McGraw-Hill, New York, 1994, pp 589–594.

36. Lubbe WF, Podzuweit T, Opie LH. Potential arrhythmogenic role of cyclic AMP and cytosolic calcium overload: Implications for antiarrhythmic effects of beta-blockers and proarrhythmic effects of phosphodiesterase inhibitors. J Am Coll Cardiol 1992; 19:1622–1633.

37. Lynch JJ, Simpson PJ, Gallagher KP, et al. Increase in experimental infarct size with digoxin in a canine model of myocardial ischemia-reperfusion injury. Am Heart J 1988; 115:1171–1182.

38. Marcus FI. Use and toxicity of digitalis. Heart Disease and Stroke 1992; 1:27–31.

39. Marcus FI. Digoxin is effective, but is it safe? Cardiovasc Drugs Ther 1993; 7:893–896.

40. Marcus FI. Digitalis. In: Schlant RC, Alexander RW, O'Rourke RA, et al (eds). The Heart, Eighth Edition. McGraw-Hill, New York, 1994, pp 573–588.

41. Matsuda M, Matsuda Y, Yamagishi T, et al. Effects of digoxin, propranolol, and verapamil on exercise in patients with chronic isolated atrial fibrillation. Cardiovasc Res 1991; 25:453–457.

42. Murgatroyd FD, Xie B, Gibson SM, et al. The effects of digoxin in patients with paroxysmal atrial fibrillation: Analysis of Holter data from the CRAFT-1 trial (abstr). J Am Coll Cardiol 1993; 21:203A.

43. Myers ML, Li G-H, Yaghi A, McCormack D. Human internal thoracic artery reactivity to dopaminergic agents. Circulation 1993; 88 (part 2):110–114.

44. Nul DR, Doval H, Grancelli H, et al. Amiodarone reduces mortality in severe heart failure (abstr). Circulation 1993; 88 (Suppl I):I–603.

45. PROMISE Study Research Group—Packer M, Carver JR, Rodeheffer RJ, et al., for the PROMISE Study Research Group. Effect of oral milrinone on mortality in severe chronic heart failure. N Engl J Med 1991; 325:1468–1475.

46. PROVED study—Uretsky BF, Young JB, Shahidi E, et al., on behalf of the PROVED Investigative Group. Randomized study assessing the effect of digoxin withdrawal in patients with mild to moderate chronic congestive heart failure: Results of the PROVED trial. J Am Coll Cardiol 1993; 22:955–962.

47. RADIANCE study—Packer M, Gheorghiade M, Young JB, et al., for the RADI-ANCE study. Withdrawal of digoxin from patients with chronic heart failure treated with angiotensin-converting enzyme inhibitors. N Engl J Med 1993; 329:1–7.

48. Ribner HS, Plucinski DA, Hsieh A-M, et al. Acute effects of digoxin on total systemic vascular resistance in congestive heart failure due to dilated cardiomyopathy: A hemodynamic-hormonal study. Am J Cardiol 1985; 56:896–904.

49. Rich MW. Congestive heart failure in the elderly. Cardiol in Elderly 1993; 1:372–380.

50. Ruffolo RR. The mechanism of action of dobutamine. Ann Intern Med 1984; 100:313–314.

51. Schafers RF, Adler S, Daul A, et al. Positive inotropic effects of the beta$_2$-adrenoceptor agonist terbutaline in the human heart: Effects of long-term beta$_1$-adrenoceptor antagonist treatment. J Am Coll Cardiol 1994; 23:1224–1233.

52. Schmidt TA, Holm-Nielsen P, Kjeldsen K. Human skeletal muscle digitalis glycoside receptors (Na,K-ATPase)—importance during digitalization. Cardiovasc Drugs Ther 1993; 7:175–181.

53. Schobel HP, Oren RM, Roach PJ, et al. Contrasting effects of digitalis and dobutamine on baroreflex sympathetic control in normal humans. Circulation 1991; 84:1118–1129.

54. Setaro JF, Zaret BL, Schulman DS, et al. Usefulness of verapamil for congestive heart failure associated with abnormal left ventricular diastolic filling and normal left ventricular systolic performance. Am J Cardiol 1990; 66:981–986.

55. Smith TW. Digoxin in heart failure. N Engl J Med 1993; 329:51–53.

56. Steimle AE, Stevenson LW, Fonarow GC, et al. Prediction of improvement in recent onset cardiomyopathy after referral for heart transplantation. J Am Coll Cardiol 1994; 23:553–559.

57. Taylor DO, Thompson JA, Ayres SM, Hess ML. Dobutamine. In: Messerli FH (ed). Cardiovascular Drug Therapy. WB Saunders, Philadelphia, 1990, pp 1072–1082.

58. Unverferth DV, Blanford M, Kates RE, Leier CV. Tolerance to dobutamine after a 72 hour continuous infusion. Am J Med 1980; 69:262–266.

59. Woldow A, Wang RY, Rajagopal DE, Cohen JJ. The use of digoxin 0.125 mg versus 0.25 mg daily as maintenance dosage in patients older than 75 years of age. Cardiol in Elderly 1993; 1:3–7.

60. Young JB, Gheorghiade M, Packer M, et al., on behalf of the PROVED and RADIANCE Investigators. Are low serum levels of digoxin effective in chronic heart failure? Evidence challenging the accepted guidelines for a therapeutic serum level of the drug (abstr). J Am Coll Cardiol 1993; 21:378A.

61. Zeppellini R, Bolognesi R, Javernaro A, et al. Effect of dobutamine on left ventricular relaxation and filling phase in patients with ischemic heart disease and preserved systolic function. Cardiovasc Drugs Ther 1993; 7:325–331.

# Notes

# 7  Antihypertensive Drugs

N.M. Kaplan  ◆  L.H. Opie

*"Over the past decade the goals of treatment have gradually shifted from efficacy in lowering blood pressure, which is taken for granted, toward patient well-being and potential for protection from future target-organ damage."*[68]

The blood pressure (BP) is the product of the cardiac output (CO) and the peripheral vascular resistance (PVR):

$$BP = CO \times PVR$$

Hence all antihypertensive drugs must act either by reducing the CO (beta-blockers) or the peripheral vascular resistance (all the others, and perhaps a late effect of beta-blockade). Diuretics act chiefly by volume depletion, thereby reducing the CO, and also as indirect vasodilators. All antihypertensive drugs, except the centrally active agents and ganglion blockers, have other uses and have therefore already been discussed in earlier chapters of this book. Despite the host of potential agents, the therapy of hypertension is usually simple, since many patients have minimally or moderately elevated pressures that usually respond adequately to lifestyle modification and to one or two drugs (Table 7–1). More effective, less bothersome, and longer-acting agents have become available so that for most hypertensives one or two pills every morning work quite well. Asymptomatic patients, however, often will not stay on therapy, particularly if it makes them feel weak, sleepy, forgetful or impotent. Fortunately, with most currently used modern antihypertensive agents, the quality of life improves rather than deteriorates.[74,112] A small proportion of patients have resistant hypertension, which may only respond to multiple therapies. It must constantly be considered that hypertension is usually multifactorial in etiology, that different drugs act by different mechanisms (Fig. 7–1) and that the aim is to match the drug to the patient.

## Principles of Treatment

### The Decision to Treat: Non-Drug Therapy

Before any drug is begun, persistence of the patient's hypertension should be ascertained by multiple measurements over at least a few weeks, preferably at home and at work, unless the pressure is so high (eg., > 180/110 mmHg) as to mandate immediate therapy. Non-drug therapies should be standard in all hypertensives, particularly weight reduction for the obese and moderate dietary **sodium restriction** such as 80 to 100 mmole/day or about 5 to 6 g sodium chloride or 2 g sodium,[13] which should be used before drugs in those with marginal elevations. To achieve the ideal low-sodium intake of below 70 mmole/day[110] is not easy. **Weight reduction** will reduce blood pressure and improve the quality of life,[110] and can be crucial in offsetting the increased cardiovascular risk from the cholesterol rise associated with diuretic use.[22,112] Weight reduction may specifically

174

**TABLE 7–1**    SPECIFICS ABOUT ORALLY EFFECTIVE ANTIHYPERTENSIVES

| DRUG | REGISTERED TRADE NAME (in USA) | DOSE RANGE (mg/DAY) | DOSES/DAY |
|---|---|---|---|
| **Diuretics** (see Table 6–3) | | | |
| Hydrochloro-thiazide | Hydrodiuril, Esidrix | 12.5–25 | 1 |
| Chlorthalidone | Hygroton | 12.5–25 | 1 |
| Indapamide | Lozol | 1.25–2.5 | 1 |
| Combination agents | Dyazide, Maxzide-25, Moduretic, Maxzide | ½–1 tablet ¼–½ tablet | 1 1 |
| Torsemide | Demadex | 5–10 | 1 |
| **Beta-blockers** | | | |
| Acebutolol | Sectral | 200–800 | 1 |
| Atenolol | Tenormin | 25–100 | 1 |
| Betaxolol | Kerlone | 5–20 | 1 |
| Bisoprolol | Zebeta | 5–10 | 1 |
| Carteolol | Cartrol | 2.5–10 | 1 |
| Metoprolol | Lopressor | 100–400 | 1–2 |
| Nadolol | Corgard | 40–320 | 1 |
| Penbutolol | Levatol | 10–20 | 1 |
| Pindolol | Visken | 10–60 | 2 |
| Propranolol | Inderal | 80–480 | 2 |
| Timolol | Blocadren | 20–60 | 2 |
| **Combined alpha-beta-blocker** | | | |
| Carvedilol | (not approved) | 25–50 | 1 |
| Labetalol | Normodyne, Trandate | 200–800 | 2 |
| **ACE inhibitors** | | | |
| Benazepril | Lotensin | 5–40 | 1 |
| Captopril | Capoten | 25–150 | 2 |
| Enalapril | Vasotec | 5–40 | 1–2 |
| Fosinopril | Monopril | 10–40 | 1 |
| Lisinopril | Prinivil, Zestril | 5–40 | 1 |
| Quinapril | Accupril | 5–80 | 1 |
| Ramipril | Altace | 2.5–20 | 1 |
| **Calcium antagonists** | | | |
| Verapamil SR | Isoptin SR, Calan SR, Verelan | 240–480 240–480 | 1–2 1 |
| Amlodipine | Norvasc | 2.5–10 | 1 |
| Diltiazem SR, CD or XR | Cardizem SR, CD Dilacor XR | 180–360 180–360 | (SR) 2 (CD, XR) 1 |
| Felodipine | Plendil ER | 5–20 | 1 |
| Isradipine | Dynacirc | 5–20 | 2 |
| Nicardipine | Cardene | 60–120 | 3 |
| Nifedipine XL, CC | Procardia XL, Adalat CC | 30–90 | 1 |
| Nifedipine | Procardia, Adalat | 20–120 | 2–3 |
| **Alpha-blockers** | | | |
| Prazosin | Minipress | 2.0–20.0 | 2 |
| Terazosin | Hytrin | 1–20 | 1 |
| Doxazosin | Cardura | 1–16 | 1 |
| **Direct vasodilators** | | | |
| Hydralazine | Apresoline | 50–200 | 2–3 |
| Minoxidil | Loniten | 5–40 | 1 |
| **Non-receptor adrenergic inhibitors** | | | |
| Reserpine | Serpasil | 0.05–0.25 | 1 |
| Rauwolfia root | Raudixin | 50–100 | 1 |
| **Centrally active:** | | | |
| Methyldopa | Aldomet | 500–1500 | 2 |
| Clonidine | Catapres | 0.5–1.5 | 1–2 |
| Clonidine transdermal | Catapres-TTX | 1 patch | (Once weekly) |
| Guanabenz | Wytensin | 8–64 | 2 |
| Guanfacine | Tenex | 1–3 | 1 |
| **Peripheral:** | | | |
| Guanethidine | Ismelin | 10–150 | 1 |
| Guanadrel | Hylorel | 10–75 | 2 |

## SITES OF ACTION OF ANTIHYPERTENSIVE AGENTS

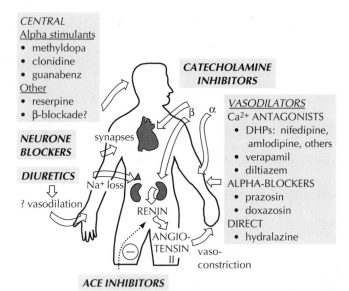

FIGURE 7–1. Different types of antihypertensive agents act at different sites. Because hypertension is frequently multifactorial in origin, it may be difficult to find the ideal drug for a given patient and drug combinations are often used. DHPs, dihydropyridines. Fig. copyright L.H. Opie.

benefit those with left ventricular hypertrophy.[57] The **ideal diet** is low in calories, rich in fresh rather than processed foods, and high in fruits and vegetables besides being low in sodium.[119] Other measures include increased **aerobic exercise,**[80] cessation of smoking, and decreased alcohol. Smoking may directly elevate systolic and diastolic blood pressure[70] particularly when combined with caffeine. Smoking may increase the swings in blood pressure that are thought to be damaging to the endothelium.[41] Smoking is an independent risk factor for coronary heart disease and stroke, besides increasing the risk of malignant hypertension (via accelerated renal artery damage).

Drugs should be reserved for those with higher blood pressure levels, especially in the presence of additional risk factors.

In the USA, an aggressive approach to the active drug therapy of even **minimally elevated pressures,** such as diastolics in the 90 to 100 mmHg range, has become "accepted medical practice." In most of the rest of the world, drug therapy is usually reserved for those with diastolics of 95 or 100 mmHg.[108] When in doubt about a marginal blood pressure level, multiple out-of-the-office readings should be obtained, either by inexpensive **home blood pressure** devices or by **ambulatory blood pressure monitoring.** As hypertension is merely one of several risk factors for coronary artery disease or stroke, it makes sense to treat at lower blood pressure values in the presence of higher blood cholesterols or in smokers or diabetics. It also makes sense to treat at lower blood pressure levels in patients with angina. Conversely, in very low risk groups (nonsmoking middle-aged white females) there may not be much advantage in drug treatment of mild to moderate hypertension. Consequently, voices for a less aggressive approach are being heard in the USA and elsewhere, and the current therapeutic overenthusiasm may cool.

The efficacy of antihypertensive treatment depends not only on the control of the blood pressure, but also on the control of coexisting risk factors, especially those for coronary heart disease which is the major cause of mortality in hypertension. Whereas in low-risk groups, many hundreds of patients must be treated to prevent one stroke, in very high-risk groups, such as the elderly, only 20 to 40 patients need to be treated for 1 year to prevent one cardiovascular event, including stroke because the majority of patients with mild to moderate hypertension are entirely asymptomatic, it is essential to match the drug to the patient. At least in some individuals drug treatment may impair the quality of life or induce adverse changes in blood chemistry and blood lipids. *Although virtually all recommendations for treatment, including those of the International Society of Hypertension, are based on a cut-off diastolic blood pressure level, it clearly makes sense to alter that level according to the degree of estimated risk for concomitant coronary artery disease, stroke or renal failure.*[76] *Moreover, systolic levels should be considered, particularly in the elderly. At all ages, they are even more predictive of risk than are diastolic levels.*

## Overall Aims of Treatment

Lowering the blood pressure should never be the sole aim of therapy. Ideally all abnormalities associated with hypertension, including shortened life expectancy, should be reverted to normal. Overall cardiovascular mortality has been reduced by therapy, primarily through a decrease in stroke mortality.[5] *Yet thus far in no single trial has mortality from coronary disease been convincingly improved,* although borderline decreases have been achieved in trials in the elderly.[91,105] Why are excess risks for coronary disease associated with elevated blood pressure not fully removed by reduction of the pressure to levels seen in untreated people? There are several possibilities including (1) the multifactorial nature of coronary heart disease, (2) the short duration of treatment, (3) the lack of adequate control of blood pressure, (4) the metabolic side-effects or other hazards of the drugs used, and (5) overtreatment in susceptible patients. Several trials have suggested a **J-shaped curve** indicating an increase of coronary complications in patients whose diastolic blood pressure was reduced to 85 mmHg or lower (or about 95 mmHg in the elderly). Reduction of diastolics below 95 mmHg during treatment has been associated with only a marginally lower incidence of stroke or coronary events than a reduction to higher values.[1] Therefore, at least in some patients, the effort involved, the discomfort to the patient, and the cost in achieving lower diastolics might not be worth it, especially because a fall of only 5 mmHg of the usual diastolic blood pressure removes at least one-third of the risk of stroke and one-fifth that of coronary heart disease.[5] Nonetheless, in patients at higher risk, or in diabetics, or those with end-organ damage, vigorous pursuit of blood pressure lowering to below 90 mmHg is warranted, unless the drop of diastolic blood pressure provokes symptoms such as angina.

## Choice of Initial Drug

Traditionally, a **diuretic** has been the first drug advocated by authorities and chosen by most practitioners.[1] Next, beta-blockers gained in popularity and these two categories are preferred for first-choice therapy by the Joint National Committee.[28] Even more recently, ACE inhibitors and calcium antagonists have become widely used, also in the elderly.[99] Although an overall meta-analysis of 14 major trials involving over 37,000 patients has demonstrated a modest protection against coronary disease by traditional treatment based on diuretics and beta-blockers, these agents were nevertheless only about half as effective as they should have been, taking into account the blood pressure reduction found (Fig. 7–2).[5] The reason for this discrepancy is not clear, but may include metabolic side-effects of diuretics[46A] and beta-blockers (Table 7–2).

METABOLIC CONSIDERATIONS.   A complex interrelation between hypertension, obesity and maturity onset diabetes may be explained by **insulin-resistance** as the common denominator (Fig. 7–3). The fear is that diuretics and beta-blockers, separately or especially together, may further impair insulin sensitivity with risk of overt diabetes

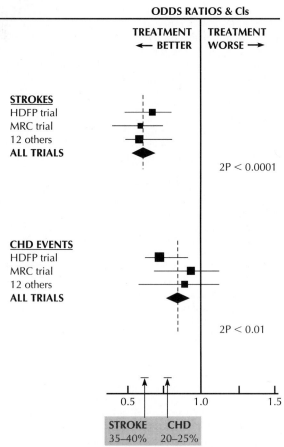

**FIGURE 7–2.** Results of meta-analysis of 4 large and 13 smaller trials showing uniform reduction of stroke and borderline reduction of CHD (coronary heart disease). Reproduced with permission from Collins and Peto, 1994. In: Swales JD (ed), Textbook of Hypertension, Blackwell Scientific Publications, Oxford, pp 1156–1164.

and/or lipid abnormalities. In contrast, other classes of antihypertensives, such as ACE inhibitors and alpha-blockers, seem to improve insulin sensitivity. Thus, these categories are logical first choice agents, as also recognized by the International Society of Hypertension[108]—yet there are unfortunately no long-term trials to prove their efficacy on morbidity or mortality.

CHOICE OF DRUGS. This should not be automatic, based upon habit (eg., the continued widespread use of methyldopa) or based upon the intensity of promotional advertising (eg., the minimal use of low-dose reserpine, which has no commercial advocates, or the excess use of ACE inhibitors, currently heavily promoted). Increasingly, instead of automatically going through a rigid step-care procedure, it seems logical that *the drug should be tailored to the patient* (Fig. 7–4). For example, in the presence of diabetes or gout, thiazide diuretics are usually contraindicated unless carefully given in low doses, whereas ACE inhibitors, alpha-blockers, and calcium antagonists are metabolically "neutral." In diabetic patients with renal disease, there is a special case for the use of ACE inhibitors. In black patients, ACE inhibitors and beta-blockers as monotherapy are not very effective, especially in older men. Although there can be no firm guidelines to such patient-guided therapy, some reasonable proposals can be offered (Table 7–3). A moderate dose of any of the five major groups of agents—calcium antagonists, diuretics, beta-blockers, ACE inhibitors, and alpha-blockers—when combined with lifestyle modifica-

**TABLE 7–2    CHIEF DISTINGUISHING FEATURES OF CLASSES OF ANTIHYPERTENSIVE AGENTS**

| | JNC 1ST CHOICE | WHO 1ST CHOICE | STROKE | CAD | ELDERLY | RENAL | INSULIN | BLOOD LIPIDS | PLASMA K$^+$ | PEAK EXERCISE |
|---|---|---|---|---|---|---|---|---|---|---|
| | | | OUTCOME STUDIES | | | | METABOLIC | | | |
| Diuretics | + | + | + | +/– | ++ | ? | ↓ | ↑/0 | ↓ | → |
| Beta-blockers | + | + | + | ? | + | ? | ↓ | ↑/0 | ↑ | → |
| Calcium antagonists | – | + | ? | ? | ? | ? | ↑ | ↑ | ← | ↑ |
| ACE inhibitors | – | + | ? | ? | ? | +* | ↑ | ↑→ | ↑ | ↑ |
| Alpha-blockers | – | + | ? | ? | ? | ? | → | ↓ | ↑ | ↑ |
| Central agents | – | – | ? | ? | ? | ? | ? | ↑ | ↑ | ↑ |

+ = JNC/WHO recommended; positive outcome studies.

– = not recommended; ? = not known; ↓ = decreased; ↑ = increased; → = unchanged

CAD = coronary artery disease

JNC = Joint National Council V 1993

WHO = World Health Organization—International Society of Hypertension

* renal protection in overt diabetic nephropathy

Insulin = insulin resistance

Peak exercise = capacity for maximum exercise.[88]

179

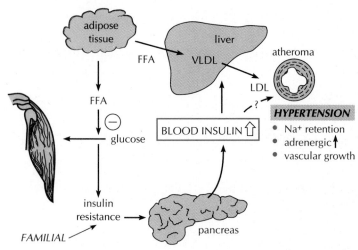

**FIGURE 7–3.** Proposed mechanisms of insulin resistance in (1) obese hypertensives (top left) and (2) familial hypertension (bottom left). Mechanisms whereby insulin evokes hypertension are still not clarified. See Salvetti et al.[101] Fig. copyright L.H. Opie.

tion will lower the blood pressure to about the same degree in most patients with mild hypertension.[112] It is in the moderately severe hypertensive patients that differences between old and young, and white and black, become more apparent,[90] at least in the case of men. A further point to consider is that the **response rate** to each of the five major groups of agents may be no more than about 50 to 60%, depending on the severity of the hypertension, so that combination therapy is often required in addition to lifestyle modification.

## Diuretics for Hypertension

The diuretic-first step-care approach has been used in most large therapeutic trials in the USA. Recently, diuretics have also been the basis of several impressive trials in the elderly in which hard end-points have been reduced. Diuretics are cheap. Thus, it is not surprising that they are still widely used either as monotherapy or in

STEP CARE: RIGID VS. LIBERAL

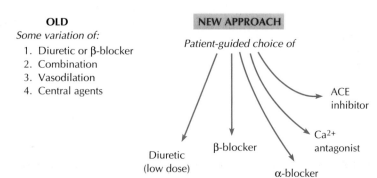

**FIGURE 7–4.** The concept of rigid step-care, almost always starting with a diuretic and going on to a beta-blocker before a vasodilator, is now being replaced by a much more liberal approach. Although the JNC has reverted back to a step-care policy based on diuretics and beta-blockers as first choice, yet according to the World Hypertension League,[119] any of five agents can be chosen as first-line therapy. Thereafter it is appropriate to proceed to combinations of those agents, progressively increasing the number of agents used, as required. Fig. copyright L.H. Opie and modified from Reference 1.

TABLE 7–3

| PATIENT-GUIDED THERAPY |
| PROPOSALS FOR FIRST CHOICE OF ANTIHYPERTENSIVE AGENTS |

| SITUATIONS FAVORING | RELATIVE CONTRAINDICATIONS AND SIDE-EFFECTS |
|---|---|
| **Diuretics** | |
| Elderly patients | Type II diabetes |
| Black ethnic group | Gout or prediabetes |
| In the obese, with weight reduction | Hyperlipidemia |
| | Pre-existing volume depletion |
| When cost is important | Young whites* |
| High salt intake | S/E: metabolic; impotence |
| Renal disease with sodium retention | |
| **Beta-blockade** | |
| Angina pectoris | Elderly blacks |
| Postinfarct prophylaxis | Left ventricular failure |
| Coexisting anxiety or tachycardia | Optimal physical activity required |
| Tense young patients | Hyperlipidemia (high TG, low HDL) |
| | Diabetes or prediabetes |
| | General contraindications (asthma) |
| | S/E: fatigue, cold extremities |
| **Calcium antagonists** | |
| Black ethnic group | Congestive heart failure |
| Elderly whites | Severe aortic stenosis |
| Physically active | Verapamil, diltiazem: |
| High salt intake | sick sinus syndrome, heart block |
| Maintenance of metabolic status | S/E: headache, flushing, |
| Associated angina, Raynaud's disease | tachycardia, ankle edema |
| **ACE inhibitors** | |
| Younger whites | Renal artery stenosis |
| High-renin status | Renal impairment |
| Low salt diet | Black ethnic group |
| Maintenance of metabolic status | S/E: hypotension, cough |
| Left ventricular hypertrophy | |
| Diabetic nephropathy | |
| Congestive heart failure | |
| **Alpha-blockers** | |
| Lipidemias | Aortic stenosis, severe |
| Prostatism | S/E: syncope, hypotension |
| Maintenance of metabolic status | |

S/E = side-effects; TG = triglycerides; HDL = high-density lipoproteins. * = see p 293

combination. Theoretically, they combine particularly well with beta-blockers or with ACE inhibitors (Fig. 7–5). The vascular complications that are more directly related to the height of the blood pressure per se (strokes and congestive heart failure) have been reduced, but the frequency of the most common cause of disease

## DIURETIC COMBINATIONS

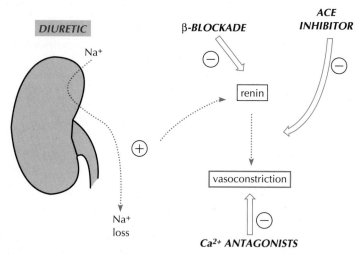

**FIGURE 7–5.** Diuretics, basically acting by sodium loss, cause an increased circulating renin which results in angiotensin-mediated vasoconstriction. Diuretics therefore combine well with beta-blockers which inhibit the release of renin, with ACE inhibitors which inhibit the formation of angiotensin-II, and with calcium antagonists which directly oppose diuretic-induced vasoconstriction. Of these combinations, that of diuretic and ACE inhibitor is particularly well tested. ACE inhibitors lessen the metabolic side-effects of diuretics. Fig. copyright L.H. Opie.

and death among hypertensives, namely coronary heart disease, has not fallen as much as anticipated (Fig. 7–2). Hypothetically, metabolic side-effects of the high doses of diuretics, particularly on lipids and insulin sensitivity, as well as potassium and magnesium depletion,[46A] may in part explain why death from coronary disease has not decreased as much as it should have. Also on the debit side, impotence seems to be a serious side-effect, although reduced by low-dose diuretics[110] when compared with standard dose.[111]

DIURETIC DOSE. Although a single morning dose of 25 mg of **hydrochlorothiazide** or its equivalent will provide a 10 mmHg fall in the blood pressure of most uncomplicated hypertensives within several weeks, even that dose is probably too high. Lower doses (12.5 mg hydrochlorothiazide) are equally effective especially when combined with beta-blockade or ACE inhibition. Nevertheless, only 12.5 mg hydrochlorothiazide may still induce early (and possibly transient) blood lipid abnormalities,[16] even though the blood sugar does not rise.[4] Such low doses of hydrochlorothiazide may require several weeks to act.[117] Even lower doses, such as 6.25 mg hydrochlorothiazide, may be antihypertensive, particularly in black patients.[66] Low-dose thiazides, if ineffective, may be combined with a calcium blocker such as verapamil[75] or diltiazem,[117] or a beta-blocker,[66] or an ACE inhibitor (p 124). Alternatively, salt restriction may be the secret in making low-dose hydrochlorothiazide work.[119] The advantage of low-dose hydrochlorothiazide (or its equivalent in other diuretics) is that adverse metabolic and lipid effects are minimized or completely avoided.[51] Logically, the lower the dose of diuretic, the fewer the metabolic side-effects, whereas the antihypertensive potency may still be adequately expressed.

Whether or not changes in blood lipids with standard doses of hydrochlorothiazide, such as 25 mg, are transient or sustained is a matter of dispute. In a recent careful placebo-controlled study of over 1,000 hypertensives, cholesterol changes found at 3 months in patients given 12.5 mg to 50 mg hydrochlorothiazide daily were no different from placebo nor from groups treated by an ACE inhibitor, an alpha-blocker, or a calcium antagonist.[55] That study was confined to males. In contrast, in a population consisting largely of middle-aged black females, thiazide treatment (25 to 50 mg daily) over 5 years still significantly increased glucose and cholesterol when compared with non-thiazide-treated groups.[61] To be safe, concurrent dietary control of cholesterol is advisable.

OTHER THIAZIDES. The longer-acting **chlorthalidone** at a lower dose of 15 mg daily is almost as good as 25 mg and less hypokalemic.[35] Chlorthalidone 15 mg daily was used in the TOMH study[111] in patients with very mild hypertension. Combined with weight loss and other measures, it was as effectively antihypertensive as other groups of agents. It gave an unexpectedly good quality of life (despite the marginally higher incidence of impotence) and at the end of 4 years blood cholesterol changes (elevated at 1 year) had reverted to normal.[112] Chlorthalidone 12.5 mg daily was the first-line treatment in the study on systolic hypertension in the elderly.[105] Thereafter the dose was doubled and atenolol 25 mg daily was added. After 4.5 years, total stroke was reduced by 36%.

The modified thiazide **indapamide (Lozol, Natrilix)** may be more lipid neutral. The previous standard dose of 2.5 mg once daily has been dropped by the manufacturers to 1.25 mg daily for at least 4 weeks, followed by a dose increase if needed. Yet the potassium may fall, and the blood glucose and uric acid rise, as warned in the package insert. Nonetheless, indapamide may be better than hydrochlorothiazide in inducing regression of left ventricular hypertrophy.[104]

Of the **loop diuretics,** the recently introduced **torsemide (Demadex)** is particularly well studied in hypertension.[43] Some reports have suggested that torsemide is free of metabolic and lipid side-effects besides being antihypertensive when used in the subdiuretic dose of 2.5 mg.[43] At the higher doses registered for use in the USA, namely 5 to 10 mg once daily, it becomes natriuretic with greater risk of metabolic changes.

**Potassium-sparing diuretics** may add a few cents to the cost but save a good deal more by the prevention of diuretic-induced hypokalemia and hypomagnesemia, and hence by lessening or avoiding associated metabolic changes. The risk of torsades-related sudden death should also be reduced.[46A] Blood lipid changes may also be lessened or avoided.[43] To be effectively antihypertensive, the potassium-sparing agents are combined with another diuretic generally a thiazide. The combinations of triamterene (**Dyazide, Maxzide**) or amiloride (**Moduretic**) with hydrochlorothiazide are usually chosen rather than spironolactone (**Aldactazide**) because the latter decreases testosterone synthesis. The dose of hydrochlorothiazide in one tablet of Dyazide is 25 mg, but only about half is absorbed. Maxzide contains 25 or 50 mg hydrochlorothiazide. Standard Moduretic contains 50 mg (far too much), but in Europe, a "mini-Moduretic" (**Moduret**) with half the standard thiazide dose is now marketed to overcome this objection. However, even these doses may be too high.

COMBINATION WITH OTHER ANTIHYPERTENSIVES. Diuretics may add to the effect of almost all other types of antihypertensives, with the possible exception of the dihydropyridine calcium antagonists. Combination with ACE inhibition is particularly logical (p 124). A number of well-designed factorial studies have varied the dose of hydrochlorothiazide from 6.25 mg to 25 mg and studied the interaction with a beta-blocker,[66,84] or diltiazem[4] or an ACE inhibitor.[49] In general, a surprising blood pressure reduction can be obtained from only 6.25 mg thiazide when combined with only a low dose of the second agent. For diltiazem the same principle holds, but the lowest thiazide dose tested was 12.5 mg daily. Previous evidence also argues for 6.25 mg hydrochlorothiazide in combination with enalapril.[39] In general, somewhat greater antihypertensive effects were obtained with 25 mg hydrochlorothiazide, yet the difference between the high and

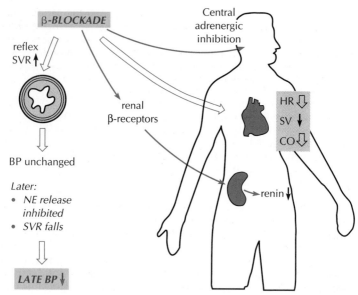

FIGURE 7-6. Proposed antihypertensive mechanisms of beta-blockade. An early fall in cardiac output (CO) does not lead to a corresponding fall in blood pressure because of baroreflex-mediated increased peripheral alpha-adrenergic vasoconstriction. Within a few days beta-blockade of prejunctional receptors on the terminal neurone with consequent inhibition of release of norepinephrine (NE) may explain why the systemic vascular resistance (SVR) falls to normal. The blood pressure (BP) now falls. In the case of vasodilatory beta-blockers, especially those with added alpha-blockade, there is an early decrease in SVR and a rapid fall in BP.[88] HR = heart rate; SV = stroke volume. Fig. copyright L.H. Opie.

the low doses of thiazide were negligible when the alternate agent was given at higher doses. Thus there is a good argument for starting combination therapy with 6.25 mg hydrochlorothiazide, a dose which effectively prevents hypokalemia.

DIURETICS: CONCLUSIONS. Despite reservations about metabolic side-effects, diuretics remain among the preferred initial treatment in the elderly,[105,107] the obese and in black patients. Diuretics appear to work particularly well in elderly blacks while being much less effective in younger whites.[90] In the obese, if there is no response to low-dose diuretic therapy, weight reduction must be insisted on. The next step might be to add an ACE inhibitor or alpha-blocker rather than to increase the diuretic in view of the association of obesity with insulin insensitivity. Compared with placebo, diuretics have been shown to reduce stroke in the elderly and in patients with mild to moderate hypertension.[5,105] Strictly speaking, we do not know that the low doses of diuretics currently used really result in patient benefit except in the elderly where low-dose chlorthalidone (12.5 mg) was chosen as initial therapy in the SHEP study;[105] even there, in many patients the dose was doubled and a beta-blocker added.

## Beta-blockers for Hypertension

For initial therapy of hypertension, beta-blockade is now recommended as an alternative to diuretic therapy by the Joint National Committee. The antihypertensive mechanisms are still not well understood (Fig. 7-6). It is particularly suitable for patients with "increased adrenergic drive," those with associated angina pectoris, or in postinfarct patients. In young hypertensives (17 to 29 years old), the cardiac output is high and the systemic vascular resistance not increased,[11] so that beta-blockade should theoretically be ideal treatment, although no formal studies can prove this point. In older hypertensives (mean age 59 years), particularly in white males, beta-blockers gave good results[90] and in some outcome studies beta-blockade, mostly combined with a diuretic, reduced mortality.[106] In the MRC trial in the elderly,[91] diuretics reduced mortality from coronary heart disease, whereas beta-blockers did not.

In black patients, vasodilation or sodium loss seems to be the key to successful treatment; hence, logical first choices are diuretics,[1] or the vasodilatory beta-blocker, labetalol,[1] or centrally active agents or vasodilators apart from the ACE inhibitors. In general, black patients have low renin values and so do the elderly; thus, the ineffectiveness of atenolol and captopril in elderly black males[90] is explicable.

DOSE. It is best to start with a low dose to lessen the chances of initial fatigue, which is probably due in part to the fall in cardiac output. A low dose, in the elderly, lessens the risk of excess bradycardia. Today, standard doses are what used to be termed low. For example, with propranolol there is little, if any, additional antihypertensive effect with doses above 80 mg/day, given either once or twice per day.[1] If the response to ordinary doses of a beta-blocker is inadequate, a higher dose may sometimes work but, more generally, it is easier to change to another category of agent or to undertake combination therapy.

PHARMACOKINETICS. Dose adjustment is more likely to be required with more lipid-soluble (lipophilic) agents, which have a high "first-pass" liver metabolism that may result in active metabolites (4-hydroxypropranolol or the diacetolol metabolite of acebutolol); the rate of formation will depend on liver blood flow and function. The ideal beta-blocker for hypertension would be long-acting, cardioselective (Fig. 1–8), and usually effective in a standard dose; there would also be simple pharmacokinetics (no liver metabolism, little protein binding, no lipid-solubility, and no active metabolites). Sometimes added vasodilation should be an advantage, as in the elderly[107] or in black patients. When a vasodilatory beta-blocker was compared with atenolol over 1 year in younger hypertensives, there was no difference in the overall effects or side-effects.[2] The ideal drug would be "lipid neutral" as claimed for agents with ISA or particularly cardioselective agents with ISA, such as acebutolol.[111,112] In smaller trials, celiprolol has also been promising, yet even standard beta-blockers, such as propranolol and atenolol, tend to drop blood cholesterol in patients with initially high values.[115] In practice, once-a-day therapy is satisfactory with many beta-blockers, but it is important to check early morning blood pressure to ensure 24 hour coverage (as with all agents).

COMBINATION THERAPY WITH BETA-BLOCKADE FOR HYPERTENSION. Combinations of beta-blockers with one or another agent from all other classes have been successful in the therapy of hypertension.

In the case of **diuretics plus beta-blockers,** the total daily dose of beta-blocker plus thiazide combination should ideally contain no more than 12.5 mg hydrochlorothiazide, 2.5 mg bendrofluazide, or a similar low dose of another diuretic.[1] A combination of bisoprolol plus 6.25 mg hydrochlorothiazide (**Ziac**) is now available in the USA and licensed for initial therapy. Double the ideal diuretic doses are provided in the USA by **Timolide** (10 mg timolol, 25 mg hydrochlorothiazide) or **Corzide** (80 mg nadolol, 5 mg bendrofluazide). Neither combination agent has a potassium-retaining component, provided in Europe by **Kalten** with 50 mg atenolol, 25 mg hydrochlorothiazide, and 2.5 mg amiloride.

**Beta-blocker plus nifedipine** (or any other dihydropyridine) is a hemodynamically sound combination, with powerful afterload reduction achieved by the dihydropyridine offsetting the bradycar-

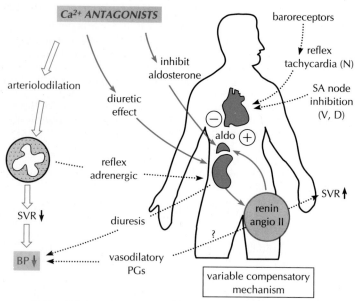

**FIGURE 7–7.** Calcium antagonists evoke counter-regulatory mechanisms, dependent on stimulation of renin and formation of angiotensin, as well as on reflex release of norepinephrine. The baroreceptor reflexes are inhibited by severe hypertension, by increasing age, and by continued use of the calcium antagonist drugs (nifedipine more so than verapamil, in turn more so than diltiazem). The concomitant use of ACE inhibitors is logical because ACE inhibitors decrease peripheral vasoconstriction and indirectly act as sympatholytic agents (Fig. 5–5). Fig. copyright L.H. Opie.

dia and negative inotropic effects of beta-blockade. There is an added hypotensive effect. Such combination therapy may be used both in mild to moderate hypertension not responding to monotherapy,[1] and in severe or refractory hypertension when further combination with a diuretic is usual.[1] In Europe, combination acebutolol with nifedipine is available, as well as atenolol-nifedipine (**Tenif** or **Beta-Adalat**), consisting of atenolol 50 mg and slow-release nifedipine 20 mg; the dose is 1–2 capsules daily for hypertension. In a large randomized controlled study, nifedipine was more effective than atenolol in lowering systolic blood pressure, both drugs were equally effective in lowering diastolic blood pressure, and when patients failed to respond to atenolol or nifedipine alone, the combination showed further reduction in blood pressure.[9]

## Calcium Antagonists for Hypertension

Calcium antagonists compare well in their hypotensive effect with the established first-line agents, diuretics or beta-blockers. Calcium antagonists act primarily to reduce peripheral vascular resistance, aided by at least an initial diuretic effect, especially in the case of nifedipine-like agents. No negative inotropic effect can be detected in patients with initially normal myocardial function. All three prototypical calcium antagonists, especially nifedipine, tend to increase plasma catecholamines modestly with a borderline elevation of plasma renin activity caused by the counter-regulatory effect (Fig. 7–7). There are no long-term outcome studies available on calcium antagonists in hypertension. As a group, calcium antagonists and especially nifedipine and verapamil are well tested in patients with severe hypertension. These agents are particularly effective in elderly patients and are equally effective in blacks as in nonblacks. Calcium antagonists may be selected as initial monotherapy, especially if there are other indications for these agents such as angina pectoris, Raynaud's phenomenon, or supraventricular tachycardia. Several formulations are now available providing 24 hour blood pressure coverage with once-daily dosing.

CHOICE OF AGENT. Nifedipine is among the most effective antihypertensives in severe hypertension and its use for mild to moderate hypertension has increased with the introduction of extended once-daily tablets (**Procardia-XL, Adalat CC**). In the TOMH study,[111] **amlodipine** 5 mg once-daily was one of five drugs that reduced blood pressure with minimal side-effects and was the best-tolerated drug. Headache and ankle swelling are likely to remain the limiting side-effects of all dihydropyridines. The mild diuretic effect of the dihydropyridines contributes to the long-term benefit. **Verapamil** and diltiazem are also increasingly chosen as first-line antihypertensive agents, especially if angina is associated. Frequent constipation with **verapamil** is a disadvantage especially in the elderly although in those on high fiber diets, verapamil can obviate diarrhea. In the massive VA study, diltiazem (sustained-release) in a dose of 120 to 360 mg daily had the highest success rate in blacks and was second best of the tested agents in older whites.[90] Both verapamil and diltiazem are now available in once-daily preparations.

**Compared with diuretics** (also advocated for elderly or black patients), calcium antagonists are more expensive; however, calcium antagonists cause little or no metabolic disturbances in potassium, glucose, uric acid or lipid metabolism, nor does aldosterone increase, while with long-acting preparations renin rises only slightly or not at all. Patients on calcium antagonists do not require intermittent blood chemistry checks. There is no evidence that calcium antagonists cause impairment of renal function as may be found with thiazide diuretics. Experimentally, the calcium antagonists protect from glomerular injury after subtotal nephrectomy by reducing compensatory glomerular growth.[59]

**Compared with beta-blockers,** calcium antagonists cause less fatigue and little or no interference with normal cardiovascular dynamics especially during exercise.[96] Calcium antagonists have fewer contraindications and can, for example, be used safely in asthmatics, cause little or no interference with diabetic control and are not contraindicated in peripheral vascular disease. Beta-blockers have established postinfarct protection. Verapamil is, however, licensed in some European countries for postinfarct protection when beta-blockers are contraindicated. Verapamil can reduce blood pressure and reinfarction.[77] Diltiazem may also be used in those without pulmonary congestion.[21] Caution is advised with dihydropyridines postinfarction.

COMBINATIONS WITH CALCIUM ANTAGONISTS. **Calcium antagonist plus beta-blocker therapy** has been well studied and is especially safe in the case of dihydropyridines. Whether or not addition of a diuretic has added benefit may depend on the type of calcium antagonist used. In the case of verapamil[75] and diltiazem,[4] the evidence for added benefit is good, whereas in the case of nifedipine and other dihydropyridines the evidence is not.[12] Furthermore, the dihydropyridines may be effective even in the presence of a high sodium intake[8] and it is doubtful whether a low sodium diet enhances their efficacy.[119] Calcium antagonists are thought to be most effective in the same groups as diuretics (elderly, blacks) and the DHP calcium antagonists may have inherent diuretic properties. Therefore the combination of the DHP calcium antagonists with beta-blockers seems more logical than that of calcium antagonists with diuretics, unless there is a persisting high-sodium intake.[8] There are no comparative outcome studies in which calcium antagonists have been put against beta-blockers or diuretics, so that the advantages of choosing a calcium antagonist must be predicted by an equal antihypertensive efficacy and lack of metabolic adverse effects.

**Calcium antagonists and ACE inhibitors** should combine well,[33] without the hemodynamic disadvantages of beta-blockade or the

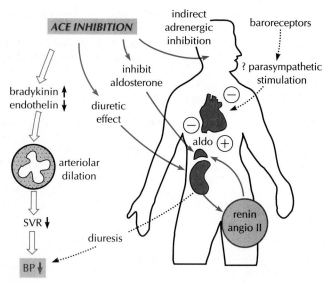

**FIGURE 7–8.** Proposed mechanisms whereby ACE inhibitors as a class may have their antihypertensive effects. Note that the major effect is on the peripheral arterioles causing vasodilation and a fall in the systemic vascular resistance (SVR), also called the peripheral vascular resistance. Indirect inhibition of adrenergic activity also promotes arteriolar dilation. Decreased angiotensin-II levels may also act by increased formation of bradykinin and vasodilatory prostaglandins as well as by inhibition of central effects of angiotensin-II. Parasympathetic activity also appears to be stimulated. PGs = prostaglandins; aldo = aldosterone. Fig. copyright L.H. Opie.

metabolic problems caused by diuretics. ACE inhibitors oppose the negative counterregulation induced by the powerful vasodilatory calcium antagonists (Fig. 7–7). In the case of hypertensives with early renal disease, verapamil and ACE inhibitor reduced microalbuminuria more than did either agent singly.[42,65] More information is needed on this combination, particularly outcome studies.

OUTCOME STUDIES WITH CALCIUM ANTAGONISTS. These are still missing. The first home will probably be the SystEur study[36] in which nitrendipine is the basic agent in elderly hypertensives. Others under way are the second STOP (Swedish Trial in Old Patients) study in which one of the three arms will be the calcium antagonists, felodipine and isradipine, compared with diuretics and beta-blockers. In the HOT (Hypertension Optimal Treatment) study, the effect of felodipine on cardiovascular morbidity and mortality will be evaluated at various diastolic blood pressure therapeutic goals (DBP equal to or less than 90, 85 or 80 mmHg). Whether, while these trials are awaited, the current American and Canadian official recommendations[108] to use diuretics and/or beta-blockers first will influence the stampede toward ACE inhibitors and calcium antagonists remains to be seen.

## ACE Inhibitors for Hypertension

ACE inhibitors (Fig. 7–8), once reserved for refractory hypertension, especially when renal in origin, have edged their way into a prime position, where they are recognized as one of several agents of first choice. ACE inhibitors have minimal side-effects (cough), simplicity of use, a flat dose-response curve, virtual absence of contraindications except for bilateral renal artery stenosis and some related types of renal impairment, and ready combination with other modalities of treatment as well as acceptability by the elderly. Furthermore, a specific case can be made for their preferential use in diabetic hypertensives, in patients with hyperuricemia, and in post-infarction follow-up.

Captopril was the first ACE inhibitor, but multiple others are now available, one from almost every drug company. All are antihypertensive, with a few practical differences (Table 5–3), except that (1) ramipril seems to have the longest plasma half-life, and (2) lisinopril has the simplest pharmacokinetics being water soluble and not metabolized by the liver.

In **mild to moderate hypertension,** ACE inhibitors can be used as monotherapy, even in low-renin patients,[1] or in combination with other standard agents. For monotherapy, moderate dietary salt restriction is especially important.[119] The reason why only a variable percentage of mild to moderate hypertensives respond to monotherapy with ACE inhibition (from less than 50 to 75%) may be the variable sodium intake and differences between white and black patients (see p 193).

RENAL DISEASE AND ACE INHIBITORS. In **renovascular hypertension,** where circulating renin is high and a critical part of the hypertensive mechanism, ACE inhibition is logical first-line therapy. Because the hypotensive response may be dramatic, a low test dose is essential; because captopril acts quickest and is shortest in its duration of action, the **test dose** for ACE inhibitors should be 6.25 mg captopril. With standard doses of captopril or enalapril, the GFR falls acutely[1] to largely recover in cases of unilateral, but not bilateral, disease. However, blood flow to the stenotic kidney may remain depressed after removal of the angiotensin-II support, and progressive ischemic atrophy is possible.[26] This mechanism is quite different from the immune-based renal toxicity caused by captopril in the early high-dose studies. Careful follow-up of renal blood flow and function is required. Angioplasty or surgery is preferable to chronic medical therapy.

In **bilateral renal artery stenosis,** ACE inhibitors should be given only with greatest care (if at all). Similar contraindications hold for unilateral renal artery disease in a solitary kidney or when renal failure complicates renal artery stenosis.

In **acute severe hypertension,** sublingual (chewed) captopril rapidly brings down the blood pressure,[1] but it is not clear how bilateral renal artery stenosis can be excluded quickly enough to make the speed of action of captopril an important benefit. Furthermore, the safety of such sudden falls of blood pressure in the presence of possible renal impairment (always a risk in severe hypertension) has not been evaluated.

In **diabetic hypertensives,** ACE inhibitors may be better than beta-blockade or diuretics because of the benefit against progressive glomerulosclerosis[86] and because blood sugar regulation is unaltered. Diabetic hypertension may be a clear indication for preferential use of the ACE inhibitors.[23] In a comparative study, captopril decreased filtration fraction, whereas nifedipine increased it; correspondingly, captopril reduced albuminuria, whereas nifedipine increased it,[20] suggesting that the site of vasodilation might be important. Preglomerular vasodilation by calcium antagonists may increase intraglomerular pressure and albuminuria, whereas postglomerular dilation by the ACE inhibitors may be beneficial. Proper clinical study of this potential difference is needed.

In **nondiabetic hypertension with microalbuminuria,** ACE inhibitors are being tested for a possible beneficial effect, acting by reduction of intrarenal hypertension.

In **hypertensive renal failure,** ACE inhibitors appear to slow the progression to the end stage when compared with beta-blockers.[72A]

SPECIAL GROUPS OF PATIENTS. In **elderly hypertensives,** ACE inhibitors were originally thought not to work so well because of the trend to a low renin status in that group. Several studies have now documented the efficacy of ACE inhibition therapy in elderly whites,[90] although in many studies a diuretic was added.[23]

In **black hypertensives,** ACE inhibitors are not very effective unless an added diuretic is given. In **elderly black hypertensive males,** captopril was no better than placebo,[90] perhaps because there were two factors (ethnic group and age) both predisposing to a low-renin state.

In **hypertension with heart failure,** ACE inhibitors with diuretics are automatic first-line therapy.

In **pregnancy hypertension,** ACE inhibitors are contraindicated.

COMBINATIONS WITH ACE INHIBITORS. ACE inhibitors are often combined with **thiazide diuretics** to enhance hypotensive effects (see Fig. 7–3), and to lessen metabolic side-effects.[1] This combination is logical because diuretics increase renin, the effects of which are antagonized by ACE inhibitors. Combinations of several ACE inhibitors with diuretics are now available. The ideal thiazide dose should not exceed 12.5 mg hydrochlorothiazide.[1] A higher dose gives no better antihypertensive effect.[53] Such addition of a thiazide is better from the blood pressure point of view than increasing the dose of the ACE inhibitor.[31] When combined with potassium-retaining thiazide diuretics (**Dyazide, Moduretic, Maxzide**), and especially spironolactone,[1] there is a **risk of hyperkalemia** because ACE inhibitors decrease aldosterone secretion and hence tend to retain potassium (Fig. 7–8).

**ACE inhibition plus beta-blockade** is a combination widely used in hypertension, although theoretically it is not the combination of choice because both agents have an ultimate antirenin effect. Nonetheless, current studies show additive antihypertensive effects.

**ACE inhibitors plus calcium antagonists** are now increasingly used in the therapy of hypertension. This combination attacks both the renin-angiotensin system and the increased peripheral vascular resistance. There may be specific renal benefits (verapamil study). Both types of agents are free of metabolic and central nervous side-effects. Large-scale studies on the combination are lacking.

OUTCOME STUDY. The major defect with the ACE inhibitors is that there are no hard outcome data to substantiate their frequent use as first-line agents in hypertension. The CAPPP (Captopril Prevention Project) study on about 7,000 hypertensives has as end-points cardiovascular mortality and morbidity, and results will become available in 1995.

## Alpha-Adrenergic Blockers

Of the alpha$_1$-receptor blockers, **prazosin (Minipress)**, **terazosin (Hytrin)**, and **doxazosin (Cardura)** are available in the USA. Their advantages are freedom from metabolic or lipid side-effects and a more appropriate physiologic action than beta-blockers in lowering peripheral resistance. Some patients develop troublesome side-effects: drowsiness, postural hypotension, and occasional tachycardia. Tolerance, related to fluid retention, may develop during chronic therapy with alpha$_1$-blockers, requiring increased doses[1] or added diuretics. Nonetheless, these agents clearly have a place in initial monotherapy. In the TOMH studies[111,112] on mild hypertension, doxazosin 2 mg/day given over 4 years and combined with hygienic measures reduced the blood pressure as much as agents from other groups. The quality of life improved as much as with placebo, though not quite as much as with acebutolol, and blood cholesterol fell. In the VA study on more severely hypertensive males, prazosin 4 to 20 mg/day given over 1 year had a success rate (DBP fell to below 95 mmHg) in 54% versus placebo 31%.[90] There appeared to be no particularly important influences of ethnic group nor age.

Alpha-blockers are particularly chosen in those with some disturbance of the blood lipid profile, or in diabetics, or in men with benign prostatic hypertrophy. Alpha-blockers combine well with beta-blockers or diuretics. In the case of calcium antagonists there may be an excess hypotensive response, as the combination eliminates two of the three major vasoconstrictive mechanisms, the remaining one being angiotensin-mediated. Thus, when used with care, alpha-blockers are often excellent catalysts to calcium antagonists. Little is known of alpha-blockers plus ACE inhibitors. Phenoxybenzamine and phentolamine are combined alpha$_1$- and alpha$_2$-blockers used only for **pheochromocytoma.**

## Direct Vasodilators

**Hydralazine** used to be a standard third drug, its benefits enhanced and side-effects lessened by concomitant use of a diuretic and an adrenergic inhibitor. Being inexpensive, hydralazine is still widely used in the Third World. Elsewhere fear of lupus (especially with continued doses above 200 mg daily) and lack of evidence for regression of left ventricular hypertrophy has led to its replacement by the calcium antagonist vasodilators. **Minoxidil** is a potent long-acting vasodilator acting on the potassium channel. There is renal excretion without hepatic metabolism, and the biologic half-life is 1 to 4 days. It often causes profuse hirsutism so its use is usually limited to men with severe refractory hypertension or renal insufficiency (it dilates renal arterioles). Occasionally minoxidil causes pericarditis. In one series, LV mass increased by 30%.

## Central Adrenergic Inhibitors

Of the centrally-acting agents, **reserpine** is easiest to use in a low dose of 0.05 mg/day, which provides almost all of its antihypertensive action with fewer side-effects than higher doses.[1] Onset and offset of action are slow and measured in weeks. When cost is crucial, reserpine and diuretics are the cheapest combination. **Methyldopa,** still widely used despite adverse central symptoms and potentially serious hepatic and blood side-effects, acts like clonidine on central alpha$_2$-receptors, usually without slowing the heart rate.[1] **Clonidine, guanabenz** and **guanafacine** provide all of the benefits of methyldopa with none of the rare but serious autoimmune reactions (as with methyldopa, sedation is frequent). In the VA study,[90] clonidine 0.2 to 0.6 mg/day was among the more effective of the agents tested. It worked equally well in younger and older age groups and in black and whites. The major disadvantage was the highest incidence of drug intolerance (14%). A **transdermal form of clonidine (Catapres-TTS)** provides once-a-week therapy likely minimizing the risks of clonidine-withdrawal. **Guanabenz** resembles clonidine but may cause less fluid retention and reduces serum cholesterol by 5 to 10%. **Guanfacine** is a similar agent which can be given once daily.

## Patient Profiling

Ideally, the antihypertensive drug should be matched to the patient.

HYPERTENSIVES WITH LIPIDEMIAS. Although doses of diuretics previously used increased plasma cholesterol, with modern low-dose treatment the problem is less.[81] The increase of blood cholesterol found after 1 year with chlorthalidone (15 mg daily) reverted to normal after 4 years, probably because of concurrent rigid dietary fat restriction.[112] Thus the diuretic dose should be as low as possible, while maintaining antihypertensive efficacy.[81]

Regarding beta-blockade, many clinicians assume (without sure evidence) that the partial protection beta-blockers provide against recurrent heart attacks may serve to prevent initial coronary events in hypertensives, but the evidence is not clear-cut with only one of five trials showing that a beta-blocker was better than a diuretic.[27,91] Pooled data suggest a small benefit in men, especially nonsmokers. In general, beta-blockers tend to raise serum triglycerides, to lower HDL-cholesterol levels, and to impair insulin sensitivity.[25] Beta-blockers with ISA may decrease rather than increase the serum total and LDL-cholesterol. Not even conventional beta-blockers increase an initially high serum cholesterol value.[115]

In contrast to the potential problems raised by diuretics and beta-blockers, the alpha-blockers clearly improve the blood lipid profile, whereas the ACE inhibitors and calcium antagonists are "lipid neutral" in most studies, or even tend to reduce the cholesterol. All of these agents also allow a better exercise performance than beta-blockers.[96]

The ideal prevention of coronary heart disease in hypertensives with lipidemia would include not only control of blood pressure but also of the blood lipid profile and other risk factors such as smoking. Thus, strict dietary recommendations should be followed, the dose of diuretic kept low, the beta-blocker (if necessary) chosen with care, and lifestyle modifications should be followed. Exercise helps to normalize blood lipid patterns (Table 10–4) in part by specifically increasing HDL-cholesterol.

*Whatever the drug chosen, evaluation of blood cholesterol is essential in all hypertensives.* Hopefully, more vigorous treatment of associated lipid abnormalities as well as the blood pressure will in time lead to decreased coronary artery disease.[30]

HYPERTENSIVES WITH ANGINA. Here the preferred agents are beta-blockers and calcium antagonists or both. Diuretics, alpha-blockers and ACE-inhibitors do not have direct anti-anginal effects, although indirect improvements in the myocardium oxygen balance by regression of left ventricular hypertrophy and/or reduction of blood pressure should benefit. In patients with angina and lipidemia, the category of beta-blocker of choice may be cardioselective with ISA (acebutolol, celiprolol) or pindolol (nonselective), although standard beta-blockers may not be as harmful on blood lipids as commonly supposed.[115]

POSTINFARCT HYPERTENSIVES. In hypertensives, AMI often drops the blood pressure, which may then creep back in the postinfarct months. There has been no adequate prospective study to determine the best treatment of postinfarct hypertension. Retrospective analyses give some guidance.[77] Currently, the agents of choice are beta-blockers with added ACE inhibitors when there is early left ventricular dysfunction. In normotensive patients without a history of congestive heart failure, a retrospective analysis shows that verapamil reduces blood pressure and reinfarction.[77] Diltiazem should work likewise, while dihydropyridines are best avoided, judging by the failure of nifedipine to benefit normotensive postinfarct patients.[77]

HYPERTENSION IN THE ELDERLY. What constitutes hypertension in the elderly and who constitute the elderly are moot questions. Nonetheless, four large and three smaller trials have documented even better protection against strokes and congestive heart failure by treatment of the elderly than reported in the middle-aged in prior trials.[78] Thus, an equivalent blood pressure reduction will produce a greater benefit in the elderly than in younger patients.[93] Although reduction of coronary events is a more elusive goal, it was achieved in several studies.[62,105] The overall death rate fell in the STOP study,[105] and in others the trend was downwards.[44]

Which age groups? The largest studies[91,105] chose 65 to 74 and 60 to 80 years. Concern remains about the very old, over age 75, since increased mortality can occur with even as little as 5 mmHg reduction in diastolic blood pressure.[85] In this age group, treatment, if at all, should be gentle.

Which blood pressure limits? There is compelling evidence to suggest that sustained systolic blood pressure elevations above 160 mmHg require treatment,[44,100] even in the absence of any rise in diastolic blood pressure, so that **isolated systolic hypertension** is now actively treated. With lower systolic values, sustained diastolic blood pressure values of 100 mmHg or more **(isolated diastolic hypertension)** are often taken as an indication for therapy, although trial-based data suggest a value of 105 mmHg.[100] In the presence of end-organ damage, including abnormalities of the thoracic or abdominal aorta, lower blood pressure values should be taken.

Which drug? Again, whenever possible, treatment includes non-pharmacological measures as in younger patients, including exercise training.[48] Elderly females are especially salt-sensitive.[95] Besides salt restriction, an increased dietary potassium and magnesium may be protective.[67A]

**Diuretics** in low doses remain the first-line drug choice in the elderly, because they have been used in virtually all the major trials[93] and perhaps, equally important, because they help to prevent osteoporosis (p 100), a condition that is often disabling in the elderly.

**Beta-blockers** do reduce blood pressure in the elderly, although with disappointing data for hard end-points in the MRC trial.[91] The data for blood pressure reduction in elderly white males given atenolol are particularly good.[90] In the STOP study,[107] beta-blockade was usually combined with diuretics after 2 months to achieve the desired blood pressure reduction, and it was the combination that reduced stroke mortality. Risks of beta-blockade in the elderly include excess sinus or AV node inhibition and a decreased cardiac output, which in the senescent heart could more readily precipitate failure. In the elderly, the vasodilatory beta-blockers may be better because they maintain a higher heart rate and cardiac output.

**Calcium antagonists** are popular[99] without proof of reduction of hard end-points. In the Syst-Eur study,[36] nitrendipine is the initial drug being used.

**ACE inhibitors** are also often used in the elderly again without hard outcome data. Logically, they should become more effective with dietary salt restriction, or low-dose diuretics, or both. ACE inhibitors improve insulin sensitivity in the elderly,[97] which may help protect from adverse metabolic effects of concurrent diuretics.

To avoid **tissue under-perfusion,** low initial doses of drugs may be followed by a cautious increase. Indiscriminate reduction of diastolic blood pressure below a certain optimal value, perhaps around 90 mmHg, may actually increase mortality.[34] This is the so-called **J-shaped curve,** perhaps of particular significance in hypertensive men with ischemia or left ventricular hypertrophy.[87] Nevertheless, in systolic hypertension where the diastolic is not elevated to start with, a reduction of diastolic blood pressure from a mean of 77 mmHg to 69 mmHg over 4 years was associated with reduced not increased cardiovascular events.[105] Perhaps those elderly prone to poor myocardial perfusion from a low diastolic blood pressure had already eliminated themselves from entering the trial by suffering from a myocardial infarction.

BLACK PATIENTS. "Within the criteria of the individualized patient profile, the race of the patient should be considered."[32] Black patients seem to respond better to monotherapy with a diuretic,[1] a vasodilatory beta-blocker (labetalol),[1] or to a calcium antagonist[15] than to an ACE inhibitor.[90] Younger blacks, however, react surprisingly well to a beta-blocker.[90] In elderly blacks, a beta-blocker and an ACE inhibitor were only marginally better than placebo.[90] The common denominator might be the low renin status of elderly black patients taken as a group. Overall evidence suggests that combination with a diuretic increases sensitivity to a beta-blocker or an ACE inhibitor,[92] perhaps because the diuretic increases renin.

When cost is crucial, it is important to know that reserpine plus diuretic is as effective as beta-blocker plus diuretic in black patients.[32]

SMOKERS. It is imperative that the patient stops smoking. Smoking, besides being an independent risk factor for coronary artery disease and for stroke (the latter often forgotten), also interacts adversely with hypertension. First, smoking helps to promote renovascular and malignant hypertension. Second, smoking damages the vascular endothelium, the integrity of which is now thought to be important in maintaining a normal blood pressure.[52] Third, heavy smoking results in a sustained rise in blood pressure or intense swings to high systolic values, as revealed by ambulatory measurements.[41,70] Apparently normal casual office blood pressure values while the patient is not smoking mask the adverse effects of smoking on the blood pressure. Smoking may also interfere with the effects of propranolol, perhaps by induction of the liver enzymes concerned with its metabolism.[14,18] Therefore, in a confirmed smoker requiring a beta-blocker, an agent such as atenolol that is not metabolized by the liver would be preferable.

OBESE HYPERTENSIVES. The characteristics of obesity hypertension are a high cardiac output, a low peripheral vascular resistance, and an increased plasma volume.[19,28,64] The basic mechanisms are complex but include an increased tubular reabsorption of sodium and increased sympathetic outflow.[71] Weight reduction, although a laudable and crucial goal, which in itself reduces the blood pressure[17,113] and improves the quality of life[110,112] is not easy to achieve and may require multiple visits to the dietician and group counseling as well as increased exercise. The mechanism whereby weight loss works is in part related to changes in blood volume and cardiac output[116] and in part due to decreased sympathetic outflow.[38]

Because of the association between **insulin resistance** and obesity, and the potential adverse effects of diuretics on insulin, the dose of diuretic should be kept low. Vigorous dietary restriction of calories, salt and fat is able to improve blood lipid profiles and insulin sensitivity in the obese,[63] so that such measures should be combined with low-dose diuretic as in the TOMH study.[112] Left ventricular hypertrophy is a particular hazard, which obesity and insulin resistance promote independently of the blood pressure.[57,103]

Regarding further drug choice, in the absence of good trial data, a logical selection would be an agent that is metabolically neutral and known to combine well with a diuretic such as an ACE inhibitor. Beta-blockade is also logical[110] to limit the enhanced sympathetic outflow. There would be less argument for calcium antagonists which cause peripheral vasodilation and increase the cardiac output, already high in the obese.

DIABETIC OR PREDIABETIC HYPERTENSIVES. Again, treatment starts with lifestyle modification now including control of hyperglycemia.[94] Both diabetes (type II; maturity onset; non-insulin-dependent) and hypertension are associated with insulin resistance.[7] Both high-dose thiazides and beta-blockers can impair insulin sensitivity in nondiabetic hypertensives.[25,109] Therefore, it makes sense to avoid high-dose diuretics and beta-blockers in the therapy of those prone to diabetes by a personal or family history or in non-insulin-dependent diabetics. Rather, there are arguments for the use of ACE inhibition. ACE inhibitors lessen the hypokalemic effects of insulin, thereby improving glucose tolerance.[102] In nondiabetic hypertensives with marked insulin resistance, changing therapy from a beta-blocker (usually atenolol) to an ACE inhibitor (captopril) improved insulin resistance over 1 year.[45]

Calcium antagonists generally leave diabetic control unaltered although rarely deterioration occurs. In the specific case of verapamil, fasting blood glucose may actually fall.[89] Alpha-blockers also work. Although there is no conclusive evidence that such "metabolic management" is beneficial for hypertensive type II diabetics or for prediabetics, the approach is nonetheless logical, because defects in glucose metabolism and insulin resistance develop over many years into overt diabetes.

DIABETIC HYPERTENSIVES WITH MICROALBUMINURIA. Apparently trivial leaks of protein into the urine can presage overt proteinuria and later renal failure, both in insulin-dependent and in non-insulin-dependent diabetics.[47,67] In **nonhypertensive diabetics,** ACE inhibitors may bring about specific benefit in those with albuminuria,[72] acting perhaps by a specific effect on glomerular pore size. Furthermore, captopril is better than nifedipine in lessening exercise-induced microalbuminuria in diabetics.[29]

Do similar principles hold for **hypertensive diabetics with microalbuminuria**? Captopril over 3 years, alone or in combination with hydrochlorothiazide, prevented the development of macroalbuminuria,[83] but it was not clear whether the renoprotection was a specific effect of the ACE inhibitor or the result of vigorous blood pressure control. Another study, this time with perindopril, also over 3 years, gave similar conclusions.[73] In a small prospective study on patients with biopsy-proven diabetic glomerulopathy and microalbuminuria, either enalapril or the calcium antagonist nitrendipine improved the glomerular filtration rate without altering the rather low rates of urinary albumin excretion.[37] Of interest is that the combination of verapamil and an ACE inhibitor decreased microalbuminuria in insulin-dependent diabetics more than did either agent alone.[65]

INSULIN-DEPENDENT DIABETICS WITH OVERT NEPHROPATHY. In a landmark study, Lewis et al.[86] gave captopril for 3 years to 207 diabetics with overt proteinuria and renal insufficiency (elevated serum creatinine) Compared with 202 placebo-treated patients, captopril reduced hard end-points such as death, dialysis and renal transplantation. The majority of the patients were mildly hypertensive, yet the effects of captopril were independent of any blood pressure lowering.

DIABETIC HYPERTENSIVES WITH RENAL DISEASE: CONCLUSIONS. Taking together the available information on those with only microalbuminuria and those with overt nephropathy, ACE inhibitors emerge as the preferable class of drug to control hypertension. They will, however, often have to be combined with other drugs and of these the calcium antagonists seem to be best. Vigorous blood pressure control is essential and may be the clue to at least part of the benefit achieved by the ACE inhibitors. Because of the serious long-term significance of microalbuminuria and because increased blood pressure is a major risk factor for renal protein leakage in diabetics, *the cornerstone to the management of diabetic hypertensives is to reduce the blood pressure to well below 140/90 mmHg.*

EXERCISING HYPERTENSIVES. Several studies show that low- to moderate-intensity aerobic exercise training helps to reduce the resting blood pressure, so that increased exercise is often part of lifestyle modification in the treatment of hypertension. Practical advice, not substantiated by any long-term prospective studies, is to exercise vigorously (eg., running or cycling, 20 minutes 3 times a week), or to undertake 40 minutes of moderate activity (eg., brisk walking).[40] The benefits of exercise also extend to the elderly.[60] When, besides lifestyle modification and exercise, drug treatment is required, then the best category of drug might be that which leaves the increased cardiac output of exercise unchanged while blunting the simultaneous blood pressure rise. This goal is best attained by vasodilators such as the alpha-blockers, ACE inhibitors or calcium antagonists (especially the dihydropyridines).[96] Beta-blockade, in contrast, limits the cardiac output by decreasing the heart rate, even in the case of vasodilatory beta-blockers. Furthermore, beta-blockade tends to decrease HDL-cholesterol despite exercise training.[79]

PREGNANCY HYPERTENSION. The best tested drug is methyldopa (Category B; Table 11–8). ACE inhibitors are contraindicated (Table 11–8).

## HYPERTENSION AND CONCOMITANT DISEASE

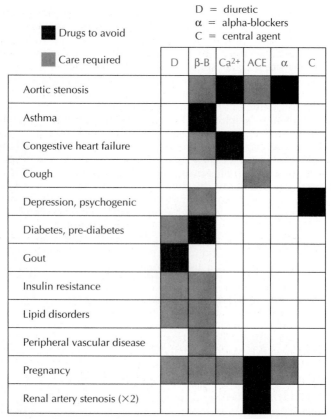

FIGURE 7–9. Effect of various concomitant diseases on choice of antihypertensive therapy. βB = beta-blocker; $Ca^{2+}$ = calcium antagonist; ACE = ACE inhibitor. For use of beta-blockers in CHF, see Chapter 1, p 14. Fig. copyright L.H. Opie.

CONCOMITANT DISEASES. The drugs to avoid and those for which care is required are shown in Fig. 7–9.

## Specific Aims of Antihypertensive Therapy

REGRESSION OF LEFT VENTRICULAR HYPERTROPHY (LVH). Preferably diagnosed by echocardiography, LVH is increasingly seen as an important adverse complication of hypertension. Apart from being an independent cardiovascular risk factor, LVH is associated with abnormalities of diastolic function, which can result in dyspnea or even overt left ventricular failure. An important point is that regression of the blood pressure does not automatically result in decreased LVH. Although several important retrospective analyses[54,56] support the concept that the most effective agents in achieving left ventricular regression are ACE inhibitors, calcium antagonists or beta-blockers rather than the diuretics, yet in the recent multicenter VA trial extending over 2 years (currently only available in abstract form), hydrochlorothiazide was the best of six agents.[69] The best policy in relation to LVH is therefore not clear. Among lifestyle measures, reduction of obesity and salt intake may be especially important.[82] Logically, because increased myocardial stretch following systemic hypertension is at least one factor provoking protein synthesis, meticulous blood pressure control over 24 hours would seem important. Of interest is the concept that it is not only the daytime blood pressure that governs LVH,[118] but also the absence of a normal nocturnal blood pressure fall.[114] (see also p 119)

EARLY MORNING BLOOD PRESSURE RISE. The highest blood pressure is often soon after rising, and the early morning hours are associated with the largest proportion of sudden death, AMI and stroke. Logically, there has been a drive for the use of ultralong-acting agents to blunt this early morning rise. In reality, the optimal management of early morning hypertension is still not clear and few, if any, comparative prospective trials address this point. The danger of bringing down the blood pressure excessively over 24 hours is nocturnal ischemia. On the other hand, a normal fall in blood pressure at night is desired to help avoid LVH (114). Thus, the ideal remedy, especially in those at risk of cardiac complications and/or with LVH, is to achieve a normal blood pressure in the morning, a normal blood pressure at night and a normal diurnal rhythm, all as measured by ambulatory blood pressure monitors.

VENTRICULAR ARRHYTHMIAS. Although often associated with LVH, such ventricular ectopic activity seems relatively harmless and does not warn of sudden cardiac death.[58] Rather, persistent and significant ventricular tachycardia may reflect accompanying coronary artery disease. Severe life-threatening arrhythmias in a hypertensive may require the beta-blocker sotalol (p 233), taking care to avoid diuretic-induced hypokalemia with risk of torsades. In any hypertensive patient with arrhythmias, plasma potassium and magnesium should be monitored.[46A]

PREVENTION OF SEXUAL DYSFUNCTION. Sexual dysfunction has been reported with almost every antihypertensive drug, probably a consequence of reduction of blood flow through genital vessels already sclerotic from the ravages of smoking, hypercholesterolemia, and diabetes.[3] As impotence often has a psychogenic component, it can do no harm to tell the patient that vasodilators will bring more blood to the penis. At the same time, any diuretic therapy should be phased out; it is this category of drugs that most consistently causes impotence.[110] The centrally acting alpha-agonists (such as clonidine) are the other chief offenders.[46]

OPTIMAL INTELLECTUAL ACTIVITY. In general, antihypertensives with the exception of centrally active agents should be free of central side-effects. Nevertheless, it is now becoming clear that beta-blockers may have subtle effects on the intellect. Although propranolol is the major culprit, even the lipid-insoluble agent atenolol is not blameless. To be sure of unimpaired intellectual activity, calcium antagonists or ACE inhibitors seem to be the agents of choice. For example, patients on enalapril (20 to 40 mg daily) showed no change in memory, whereas atenolol (50 to 100 mg daily) caused mild but consistent impairment.[10]

OVERALL QUALITY OF LIFE (QOL). In general, all categories of antihypertensive agents improve the quality of life[46,74] except for propranolol and methyldopa, and probably other centrally active agents such as clonidine.[1,90] Alpha-blockers are not well tested in quality of life studies. Caution is advised in the interpretation of QOL studies since drop-outs from adverse effects are not included.

COST EFFECTIVENESS. In the **Third World** and often elsewhere, expensive drugs are a luxury, and the principles of choice are governed by economic necessity. Much can be said for low-dose thiazide diuretics as initial therapy, followed by reserpine. Low-dose thiazides are relatively free of metabolic side-effects (possibly except for effects on lipids). The cost of reserpine is extremely low, it is effectively antihypertensive, and it is relatively free from significant hemodynamic or subjective side-effects. A diuretic-based therapy is also logical in black patients. When compliance is relatively limited by educational handicaps, the very long biologic half-life of reserpine, with catecholamine depletion lasting for many weeks, could be a major advantage. Furthermore, a cheap vasodilator (hydralazine) can readily be combined with diuretic-reserpine as the next step to give a poor man's equivalent of the very effective beta-blocker plus diuretic plus calcium antagonist combination.

In the USA, complex and potentially misleading computer calculations[6] suggest that in 1990 the cost of treatment for 1 year for each life saved was $10,900 for propranolol, $16,400 for hydrochlorothiazide (where the greatest cost is in the laboratory blood tests), $20,800 for atenolol, $31,600 for nifedipine, $61,900 for prazosin, and $72,100 for captopril. If, however, the impaired quality of life with propranolol was allowed for, the cost with propranolol became $33,300 per quality-adjusted life year. These figures are highly suspect in the absense of adequate morbidity and mortality data needed for valid cost-benefit analyses. The best course is to hold back on any drug therapy of many low-risk mild hypertensives.[76]

## Acute Severe Hypertension

For urgent therapy of acute severe hypertension (Table 7–4) the choice used to fall on an intravenous agent, but **nifedipine** (bite and swallow) is now almost standard therapy. It consistently reduces systolic and diastolic blood pressures by about 20% within 20 to 30 minutes.[1] Such a rapid reduction of hypertension may be safe even in the presence of cerebral symptoms.[1] *Nevertheless, it is prudent to consider whether rapid pressure reduction is really desirable in the presence of cerebral symptoms or symptoms of myocardial ischemia.* Commonsense says that even with nifedipine, which seldom causes "overshoot," rapid falls in blood pressure will occasionally have serious side-effects such as myocardial or cerebral ischemia. Therefore, carefully titrated **intravenous nicardipine** or labetalol seems preferable. For acute LV failure, enalaprilat is first choice (Table 7–5). For acute coronary syndromes, intravenous nitroglycerin is first choice.

Other parenteral agents such as **nitroprusside** are still used extensively. These all require careful monitoring to avoid overshoot. Nitroprusside reduces preload and afterload and has the risk of rebound hypertension. **Labetalol** does not cause tachycardia and gives a smooth dose-related fall in blood pressure; the side-effects of beta-blockade, such as heart failure and bronchospasm, may be countered by the added alpha-blockade of labetalol. Diazoxide is best avoided. Hydralazine and dihydralazine may cause tachycardia and are also best avoided, especially in angina, unless there is concomitant therapy with a beta-blocker.

At present, when *the ideal rate of reduction of hypertension requiring urgent therapy is not known,* the simplicity of sublingual nifedipine (10 mg) is increasingly seen as seemingly safe therapy, provided that there is no clinical evidence of cerebral or myocardial ischemia or clinically evident renal failure. When such complications are present, careful slow-monitored reduction of blood pressure is best using, for example, intravenous nicardipine.

In **severe hypertension in the elderly,** sublingual nifedipine seems as safe as in younger subjects.[1] Decreased cerebral perfusion is potentially serious, so that the risk of precipitating cerebral ischemia must be carefully considered despite the reported cerebral vasodilating effect of nifedipine. Rather, blood pressure reduction should be slow if clinically acceptable.

In **acute stroke with hypertension**, the benefits of blood pressure reduction remain conjectural.[98A] If **subarachnoid hemorrhage** is suspected, **nimodipine** may reduce the blood pressure.

## Maximal Therapy

When confronted with the occasional patient who appears to be refractory to all known forms of therapy, the following points are

**TABLE 7–4    AGENTS FOR USE IN HYPERTENSIVE EMERGENCIES (CAUTION: SEE TEXT FOR IMPORTANT RESERVATIONS)**

| AGENT | USUAL DOSE | SIDE-EFFECTS | COMMENTS | CROSS-REFERENCE |
|---|---|---|---|---|
| Captopril | 25 mg chewed* Test dose 6.25 mg | Renal failure (renal artery stenosis). Hypotension | Exclude renal artery stenosis, especially bilateral. Not in pregnancy. | Chapter 5, p 126 |
| Enalaprilat | IV 0.625–1.25 mg over 5 min every 6 h | Hypotension, renal failure | Effective for hypertensive heart failure. See captopril for exclusions. | Chapter 5, p 128 |
| Esmolol | IV 50–300 µg/kg/min | As for beta-blockade | Licensed for perioperative hypertension. | Chapter 1, p 26 |
| Furosemide | IV 40–180 mg | Hypokalemia, hyponatremia | Best for fluid retention, renal failure. | Chapter 4, p 85 |
| Hydralazine | IV 5–10 mg every 4–6 h | Tachycardia, contraindicated in angina, ischemic strokes | Avoid if possible. For tachycardia, propranolol 1–2 mg IV. | Chapter 5, p 134 |
| Labetalol | IV 2 mg/min to total of 1–2 mg/kg | May worsen cardiac failure; usually safe | Avoids tachycardia. Smooth and rapid dose-related fall in BP. | Chapter 1, p 17 |
| Nicardipine[+] | IV 5–15 mg/h | See nifedipine | Licensed for severe hypertension. | Chapter 3, p 77 |
| Nifedipine | 10–20 mg bite-and-swallow, repeat every 4–6 h | Few; "overshoot" seldom; myocardial and cerebral ischemia | Simple therapy, usually effective; needs further evaluation and caution in presence of papilledema. | Chapter 3, p 72 |
| Nitroglycerin | IV 5–100 µg/min | Headaches, unexpected bradycardia | Ideal for ischemic left ventricular failure. | Chapter 2, p 36 |
| Nitroprusside | IV 40–75 µg/min | Hypotension, must monitor; coronary steal | Especially if pulmonary edema or encephalopathy or acute stroke, otherwise avoid. | Chapter 5, p 133 |

* Tschollar and Belz. Lancet 1985; 2:34–35.

[+] Ref 82, Chapter 3. For safety a slow infusion is better than a bolus.

**TABLE 7–5**    **PREFERRED PARENTERAL DRUGS FOR SPECIFIC HYPERTENSIVE EMERGENCIES (IN ORDER OF PREFERENCE)**

| EMERGENCY | PREFERRED | AVOID (REASON) |
| --- | --- | --- |
| Hypertensive encephalopathy | Labetalol | Methyldopa (sedation) |
| | Nicardipine | Diazoxide (fall in cerebral blood flow) |
| | Nitroprusside | Reserpine (sedation) |
| Accelerated-malignant hypertension | Labetalol | Methyldopa (sedation) |
| | Enalaprilat | |
| | Nicardipine* | |
| Left ventricular failure | Enalaprilat | Labetalol, esmolol, and other beta-blockers |
| | Nitroglycerin | (decrease cardiac output) |
| | Nitroprusside | |
| Coronary insufficiency | Nitroglycerin | Hydralazine (increase cardiac output) |
| | Esmolol | Diazoxide (increase cardiac output) |
| | Nicardipine | Nitroprusside (coronary steal) |
| Dissecting aortic aneurysm | Trimethaphan* | Hydralazine (increase cardiac output) |
| | Nitroprusside | Diazoxide (increase cardiac output) |
| | Esmolol | |
| Catecholamine excess | Phentolamine | All others (less specific) |
| | Labetalol | |
| Postoperative | Labetalol | Trimethaphan (bowel and bladder atony) |
| | Nitroglycerin | |
| | Nicardipine | |

*Dose 0.5 to 5 mg/min as intravenous infusion; onset 1 to 5 min; S/E: general autonomic blockade.

Modified from Reference 120.

worth considering: (1) Is the patient really compliant with the therapy? (2) Are the blood pressure values taken in the doctor's office really representative of those with which the patient lives (there can be striking differences)? (3) Has the patient developed some complications such as atherosclerotic renal artery stenosis or renal failure? (4) Has the patient increased salt or alcohol intake, or taken sympathomimetic agents or nonsteroidal anti-inflammatory agents with sulindac and iboprufen seeming the least harmful?[98] (5) Are there temporary psychological stresses? (6) Is the therapy really maximal, particularly regarding the diuretic dose, because overfilling of dilated vasculature by reactive sodium retention may also preclude a fall in the peripheral resistance? (Note that the concept of low-dose diuretic therapy must be abandoned at this stage).

Logically, **refractory hypertension** means that the peripheral vascular resistance has failed to fall. Therefore the emphasis should be on vasodilator therapy, acting on every conceivable mechanism: calcium antagonism, alpha-blockade, ACE inhibition, $K^+$ channel-induced vasodilation by minoxidil, and high-dose diuretics. Combination of alpha-blockade and ACE inhibition together with calcium antagonism blunts the adverse baroreflex response to the calcium antagonism. Potassium channel dilation complements other vasodilatory mechanisms. In addition, a centrally active agent indirectly lessens the release of norepinephrine from the nerve terminals. Beta-blockade, by reducing the cardiac output, acts through an entirely different mechanism. Severe hypertension often has a volume-dependent component and reactive sodium retention often accompanies the fall in blood pressure induced by vasodilatory drugs; therefore the addition of more diuretics, particularly the loop agents, is an important component of maximal therapy. Of the loop diuretics, the new agent torsemide is registered for once daily use in hypertension. Occasionally, in a patient in whom blood pressure remains elevated despite the above measures, hospital admission and acute intravenous blood pressure lowering, for example by intravenous verapamil or labetalol, helps to reset the baroreflexes whereupon previously refractory hypertension yields to more standard therapy.

The **ganglion blockers** (**guanethidine** and **guandrel**), now decidedly out of fashion because of frequent orthostatic hypotension and interference with sexual activity, should therefore be reserved for the last resort.

## Summary

Since the last edition of this book there have been several major advances. In the elderly, treatment of hypertension and systolic hypertension reduces stroke and, in some studies, decreases cardiac events and mortality. In all of these studies, diuretics have been the initial therapy of choice in patients lacking specific indications for other agents. Second, the Joint National Committee in the USA has brought out new recommendations suggesting that diuretics and beta-blockers should be the agents of first choice. In contrast, the International Society of Hypertension proposes that any of five categories of drugs should be suitable, namely low-dose diuretics, beta-blockers, calcium antagonists, ACE inhibitors, or alpha-blockers. In one major comparative study, therapy of very mild hypertension by any of these five types of agents together with lifestyle modification resulted in almost equal reduction of blood pressure and improvement of quality of life with few adverse effects for any specific agent.[112]

Another important comparative trial found that younger and older patients responded differently to various antihypertensives, as did whites and blacks.[90] In younger whites, the best agent, purely from the point of view of blood pressure reduction, was an ACE inhibitor and in older whites, a beta-blocker. In both younger and older black patients, a calcium blocker was best and an ACE inhibitor (without a diuretic) virtually without effect.

Currently running are several major European-based outcome studies using either ACE inhibitors or calcium antagonists as initial therapy.

In the meantime, it makes sense to be aware of the metabolic abnormalities, including increased insulin resistance and deviations of the blood lipid profile from normal, induced by high-dose diuretics and beta-blockers more than by calcium antagonists, ACE inhibitors or alpha-blockers. In those many hypertensive patients also prone to coronary disease, optimal metabolic management should help achieve the dual aims of control of blood pressure and blood lipids, thereby hopefully helping to reduce coronary mortality. The patient-guided approach detailed in the Table 7–3 is the most appropriate way to treat hypertension.

## References

*For references from Second Edition, see Kaplan and Opie (1991)*

1. Kaplan NM, Opie LH. Antihypertensive drugs. In: Opie LH (ed), Drugs for the Heart, Third Edition. WB Saunders Company, Philadelphia, 1991, pp 155–179.

*References from Third Edition*

2. Ambrosioni E, Birkenhager W, De Leeuw PW, et al. J Hypertens 1989; 7 (Suppl 6):S266–S267.
3. Bansal S. Hypertension 1988; 12:1–10.
4. Burris JF, Weir MR, Oparil S, et al. JAMA 1990; 263:1507–1512.
5. Collins R, Peto R, MacMahon S, et al. Lancet 1990; 335:827–838.
6. Edelson JT, Weinstein MC, Tosteson ANA, et al. JAMA 1990; 263:408–413.
7. Ferrannini E, Buzzigoli G, Bonadonna R, et al. N Engl J Med 1987; 317:350–357.
8. Galletti F, Strazzullo P, Cappuccio FP, et al. Cardiovasc Drugs Ther 1989; 3:135–140.
9. Heagerty AM, Swales J, Baksi A, et al. Br Med J 1988; 296:468–472.

10. Lichter I, Richardson PJ, Wyke MA. Br J Clin Pharmacol 1986; 21:641–645.
11. Lund-Johansen P. J Hypertens 1989; 7 (Suppl 6):S52–S55.
12. MacGregor GA. Cardiovasc Drugs Ther 1990; 3:295–301.
13. MacGregor GA, Markandu ND, Sagnella GA, et al. Lancet 1989; 2:1244–1247.
14. Materson BJ, Reda D, Freis ED, Henderson WG. Arch Intern Med 1988; 148:2116–2119.
15. M'Buyamba-Kabangu J-R, Lepira B, Lijnen P, et al. Hypertension 1988; 11:100–105.
16. McKenney JM, Goodman RP, Wright JT, et al. Pharmacotherapy 1986; 6:179–184.
17. McMahon SW, Wilcken DEL, MacDonald GJ. N Engl J Med 1986; 314:334–339.
18. Medical Research Council Working Party. Br Med J 1988; 296:1565–1570.
19. Messerli FH, Ventura HO, Reisin E, et al. Circulation 1982; 66:55–60.
20. Mimran A, Insua A, Ribstein J, et al. J Hypertens 1988; 6:919–923.
21. Moss AJ, Rubison M, Oakes D, et al. Circulation 1989; 80 (Suppl II):II–268.
22. Oberman A, Wassertheil-Smoller S, Langford HG, et al. Ann Intern Med 1990; 112:89–95.
23. Perry IJ, Beevers DG. Cardiovasc Drugs Ther 1989; 3:815–819.
24. Pollare T, Lithell H, Berne C. N Engl J Med 1989; 321:868–873.
25. Pollare T, Lithell H, Selinus I, Berne C. Br Med J 1989; 298:1152–1157.
26. Postma CT, Hoefnagels WHL, Barentsz JO, et al. J Human Hypertens 1989; 3:185–190.
27. Psaty BM, Koepsell TD, LoGergo JP, et al. JAMA 1989; 261:2087–2094.
28. Raison J, Achimastos A, Asmar R, et al. Am J Cardiol 1986; 57:223–226.
29. Romanelli G, Giustina A, Ababiti-Rosei E, et al. J Hypertens 1989; 6 (Suppl 6):S312–S313.
30. Samuelsson O, Wilhelmsen L, Andersson OK, et al. JAMA 1987; 285:1768–1776.
31. Sassano P, Chatellier G, Billaud E, et al. J Cardiovasc Pharmacol 1989; 13:314–319.
32. Seedat YK. J Hypertens 1989; 7:515–518.
33. Singer DRJ, Markandu ND, Shore AC, MacGregor GA. Hypertension 1987; 9:629–633.
34. Staessen J, Bulpitt C, Clement D, et al. Br Med J 1989; 298:1552–1556.
35. Vardan S, Mehrotra KG, Mookherjee S, et al. JAMA 1987; 258:484–488.

## New References

36. Amery A, Birkenhager W, Bulpitt CJ, et al. Syst-Eur. A multicentre trial on the treatment of isolated systolic hypertension in the elderly: Objectives, protocol, and organization. Aging 1991; 3:287–302.
37. Amuchastequi CS, Casiraghi F, Mosconi L, et al. Long-term treatment with both nitrendipine (N) and enalapril (E) significantly increases glomerular filtration rate (GFR) in hypertensive microalbuminuric non-insulin-dependent diabetics (NIDDs) with biopsy-proved diabetic glomerulopathy (abstr). Clin Nephrol 1993; 4:300.
38. Andersson B, Elam M, Wallen BG, et al. Effect of energy-restricted diet on sympathetic muscle nerve activity in obese women. Hypertension 1991; 18:783–789.
39. Andren L, Weiner L, Svensson A, Hansson L. Enalapril with either a "very low" or "low" dose of hydrochlorothiazide is equally effective in essential hypertension. A double-blind trial in 100 hypertensive patients. J Hypertens 1983; 1 (Suppl 2):384–386.
40. Arroll B, Beaglehole R. Exercise for hypertension. Lancet 1993; 341:1248–1249.
41. Asmar RG, Girerd XJ, Brahimi M, et al. Ambulatory blood pressure measurement, smoking and abnormalities of glucose and lipid metabolism in essential hypertension. J Hypertens 1992; 10:181–187.
42. Bakris GL, Barnhill BW, Sadler R. Treatment of arterial hypertension in diabetic humans: Importance of therapeutic selection. Kidney Int 1992; 41:912–919.
43. Baumgart P. Torasemide in comparison with thiazides in the treatment of hypertension. Cardiovasc Drugs Ther 1993; 7:63–68.
44. Beard K, Bulpitt C, Mascie-Taylor H, et al. Management of elderly patients with sustained hypertension. Br Med J 1992; 304:412–416.
45. Berntorp K, Lindgarde F, Mattiasson I. Long-term effects on insulin sensitivity anbd sodium transport in glucose-intolerant hypertensive subjects when beta-blockade is replaced by captopril treatment. J Human Hypertens 1992; 6:291–298.
46. Beto JA, Bansal VK. Quality of life in treatment of hypertension. A metaanalysis of clinical trials. J Hypertens 1992; 5:125–133.
46A. Bigger JT Jr. Diuretic therapy, hypertension, and cardiac arrest. Editorial. N Engl J Med 1994; 330:1899–1900.
47. Borch-Johnsen K, Wenzel H, Viberti GC, Mogensen CE. Is screening and intervention for microalbuminuria worthwhile in patients with insulin-dependent diabetes? Br Med J 1993; 306:1722–1723.
48. Braith RW, Pollock ML, Lowenthal DT, et al. Moderate- and high-intensity exercise lowers blood pressure in normotensive subjects 60 to 79 years of age. Am J Cardiol 1994; 73:1124–1128.
49. Canter D, Frank GJ, Knapp LE, et al., and the Quinapril Investigator Group. Quinapril and hydrochlorothiazide combination for control of hypertension: Assessment by factorial design. J Human Hypertens 1994; 8:155–162.
50. CAPPP group. The Captopril Prevention Project: A prospective intervention trial

of angiotensin converting enzyme inhibition in the treatment of hypertension. J Hypertens 1990; 8:985–990.

51. Carlsen JE, Kober L, Torp-Pedersen C, Johansen P. Relation between dose of bendrofluazide, antihypertensive effect, and adverse biochemical effects. Br Med J 1990; 300:975–978.

52. Celermajer DS, Sorensen KE, Georgekopoulos D, et al. Cigarette smoking is associated with dose-related and potentially reversible impairment of endothelium-dependent dilation in healthy young adults. Circulation 1993; 88 (Part 1):2149–2155.

53. Chrysant SG, The Lisinopril-Hydrochlorothiazide Group. Antihypertensive effectiveness of low-dose lisinopril-hydrochlorothiazide combination. A large multicenter study. Arch Intern Med 1994; 154:737–743.

54. Cruickshank JM. The case for beta-blockers as first-line antihypertensive therapy. J Hypertens 1992; 10:S21-S27.

55. Cushman WC, Nunn SL, Lakshman MR, et al. for the VA Cooperative Study Group on Antihypertensive Agents. Monotherapy of hypertension: Effects of six classes of drugs and placebo on plasma lipids (abstr). Am J Hypertens 1993; 6:9A–10A.

56. Dahlof B, Pennert K, Hansson L. Reversal of left ventricular hypertrophy in hypertensive patients. A meta-analysis of 109 treatment studies. Am J Hypertens 1992; 5:95–110.

57. de Simone G, Devereux RB, Roman MJ, et al. Relation of obesity and gender to left ventricular hypertrophy in normotensive and hypertensive adults. Hypertension 1994; 23:600–606.

58. Dunn FG, Pringle SD. Sudden cardiac death, ventricular arrhythmias and hypertensive left ventricular hypertrophy. J Hypertens 1993; 11:1003–1010.

59. Dworkin LD, Benstein JA, Parker M, et al. Calcium antagonists and converting enzyme inhibitors reduce renal injury by different mechanisms. Kidney Int 1993; 43:808–814.

60. Ehsani AA. Physiologic adaptations to exercise in the hypertensive elderly. Cardiology in the Elderly 1993; 1:558–563.

61. Elliot WJ. Glucose and cholesterol elevations from diuretic therapy: Intention to treat vs. actual on-therapy experience (abstr). Am J Hypertens 1993; 6:9A–10A.

62. EWPHE study—Amery A, Birkenhager W, Brixko P, et al. Mortality and morbidity results from the European Working Party on high blood pressure in the elderly (EWPHE) trial. Lancet 1985; 1:1349–1354.

63. Fagerberg B, Berglund A, Andersson OK, Berglund G. Weight reduction versus antihypertensive drug therapy in obese men with high blood pressure: Effects upon plasma insulin levels and association with changes in blood pressure and serum lipids. J Hypertens 1992; 10:1053–1061.

64. Ferranini E. The haemodynamics of obesity: A theoretical analysis. J Hypertens 1992; 10:1417–1423.

65. Fioretto P, Frigato F, Velussi M, et al. Effects of angiotensin-converting enzyme inhibitors and calcium antagonists on atrial natriuretic peptide release and action and on albumin excretion rate in hypertensive insulin-dependent diabetic patients. Am J Hypertens 1992; 5:837–846.

66. Frishman WH, Bryzinski BS, Coulson LR, et al. A multifactorial trial design to assess combination therapy in hypertension: Treatment with bisoprolol and hydrochlorothiazide. Arch Intern Med 1994; 154:1461–1468.

67. Gall M-A, Borch-Johnsen K, Nielsen FS, et al. Micro- and macroalbuminuria as predictors of mortality in non-insulin-dependent diabetes (NIDD)(abstr). Clin Nephrol 1993; 4:303.

67A. Geleijnse JM, Witteman JCM, Bak AAA, et al. Reduction in blood pressure with a low sodium, high potassium, high magnesium salt in older subjects with mild to moderate hypertension. Br Med J 1994; 309:436–440.

68. Gavras H, Gavras I. On the JNC V Report. A different point of view. Am J Hypertens 1994; 7:288–293.

69. Gottdiener J, Reda D, Notargiacomo A, Matersen B. VA Cooperative Study Group on Antihypertensive Agents. Comparison of monotherapy effects on LV mass regression in mild-to-moderate hypertension: Differences between short- and long-term therapy (abstr). J Am Coll Cardiol 1992; 19:85A.

70. Groppelli A, Giorgi DMA, Omboni S, et al. Persistent blood pressure increase induced by heavy smoking. J Hypertens 1992; 10:495–499.

71. Hall JE. Renal and cardiovascular mechanisms of hypertension in obesity. Hypertension 1994; 23:381–394.

72. Hallab M, Gallois Y, Chatellier G, et al. Comparison of reduction in microalbuminuria by enalapril and hydrochlorothiazide in normotensive patients with insulin-dependent diabetes. Br Med J 1993; 306:175–182.

72A. Hannedouche T, Landais P, Goldfarb B, et al. Randomised controlled trial of enalapril and beta-blockers in non-diabetic chronic renal failure. Br Med J 1994; 309:833–837.

73. Hermans MP, Brichard SM, Colin I, et al. Long-term reduction of microalbuminuria after 3 years of angiotensin-converting enzyme inhibition by perindopril in hypertensive insulin-treated diabetic patients. Am J Med 1992; 92:102S-107S.

74. Hjemdahl P, Wiklund IK. Quality of life on antihypertensive drug therapy: Scientific end-point or marketing exercise? J Hypertens 1992; 10:1437–1446.

75. Holzgreve H, Distler A, Michaelis J, et al., on behalf of the Verapamil versus Diuretic (VERDI) Trial Research Group. Verapamil versus hydrochlorothiazide in the treatment of hypertension: results of long-term double-blind comparative trial. Br Med J 1989; 299:881–886.

76. Jackson R, Barham P, Bills J, et al. Management of raised blood pressure in New Zealand: A discussion document. Br Med J 1993; 307:107–110.

77. Jespersen CM, Fischer Hansen J, and the Danish Study Group on Verapamil in Myocardial Infarction. Effect of verapamil on reinfarction and cardiovascular events in patients with arterial hypertension included in the Danish Verapamil Infarction Trial II. J Human Hypertens 1994; 8:85–88.

78. Joint National Committee. The fifth report of the Joint National Committee on detection, evaluation, and treatment of high blood pressure (JNC V). Arch Intern Med 1993; 153:154–183.

79. Keleman MH, Effron MB, Valenti SA, Stewart KJ. Exercise training combined with antihypertensive drug therapy. Effects on lipids, blood pressure, and left ventricular mass. JAMA 1990; 263:2766–2771.

80. Kelley G, McClellan P. Antihypertensive effects of aerobic exercise. A brief meta-analytic review of randomized controlled trials. Am J Hypertens 1994; 7:115–119.

81. Kochar MS, Landry KM, Ristow SM. Effects of reduction in dose and discontinuation of hydrochlorothiazide in patients with controlled essential hypertension. Arch Intern Med 1990; 150:1009–1011.

82. Kupari M, Koskinen P, Virolainen J. Correlates of left ventricular mass in a population sample aged 36 to 37 years. Focus on lifestyle and salt intake. Circulation 1994; 89:1041–1050.

83. Lacourciere Y, Nadeau A, Poirier L, Tancrede G. Captopril or conventional therapy in hypertensive Type II diabetics. Three year analysis. Hypertension 1993; 21:786–794.

84. Lacourciere Y, Lefebvre J, Poirier L, et al. Treatment of ambulatory hypertensives with nebivolol or hydrochlorothiazide alone and in combination. A randomized, double-blind, placebo-controlled, factorial-design trial. Am J Hypertens 1994; 7:137–145.

85. Langer RD, Criqui MH, Barrett-Connor EL, et al. Blood pressure change and survival after age 75. Hypertension 1993; 22:551–559.

86. Lewis EJ, Hunsicker LG, Bain RP, Rohde RD for the Collaborative Study Group. The effect of angiotensin-converting enzyme inhibition on diabetic nephropathy. N Engl J Med 1993; 329:1456–1462.

87. Lindblad U, Rastam L, Ryden L, et al. Control of blood pressure and risk of first acute myocardial infarction: Skaraborg hypertension project. Br Med J 1994; 308:681–686.

88. Lund-Johansen P, Omvik P. Acute and chronic hemodynamic effects of drugs with different actions on adrenergic receptors: A comparison between alpha-blockers and different types of beta-blockers with and without vasodilating effect. Cardiovasc Drugs Ther 1991; 5:605–616.

89. Lyngsoe J, Sorensen MB, Sjostrand H, et al. The effect of sustained release verapamil on glucose metablism in patients with non-insulin-dependent diabetes mellitus. Drugs 1992; 44 (Suppl 1):85–87.

90. Materson BJ, Reda DJ, Cushman WC, et al. Single-drug therapy for hypertension in men. A comparison of six antihypertensive agents with placebo. N Engl J Med 1993; 328:914–921. **See also Materson BJ, Reda DJ. Correction. N Engl J Med 1994; 330:1689.**

91. Medical Research Council Working Party. Medical Research Council trial of treatment of hypertension in older adults: Principal results. Br Med J 1992; 304:405–412.

92. Middlemost SJ, Tager R, Davis J, Sareli P. Effectiveness of enalapril in combination with low-dose hydrochlorothiazide versus enalapril alone for mild to moderate systemic hypertension in black patients. Am J Cardiol 1994; 73:1092–1097.

93. National High Blood Pressure Education Program Working Group Report on Hypertension in the Elderly. Hypertension 1994; 23:275–285.

94. National High Blood Pressure Education Program Working Group Report on Hypertension in Diabetes. Hypertension 1994; 23:145–158.

95. Nestel PJ, Clifton PM, Noakes M, et al. Enhanced blood pressure response to dietary salt in elderly women, especially those with small waist:hip ratio. J Hypertens 1993; 11:1387–1394.

96. Omvik P, Lund-Johansen P. Long-term hemodynamic effects at rest and during exercise of newer antihypertensive agents and salt restriction in essential hypertension: Review of epanolol, doxazosin, amlodipine, felodipine, diltiazem, lisinopril, dilevalol, carvedilol, and ketanserin. Cardiovasc Drugs Ther 1993; 7:193–206.

97. Paolisso G, Gambardella A, Verza M, et al. ACE inhibition improves insulin-sensitivity in aged insulin-resistant hypertensive patients. J Human Hypertens 1992; 6:175–179.

98. Pope JE, Anderson JJ, Felson DT. A meta-analysis of the effects of nonsteroidal anti-inflammatory drugs on blood pressure. Arch Intern Med 1993; 153:477–484.

98A. Powers WJ. Acute hypertension after stroke: The scientific basis for treatment decisions. Neurology 1993; 43:461–467.

99. Psaty BM, Savage PJ, Tell GS, et al. Temporal patterns of antihypertensive medication use among elderly patients. JAMA 1993; 270:1837–1841.

100. Reeves RA, Fodor JG, Gryfe CI, et al. Report of the Canadian Hypertension Society

Consensus Conference: 4. Hypertension in the elderly. Can Med Assoc J 1993; 149:815–820.

101. Salvetti A, Brogi G, Di Legge V, Bernini GP. The inter-relationship between insulin resistance and hypertension. Drugs 1993; 46 (Suppl 2):149–159.

102. Santoro D, Natali A, Palombo C, et al. Effects of chronic angiotensin-converting enzyme inhibition on glucose tolerance and insulin sensitivity in essential hypertension. Hypertension 1992; 20:181–191.

103. Sasson Z, Rasooly Y, Bhesania T, Rasooly I. Insulin resistance is an important determinant of left ventricular mass in the obese. Circulation 1993; 88 (Part 1):1431–1436.

104. Senior R, Imbs JL, Bory M, et al. Comparison of the effects of indapamide with hydrochlorothiazide, nifedipine, enalapril and atenolol on left ventricular hypertrophy in hypertension: A double-blind parallel study (abstr). J Am Coll Cardiol 1993; 21:57A.

105. SHEP Cooperative Research Group. Prevention of stroke by antihypertensive drug treatment in older persons with isolated systolic hypertension. Final results of the Systolic Hypertension in the Elderly Program (SHEP). JAMA 1991; 265:3255–3264.

106. STOP study—Dahlof B, Lindholm LH, Hansson L, et al. Morbidity and mortality in the Swedish Trial in Old Patients with Hypertension (STOP-Hypertension). Lancet 1991; 338:1281–1285.

107. STOP study—Ekbom T, Dahlof B, Hansson L, et al. Antihypertensive efficacy and side-effects of three beta-blockers and a diuretic in elderly hypertensives: A report from the STOP-Hypertension study. J Hypertens 1992; 10:1525–1530.

108. Swales JD. Guidelines on guidelines. J Hypertens 1993; 11:899–903.

109. Swislocki ALM, Hoffman BB, Reaven GM. Insulin resistance, glucose intolerance and hyperinsulinemia in patients with hypertension. Am J Hypertens 1989; 2:419–423.

110. TAIM study—Wassertheil-Smoller S, Oberman A, Blaufox MD, et al. The Trial of Antihypertensive Interventions and Management (TAIM) Study. Final results with regard to blood pressure, cardiovascular risk, and quality of life. Am J Hypertens 1992; 5:37–44.

111. TOMH study—Treatment of Mild Hypertension Research Group (TOMH). The treatment of mild hypertension study. A randomized, placebo-controlled trial of a nutritional-hygienic regimen along with various drug monotherapies. Arch Intern Med 1991; 151:1413–1423.

112. TOMH study—Neaton JD, Grimm RH, Prineas RJ, et al., for the Treatment of Mild Hypertension (TOMH) Study Research Group. Treatment of mild hypertension study. Final results. JAMA 1993; 270:713–724.

113. Trials of Hypertension Prevention Collaborative Research Group. The effects of nonpharmacologic interventions on blood pressure of persons with high normal levels. Results of the Trials of Hypertension Prevention, Phase I. JAMA 1992; 267:1213–1220.

114. Verdecchia P, Schillaci G, Guerrieri M, et al. Circadian blood pressure changes and left ventricular hypertrophy in essential hypertension. Circulation 1990; 81:528–536.

115. Vyssoulis GP, Karpanou EA, Pitsavos CE, et al. Differentiation of beta-blocker effects on serum lipids and apolipoproteins in hypertensive patients with normolipidaemic or dyslipidaemic profiles. Eur Heart J 1992; 13:1506–1513.

116. Weinsier HL, James LD, Darnell BE, et al. Obesity-related hypertension: Evaluation of the separate effects of energy restriction and weight reduction on hemodynamic and neuroendocrine status. Am J Med 1991; 90:460–468.

117. Weir MR, Weber MA, Punzi HA, et al. A dose escalation trial comparing the combination of diltiazem SR and hydrochlorothiazide with the monotherapies in patients with essential hypertension. J Human Hypertens 1992; 6:133–138.

118. White WB. Methods of blood pressure determination to assess antihypertensive agents: Are causal measurements enough? Clin Pharmacol Ther 1989; 45:581–586.

119. World Hypertension League. Nonpharmacological interventions as an adjunct to the pharmacological treatment of hypertension: A statement by WHL. J Human Hypertens 1993; 7:159–164.

## Book

120. Kaplan NM. Clinical Hypertension, Sixth Edition. Williams and Wilkins, Baltimore, 1994.

# Notes

# 8 Antiarrhythmic Agents

F.I. Marcus ♦ L.H. Opie

Arrhythmias require treatment either for alleviating symptoms or for prolonging survival. The wisdom of treating arrhythmias "prophylactically" has been severely questioned by the results of the CAST Study[8] and by a meta-analysis of nearly 100,000 patients with acute myocardial infarction (AMI) treated with antiarrhythmic drugs.[87] Although it is chiefly the Class I and especially the Class IC agents that are proarrhythmic, the principle raised is important in that arrhythmias need treatment only when they are symptomatically significant, or when the prophylactic power of the drug outweighs the adverse effects, as may be the case for beta-blockers and possibly some Class III agents.

## Class IA: Quinidine and Similar Compounds

There are four established classes of antiarrhythmic agents (Table 8–1). This classification, originally purely descriptive, now incorporates the ionic mechanisms which are the basis of the much more complex Sicilian Gambit.[86]

Class IA agents are those that act chiefly by inhibiting the fast sodium channel (phase 0 of the action potential). Class IA agents (quinidine, disopyramide, procainamide) lengthen the effective refractory period by two mechanisms in the usual therapeutic concentrations. First, by definition, they inhibit the fast sodium channel; second, they prolong the action potential duration and thereby have a mild Class III effect (Figs. 8–1 and 8–2). Such compounds can cause proarrhythmic complications by prolonging the QT-interval in certain predisposed individuals or by depressing conduction and promoting re-entry.

### Quinidine

Despite newly reported serious side-effects, quinidine is still one of the most widely used antiarrhythmic drugs in the USA.[61] This is probably because of lack of awareness of the potentially life-threatening side-effects of the drug, and because other drugs with a similar wide antiarrhythmic spectrum, such as flecainide and amiodarone, are not without their problems. Quinidine may exert its harmful effects by proarrhythmic activity and by numerous drug interactions. Ideally long-term prospective studies are required to settle whether the benefits balance the hazards.

ELECTROPHYSIOLOGY. Quinidine (Fig. 8–3) is the prototype of Class I agents. It has a wide spectrum of activity against re-entrant as well as ectopic atrial and ventricular tachyarrhythmias. It slows conduction and increases refractoriness in the retrograde limb of AV nodal tachycardias and over the anterograde or retrograde limbs of the accessory

TABLE 8–1    ANTIARRHYTHMIC DRUG CLASS

| CLASS | CHANNEL EFFECTS | REPOLARIZATION TIME | DRUG EXAMPLES |
|-------|-----------------|---------------------|---------------|
| IA | Sodium block Effect + + | Prolongs | Quinidine Disopyramide Procainamide |
| IB | Sodium block Effect + | Shortens | Lidocaine Phenytoin Mexiletine Tocainide |
| IC | Sodium block Effect + + + | Unchanged | Flecainide Propafenone Moricizine* |
| II | Phase IV (depolarizing current); calcium channel | Unchanged | Beta-blockers including sotalol |
| III | Repolarizing $K^+$ currents | Markedly prolongs | Amiodarone* Sotalol* Bretylium |
| IVA | AV nodal $Ca^{2+}$ block | Unchanged | Verapamil Diltiazem |
| IVB | $K^+$ channel openers (hyperpolarization) | Unchanged | Adenosine ATP |

* "Mixed" class IC and IB properties.
   + = inhibitory effect
  + + = markedly inhibitory effect
+ + + = very major inhibitory effect

paths of the Wolff-Parkinson-White (WPW) syndrome (Fig. 8–4). Quinidine slows the ventricular response to atrial fibrillation in WPW.

RECEPTOR EFFECTS. Quinidine inhibits peripheral and myocardial alpha-adrenergic receptors[66] explaining hypotension with intravenous administration. Quinidine also causes a reflex increase in sympathetic tone by its vagolytic effects because it inhibits muscarinic receptors. Thus it may cause sinus tachycardia[1] and facilitate AV conduction to increase the ventricular rate in atrial flutter or fibrillation. The increased sympathetic tone may explain part of the proarrhythmic effect.

PHARMACOKINETICS AND THERAPEUTIC LEVELS (Table 8–2). Quinidine is metabolized primarily by hydroxylation in the liver and a small amount is excreted by the kidneys; mean bioavailability is about 90% but varies greatly. Quinidine elimination is grossly normal in heart or renal failure, but not in hepatic failure which results in higher blood levels. The plasma half-life increases with age so that the dose should be reduced. Therapeutic blood levels are 2.3 to 5.0 μg/ml (= 3 to 5.5 μM/L) with specific assays.

INDICATIONS. The attempted pharmacological conversion of atrial flutter or fibrillation by quinidine has largely been replaced by cardioversion. When using quinidine for chemical cardioversion, it should be combined with verapamil or digoxin to prevent increased conduction through the AV node as the atrial rate falls and the anticholinergic effect of quinidine becomes evident. Post-cardioversion quinidine helps to maintain sinus rhythm seemingly at the cost of reducing long-term survival.[47] It is reasonably effective but not the ideal drug for reducing recurrences of supraventricular tachycardias, including those of the bypass tract, and recurrent ventricular tachycardia.

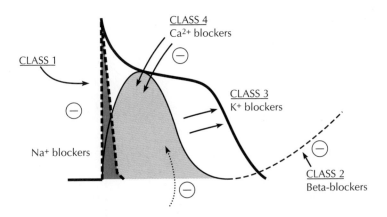

**FIGURE 8–1.** The classical four types of antiarrhythmic agents. Class I agents decrease phase zero of the rapid depolarization of the action potential (rapid sodium channel). Class II agents, beta-blocking drugs, have complex actions including inhibition of spontaneous depolarization (phase 4) and indirect closure of calcium channels, which are less likely to be in the "open" state when not phosphorylated by cyclic AMP. Class III agents block the outward potassium channels to prolong the action potential duration and hence refractoriness. Class IV agents, verapamil and diltiazem, and the indirect calcium antagonist adenosine, all inhibit the inward calcium channel which is most prominent in nodal tissue, particularly the AV node. Most antiarrhythmic drugs have more than one action. Fig. copyright L.H. Opie. Modified from Fig. 23–10, L.H. Opie, The Heart: Physiology, Metabolism, Pharmacology and Therapy, Grune and Stratton, Orlando, 1984.

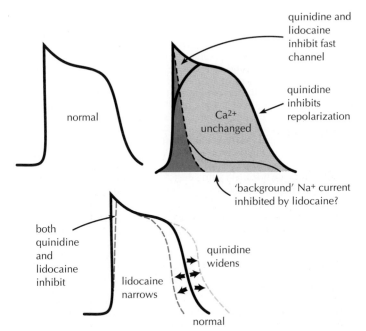

**FIGURE 8–2.** Both quinidine and lidocaine inhibit the fast sodium channel (Class I effect.). The effect on upstroke velocity is much exaggerated for diagrammatic purposes. Lidocaine maximally inhibits the fast channel when it is in the inactivated state, as found in ischemic tissue. In normal tissue, lidocaine promotes repolarization to narrow the action potential duration, possibly through inhibition of a "background" sodium current; in ischemic tissue it may prolong depolarization. In contrast, quinidine readily inhibits the sodium channel in its open state, hence explaining the more marked inhibition of the upstroke velocity of the action potential. Quinidine also prolongs the action potential duration, by inhibition of the repolarizing $K^+$ currents. Fig. copyright L.H. Opie. Modified from Fig. 23–11, L.H. Opie, The Heart: Physiology, Metabolism, Pharmacology and Therapy, Grune and Stratton, Orlando, 1984.

## QUINIDINE EFFECTS

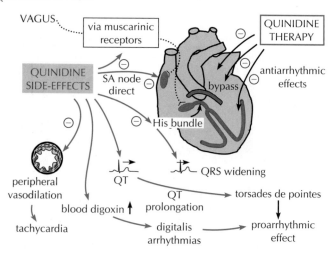

**FIGURE 8–3.** Schematic proposal for therapeutic and serious side-effects of quinidine. Note multiple mechanisms including antiarrhythmic effects by inhibition of the sodium channel (Fig. 8–1), direct inhibition of the SA node and the His bundle, a vagolytic effect via the muscarinic receptors, peripheral vasodilation via alpha-receptor blockade, and an increased blood digoxin level. Note serious risk of proarrhythmic effects. Fig. copyright L.H. Opie.

**DOSE.** Conventionally, the patient is hospitalized and monitored for 72 hours when the proarrhythmic effects may be most evident, including an early increase in PVCs.[91] Traditionally, a test of 0.2 g of quinidine sulfate is given to check for drug idiosyncrasy, including cardiovascular collapse, although such serious side-effects are seldom seen. Then sustained oral therapy is started. Conventional dosing is 300 mg or 400 mg **quinidine sulfate** 4 times daily or every 6 hours with a usual total dose of 1.2 to 1.6 g/day with a maximum of 2 g.[1] Long-acting quinidine preparations (similar dose limits) are **quinidine gluconate** (multiples of 330 mg or 325 mg) and **quinidine polygalacturonate** (multiples of 275 mg as Cardioquin 8- to 12-hourly). The systemic availability is nearly equivalent for the above doses of these three preparations. Marked individual variations in half-life may require monitoring by plasma levels. When a long-acting preparation is started, a loading dose of quinidine sulfate 0.6 to 0.8 g, given 1 hour before the first long-acting dose, will produce an adequate blood level in 3 hours. Intravenous quinidine is now rarely used because of hypotension (vasodilator effect).

**PRECAUTIONS.** Quinidine excess is best prevented by serial measurements of QRS-duration and QT-interval on the ECG. **Conduction delay and proarrhythmic effects** are potentially serious. Reduce dose or reassess therapy if QRS duration widens by 50% or 25% in presence of intraventricular conduction defects, or if the total QRS duration exceeds 140 msec, or if QT- or QTU-prolongation occurs beyond 500 msec. These guidelines although reasonable are not well documented. Besides monitoring QRS and QT-intervals throughout, avoid hypokalemia which predisposes to torsades de pointes which is the probable explanation of quinidine syncope. In patients with the **sick sinus syndrome,** a direct depressant effect of quinidine may be seen (Table 8–3); in others nodal depression is overriden by the vagolytic effect.

**SIDE-EFFECTS.** Serious side-effects may develop soon after the first dose if there is idiosyncrasy, or gradually from cumulative overdosage. Check QRS and QT. **Subjective side-effects** were studied in a double-blind trial when 139 patients took quinidine 300 to 400 mg every 6 hours. Most common were diarrhea (33%), nausea (18%), headache (13%), and dizziness (8%). Twenty-one patients discontinued the drug because of these side-effects. Long-term tolerance in those without early side-effects is excellent. Hypersensitivity reactions to quinidine include fever, skin rash, angioedema, thrombocytopenia, agranulocy-

## AV Nodal Re-entry With or Without WPW

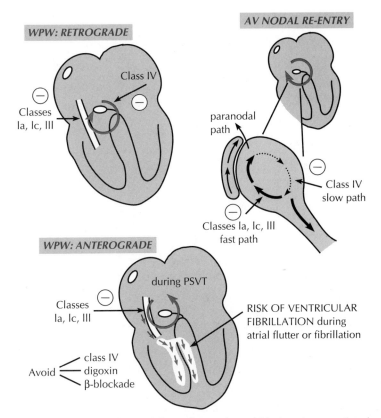

**WPW: RETROGRADE**

Class IV

Classes Ia, Ic, III

**AV NODAL RE-ENTRY**

paranodal path

Class IV slow path

Classes Ia, Ic, III fast path

**WPW: ANTEROGRADE**

during PSVT

Classes Ia, Ic, III

RISK OF VENTRICULAR FIBRILLATION during atrial flutter or fibrillation

Avoid
— class IV
— digoxin
— β-blockade

**FIGURE 8–4.** Site of effects of slow calcium channel blockers (verapamil and diltiazem) and of fast channel blockers in AV nodal re-entry tachycardia (panel A) or bypass re-entry (panel B). In top right panel, AV conduction is anterograde (dashed line) followed by retrograde (solid line). Note that disopyramide, a Class IA agent, does not inhibit the AV node, nor acts on intranodal re-entry, but rather acts on atrial tissue. In general, slow channel blockers are used in most cases of paroxysmal supraventricular nodal tachycardia with or without overt bypass conduction, unless anterograde conduction down the bypass tract is expected (panel C). Due to the proarrhythmic effect of Class IA and Class IC agents, there is currently a choice for Class III agents or for ablation therapy. Fig. copyright L.H. Opie. Modified from Figs. 23–4, 23–11 and 23–15, L.H. Opie, The Heart: Physiology, Metabolism, Pharmacology and Therapy, Grune and Stratton, Orlando, 1984.

tosis, hepatitis, and lupus erythematosus. Proarrhythmic side-effects may increase mortality.[47]

**CONTRAINDICATIONS.** Quinidine is contraindicated when ventricular tachyarrhythmias are associated with or caused by QT-prolongation or if there is already therapy by drugs known to predispose to torsades de pointes. Caution is required with a pre-existing prolonged QT-interval or pre-existing QRS duration or clinical congestive heart failure (CHF), with low initial doses and close monitoring. Other relative contraindications are sick sinus syndrome, bundle branch block, myasthenia gravis (see next section) and severe liver failure (altered pharmacokinetics; also ulcerative colitis and regional enteritis.[51] Watch for drug interactions. Periodic blood counts are advisable during long-term therapy.

**DRUG INTERACTIONS** (Table 8–4). *Quinidine increases blood digoxin levels (decrease dose of digoxin, reassess blood levels). Quinidine may enhance the effects of other hypotensive agents, or agents inhibiting the sinus node (beta-blockers and some calcium antagonists).* The effect of warfarin may be enhanced by a hepatic interaction. Drugs such as phenytoin, barbiturates, and rifampin (rifampicin), that induce hepatic enzymes, may

**TABLE 8–2  ANTIARRHYTHMIC DRUGS USED IN THERAPY OF VENTRICULAR ARRHYTHMIAS**

| AGENT | DOSE<br>(IV = INTRAVENOUS;<br>IM = INTRAMUSCULAR) | PHARMACOKINETICS AND METABOLISM<br>(t½ = PLASMA HALF-LIFE IN NORMALS;<br>LEVEL = THERAPEUTIC BLOOD LEVEL) | SIDE-EFFECTS AND CONTRAINDICATIONS | INTERACTIONS AND PRECAUTIONS |
|---|---|---|---|---|
| Quinidine<br>(Class IA) | Orally 1.2–1.6 g/day in divided doses, 4–12 hourly depending on preparation.<br>Not IV (risk of hypotension). | t½ 7–9 h. Level: 2.3–5 µg/mL. Hepatic hdroxylation. Reduce dose in liver disease. | Many side-effects including diarrhea, nausea; torsades de pointes and hypotension. Vagolytic. Monitor QRS, QT, plasma K. | Increases digoxin level. Enzyme inducers; cimetidine; Class III agents (torsades); diuretics. Warfarin (risk of bleeding). |
| Procainamide<br>(Class IA) | IV 100 mg bolus over 2 min up to 25 mg/min to 1 g in first h; then 2–6 mg/min.<br>Oral 1 g, then up to 500 mg 3 hourly. | t½ 3.5 h. Level 4–10 µg/mL. Plasma metabolism to NAPA. Rapid renal elimination. | Hypotension with IV dose. Limit oral use to 6 months (lupus).<br>Torsades de pointes rare. | No digoxin interaction. Class III agents (torsades). |
| Disopyramide<br>(Class IA) | Oral dose 100–200 mg 6-hourly. Loading dose 300 mg (less if CHF). | t½ 8 h. Level 3–6 µg/mL; toxic > 7 µg/mL<br>Hepatic metabolism (50%), unchanged urinary excretion (50%). | Prominent vagolytic (urinary retention, dry mouth) and negative inotropic effects. Hypotension, torsades, congestive heart failure. | No digoxin interaction; Class III agents (torsades). |
| Lidocaine<br>(Class IB) | IV 75–100 mg; then 2–4 mg/min for 24–30 h.<br>(No oral use) | Effect of single bolus lasts only few min, then t½ about 2 h. Rapid hepatic metabolism. Level 1.4–5.0 µg/mL; toxic > 9 µg/mL | Reduce dose by half if liver blood flow low (shock, beta-blockade, cirrhosis, cimetidine, severe heart failure). High-dose CNS effects. | Beta-blockers decrease hepatic blood flow and increase blood levels. Cimetidine (decreased hepatic metabolism of L). |
| Tocainide<br>(Class IB) | *IV 0.5–0.75 mg/kg/ min for 15 min.<br>Oral loading 400–800 mg, then 2–3 times daily. | t½ 13.5 h. Level 4–10 µg/mL. Unchanged renal excretion (50%). | CNS, GI side-effects. Sometimes immune-based problems (lung fibrosis, blood dyscrasias). | None known. |

**TABLE 8-2    ANTIARRHYTHMIC DRUGS USED IN THERAPY OF VENTRICULAR ARRHYTHMIAS**

| AGENT | DOSE (IV = INTRAVENOUS; IM = INTRAMUSCULAR) | PHARMACOKINETICS AND METABOLISM ($t_{1/2}$ = PLASMA HALF-LIFE IN NORMALS; LEVEL = THERAPEUTIC BLOOD LEVEL) | SIDE-EFFECTS AND CONTRAINDICATIONS | INTERACTIONS AND PRECAUTIONS |
|---|---|---|---|---|
| Mexiletine (Class IB) | *IV 100–250 mg at 12.5 mg/min, then 2.0 mg/kg/h for 3.5 h, then 0.5 mg/kg/h. Oral 100–400 mg 8-hourly; loading dose 400 mg. | $t_{1/2}$ 10–17 h. Level 1–2 µg/mL. Hepatic metabolism, inactive metabolites. | CNS, GI side-effects. Bradycardia, hypotension especially during cotherapy. | Enzyme inducers; dispryamide and beta-blockade; increases the theophylline levels. |
| Phenytoin (Class IB) | IV 10–15 mg/kg over 1 h. Oral 1 g; 500 mg for 2 days; then 400–600 mg daily. | $t_{1/2}$ 24 h. Level 10–18 µg/mL. Hepatic metabolism. Hepatic or renal disease requires reduced doses. | Hypotension, vertigo, dysarthria, lethargy, gingivitis, macrocytic anemia, lupus, pulmonary infiltrates | Hepatic enzyme inducers. |
| Flecainide (Class IC) | *IV 1–2 mg/kg over 10 min, then 0.15–0.25 mg/kg/h. Oral 100–400 mg 2 times daily. Hospitalize. | $t_{1/2}$ 13–19 h. Hepatic (⅔); ⅓ renal excretion unchanged. Keep trough level below 1.0 µg/mL. | QRS prolongation. Proarrhythmia. Depressed LV function. CNS side-effects. Increased incidence of death postinfarct. | Many, especially added inhibition of conduction and nodal tissue. |
| Moricizine (Class IC) | 200–300 mg 3 times daily | $t_{1/2}$ 6–13 h. Numerous hepatic metabolites; long-lasting. | Proarrhythmia especially if pre-existing congestive heart failure. | Little experience in hepatic or renal failure. |
| Propafenone (Class IC) | *IV 2 mg/kg then 2 mg/min. Oral 150–300 mg 3 times daily. | $t_{1/2}$ variable 2–10 h, up to 32 h in nonmetabolizers. Level 0.2–3.0 µg/mL. Variable hepatic metabolism (P-450 deficiency slows). | QRS prolongation. Modest negative inotropic effect. GI side-effects. proarrhythmia. | Digoxin level increased. Hepatic inducers. |

| Drug | Dose | Pharmacokinetics | Side-effects | Notes |
|---|---|---|---|---|
| Sotalol (Class III) | 160–640 mg daily, occasionally higher in two divided doses. | t½ 15–17 h. Not metabolized. Hydrophilic. Renal loss. | Myocardial depression, sinus bradycardia, AV block. Torsades if hypokalemic. | Added risk of torsades with IA agents or diuretics. Decrease dose in renal failure. |
| Amiodarone (Class III) | Oral loading dose 1200–1600 mg daily; maintenance 200–400 mg daily, sometimes less. *Occasional IV use (see text) | t½ 25–110 days. Level 1.0–2.5 µg/mL. Hepatic metabolism. Lipid soluble with extensive distribution in body. Excretion by skin, biliary tract, lacrimal glands. | Complex side-effects including pulmonary fibrosis. QT-prolongation. Torsades uncommon. | Class IA agents predispose to torsades. Beta-blockers predispose to nodal depression. |
| Betylium tosylate (Class III) | IV 5–10 mg/kg, lifting arm, repeat to max 30 mg/kg, then IV 1–2 mg/min or IM 5–10 mg/kg 8-hourly at varying sites (local necrosis). | t½ 7–9 h. Level 0.5–1.0 µg/mL. | IV: hypotension. Initial sympathomimetic effects. | Decrease dose in renal failure. |

Compiled by LH Opie and modified from previous edition. Moricizine data from Clyne et al.[46]

* Not in the USA

IV = intravenous; IM = intramuscular; t½, plasma half-life; level = therapeutic blood level.

Enzyme hepatic inducers = barbiturates, phenytoin, rifampin which induce hepatic enzymes thereby decreasing blood levels of the drug.

TABLE 8–3    EFFECTS AND SIDE-EFFECTS OF SOME VENTRICULAR ANTIARRHYTHMIC AGENTS ON ELECTROPHYSIOLOGY AND HEMODYNAMICS

| AGENT | SINUS NODE | SINUS RATE | A-HIS | PR | AV BLOCK | H-P | WPW | QRS | QT | SERIOUS HEMO-DYNAMIC EFFECTS | RISK OF TORSADES | RISK OF MONO-MORPHIC VT |
|---|---|---|---|---|---|---|---|---|---|---|---|---|
| Quinidine | → | ↑ | 0 | 0/→ | 0 | → | ↓A/R | ↑↑ | ↑↑ | IV use | ++ | 0, + |
| Procainamide | 0 | 0/↑ | 0/↓ | 0/→ | Avoid | → | ↓A/R | 0/→ | ↑ | Rare | + | 0, + |
| Disopyramide | → | ↑ | 0 | 0/→ | 0 | 0/↓ | ↓A/R | ↑ | ↑ | LV ↓↓↓ | + | 0, + |
| Lidocaine | 0 | 0 | 0/↓ | 0 | 0 | 0 | ↓/0 | 0 | 0 | Toxic doses | 0 | 0 |
| Phenytoin | 0 | 0 | ↑/0 | 0 | Lessens | 0 | ↓/0 | 0 | ↓ | IV hypotension | 0, + | 0, + |
| Mexiletine | 0 | 0 | ↑/0 | 0 | ↓/0 | ↓/0 | ↓/0 | 0/→ | 0 | Toxic doses | 0, + | 0, + |
| Tocainide | 0 | 0 | ↓/0 | 0 | ↓/0 | ↓/0 | ↓/0 | 0 | 0 | In CHF | 0, + | 0, + |
| Flecainide | 0/↓ | 0 | ↓↓↓ | → | Avoid | ↓↓ | ↓A/R | → | → (via QRS) | LV ↓↓ | 0 | +++ |
| Moricizine | 0 | 0 | → | → | Avoid | → | ? | → | → (via QRS) | Modest LV ↓ | 0 | ++ |
| Sotalol | ↓↓ | ↓↓ | → | → | Avoid | 0 | A/R | 0 | ↑↑ | IV use | ++ | 0, + |
| Amiodarone | → | → | → | 0/→ | Avoid | 0/↓ | A/R | 0 | ↑↑ | IV use | + | 0, + |

Table compiled by LH Opie and modified from previous edition. For moricizine, see Clyne et al.[46]

A-His = Atria-His conduction; H-P = His-Purkinje conduction; WPW = Wolff-Parkinson-White syndrome accessory pathways; LV = left ventricle; R = retrograde;

A = antegrade; BBB = bundle branch block; IV = intravenous; ↓ = depresses; ↑ = increases; → = prolongs; ← = shortens.

markedly increase the hepatic metabolism of quinidine with decreased steady-state blood levels. Conversely, cimetidine can decrease the metabolism of quinidine with opposite effects.[1] Quinidine would be expected to inhibit the hepatic metabolism of propafenone, metoprolol, flecainide, and other drugs dependent on the P-450 enzymes. Hypokalemia decreases quinidine efficacy and increases QT- or QTU-prolongation. Concomitant therapy with amiodarone or sotalol or other drugs prolonging the QT-interval requires great care and is best avoided.[1] Quinidine reduces the effects of procedures that enhance vagal activity such as carotid sinus massage by its vagolytic effect (this opposes some digitalis effects such as slowing of the heart). Quinidine also reduces the effects of anticholinesterases in myasthenia gravis (inhibition of muscarinic receptors) and enhances antibiotic-induced muscle weakness.

TREATMENT OF ACUTE TOXICITY. Stop quinidine, reduce plasma potassium if elevated, and acidify urine to encourage excretion. Torsades de pointes or severely disorganised conduction may require **temporary ventricular pacing** and/or **magnesium sulfate.**

## Procainamide

Procainamide (**Pronestyl**) is generally effective against a wide variety of supraventricular and ventricular arrhythmias, including VT. As in the case of quinidine, no effect on mortality or survival has been shown. Although usually given orally, intravenous procainamide may be tried if lidocaine fails. The oral use is limited by a short half-life and the long-term danger of the lupus syndrome. In contrast, other side-effects are less than with quinidine (GI, QRS or torsades, hypotension) and there is no interaction with digoxin.

ELECTROPHYSIOLOGY. Procainamide is a Class IA agent, like quinidine, but does not prolong the QT-interval to the same extent and has less interaction with the muscarinic receptors.[1]

RECEPTOR EFFECTS. Procainamide has less interaction with muscarinic receptors than does quinidine. There is direct sympathetic inhibition,[79] so that vasodilation occurs through a mechanism different from that with quinidine.

PHARMACOKINETICS. There is rapid renal elimination (half-life, 3.5 hours with normal renal function). In the elderly with decreased renal function, the dose of procainamide should be reduced by about 50%. In mild heart failure the dose should be reduced by a quarter. Intravenous procainamide should not be given at a dose exceeding 25 mg/min (see Side-effects). Plasma metabolism by acetylation yields the active N-acetyl procainamide (NAPA) with a half-life of 6 to 8 hours and Class III antiarrhythmic activity.

DOSE. An **oral** loading dose of procainamide 1 g is followed by up to 500 mg 3-hourly. A slow-release preparation of procainamide (**Procan SR**) appears to allow 6-hourly dosing intervals at a dose of 500 to 1,500 mg every 6 hours.[49] The **intravenous dose** is 100 mg over 2 minutes, then up to 25 mg/min to a maximum of 1 g in the first hour, then 2 to 6 mg/min.

INDICATIONS. In acute myocardial infarction (AMI), it can be used even when there is cardiac failure or low cardiac output.[1] For acute ventricular tachycardia, it can be given slowly intravenously. It is sometimes used for the prevention of ventricular tachycardia without proof of long-term benefit. Like other Class IA agents, procainamide is also effective against supraventricular tachyarrhythmias including those complicating the WPW bypass tract, and may cardiovert acute onset atrial fibrillation.

CONTRAINDICATIONS. These include shock, myasthenia gravis (see quinidine), heart block, and severe renal failure. Severe heart failure is a relative contraindicatio.[16]

SIDE-EFFECTS. During chronic oral therapy,[1] 9 of 39 patients had early

**TABLE 8-4     INTERACTIONS (KINETIC AND DYNAMIC) OF ANTIARRHYTHMIC DRUGS**

| DRUG | INTERACTION WITH | RESULT |
|---|---|---|
| Quinidine | digoxin | Increased digoxin level |
| | other Type 1 antiarrhythmics | Added negative inotropic effect and/or depressed conduction |
| | beta-blockers, verapamil | Enhanced hypotension, negative inotropic effect |
| | amiodarone | Risk of torsades; increased quinidine levels |
| | sotalol | Risk of torsades |
| | diuretics | If hypokalemia, risk of torsades |
| | verapamil | Increased quinidine level |
| | nifedipine | Decreased quinidine level |
| | warfarin | Enhanced anticoagulation |
| | cimetidine | Increased blood levels |
| | enzyme inducers | Decreased blood levels |
| Procainamide | cimetidine | Decreases renal clearance |
| | Class III agents, diuretics | Torsades |
| Disopyramide | other Type 1 antiarrhythmics | Depressed conduction |
| | amiodarone, sotalol | Torsades |
| | beta-blockers, verapamil | Enhanced hypotension |
| | anticholinergics | Increased anticholinergic effect |
| | pyridostigmine | Decreased anticholinergic effect |
| Lidocaine | beta-blockers, cimetidine, halothane | Reduced liver blood flow (increased blood levels) |
| | enzyme inducers | Decreased blood levels |
| Tocainide | None known | — |
| Mexiletine | enzyme inducers | Decreased mexiletine levels |
| | disopyramide, beta-blockers, theophylline | Negative inotropic potential |
| | | Theophylline levels increased[38] |
| Flecainide | Major kinetic interaction with amiodarone. | Increase of blood F levels; half-dose. |
| | Added SA or AV node inhibition (beta-blockers, verapamil, diltiazem, digoxin); | SA and AV nodal depression; depressed myocardium; conduction delay |

**TABLE 8–4** INTERACTION (KINETIC AND DYNAMIC) OF ANTIARRHYTHMIC DRUGS *(continued)*

| DRUG | INTERACTION WITH | RESULT |
|---|---|---|
| | Added negative inotropic effects (beta-blockers, quinidine, disopyramide) | As above |
| | Added HV conduction depression (quinidine, procainamide) | Conduction block |
| Moricizine | Digoxin, verapamil, diltiazem, beta-blockers | Added AV nodal block |
| | Cimetidine | Plasma concentration of M increased |
| Propafenone | As for flecainide (but amiodarone interaction not reported); digoxin; warfarin | Enhanced SA, AV and myocardial depression<br>Digoxin level increased<br>Anticoagulant effect enhanced[23] |
| Sotalol | Diuretics, Class 1A agents, amiodarone, tricyclics, phenothiazines | Risk of torsades; avoid hypokalemia |
| Amiodarone | As for sotalol<br>digoxin<br>phenytoin<br>flecainide<br>warfarin | Risk of torsades;<br>Increased digoxin levels<br>Double interaction, see text<br>Increased flecainide levels<br>Increased warfarin effect |
| Verapamil Diltiazem | Beta-blockers, excess digoxin, myocardial depressants, quinidine | Increased myocardial or nodal depression |
| Adenosine | Dipyridamole | Adenosine catabolism inhibited; much increased half-life |
| | Methylxanthines (caffeine, theophylline) | Inhibit receptor; decreased drug effects |

Enzyme inducers = hepatic enzyme inducers, i.e., barbiturates, phenytoin, rifampin. For references, see Table 3 in Opie.[76] Moricizine data from Clyne et al.[46]

side-effects (rash, fever) and 14 of 16 had late side-effects (arthralgia, rash); fear of the lupus syndrome (likeliest in slow acetylators) limited therapy to 6 months at the most. Despite the efficacy of procainamide, the risk of lupus is about one-third of patients treated for over 6 months. Agranulocytosis may be a late side-effect of procainamide, especially with the slow-release preparation.[1] Hypotension is a common side-effect with intravenous administration (vasodilator effect) especially with doses exceeding 25 mg/min.[1] Heart block may develop or increase. In atrial fibrillation or flutter the ventricular rate may increase as the atrial rate slows, so that concomitant digitalization is advisable. The vagolytic effect of procainamide is much weaker than that of quinidine.[1] Proarrhythmic effects including torsades de pointes may be dose-related.

Drug Interactions.   Cimetidine inhibits the renal clearance of procainamide to prolong the elimination half-life so that the procainamide dose should be reduced.[1] There is less risk of torsades de pointes than with quinidine.

Treatment of Acute Toxicity.   Treatment is the same as for quinidine.

## Disopyramide

Disopyramide is a Class IA antiarrhythmic agent, electrophysiologically like quinidine, with a similar antiarrhythmic profile. Like quinidine, it prolongs the QRS and QT-intervals, the latter involving risk of torsades. Unlike quinidine, it does not inhibit AV nodal conduction. The crucial differences lie in the side-effects. Disopyramide has fewer GI problems, yet much stronger anticholinergic side-effects such as urinary retention. Disopyramide inhibits the muscarinic receptors 40 times more effectively than does quinidine.[1] Thus, there is a relative increase of sympathetic activity, masking the direct depressant effects of disopyramide on the sinus node and conduction tissue. A prominent and largely unexplained side-effect of disopyramide is the negative inotropic effect, so marked that disopyramide is now also used in the therapy of hypertrophic obstructive cardiomyopathy;[1] presumably it interferes with excitation-contraction coupling.

Pharmacokinetics and Therapeutic Levels.   The phosphate salt (**Norpace** in the USA; **Dirythmin** elsewhere) and the free base (**Rythmodan** in the UK) have similar bioavailability and pharmacokinetics. Most of the oral dose is bioavailable. About half is metabolized by N-dealkylation and about half excreted unchanged in the urine. The usual half-life is about 8 hours. One metabolite is powerfully anticholinergic. The higher the blood level, the lower the percentage bound to plasma proteins so that potential toxicity is enhanced.

Dose.   The usual **oral dose** is 100 to 200 mg 6-hourly with an initial loading dose of 300 mg (less if CHF). Several long-acting preparations, including **Norpace CR, Rythmodan Retard** and **Dirythmin SA** need only 12-hourly dosing. The dose should be reduced in severe renal failure and in the elderly (renal excretion of disopyramide) and in CHF (prolonged half-life).

Indications.   Oral disopyramide is approved only in the USA for the treatment of life-threatening ventricular arrhythmias. In **paroxysmal VT,** disopyramide may be effective when other Class IA agents such as quinidine or procainamide fail;[1] the logic for this observation is not clear, but may include minor electrophysiological differences and a different side-effect profile.

In **supraventricular tachycardia,** oral or intravenous disopyramide (0.5 mg/kg over 5 minutes, then 1 mg/kg/h, not in the USA) may cause reversion to sinus rhythm, especially if the arrhythmia is of recent onset. Its major effect is not to inhibit the AV node itself, but rather the retrograde fast pathway,[1] thereby terminating a tachycardia with AV nodal re-entry. In the supraventricular arrhythmias of the WPW syndrome, disopyramide acts on the bypass tract to inhibit conduction and to increase the refractory period (Fig. 8–4).[1] Disopyramide is better than placebo in reducing recurrent atrial fibrillation.[1]

In **hypertrophic cardiomyopathy,** disopyramide acts hemodynamically by its negative inotropic effect.[31]

SIDE-EFFECTS. Side-effects include (1) negative inotropic effects; (2) possibly serious anticholinergic activity especially in elderly men (prostatic obstruction), in threatened glaucoma, with myasthenia gravis, or when constipation is a pre-existing problem (verapamil cotherapy); (3) occasional hypoglycemia[1] and cholestatic jaundice; and (4) excessive QT-prolongation and torsades de pointes.[1] In a meta-analysis, the anticipated proarrhythmic effect was not specifically confirmed.[87] Oral cholinesterase inhibitors may decrease side-effects (see Beneficial Drug Interactions). Dry mouth is common (anticholinergic).

CONTRAINDICATIONS. Uncompensated CHF is an absolute contraindication, as are glaucoma, hypotension, untreated urinary retention, and significant pretreatment QT-prolongation. Relative contraindications are (1) compensated CHF; (2) prostatism; (3) treated glaucoma or a family history of glaucoma; (4) severe constipation; and (5) sinus node dysfunction.[1]

PRECAUTIONS. Electrocardiographically, disopyramide can increase QT or QRS-prolongation; discontinue if QRS or QTc increases by 25% or more. Development of second or third degree AV block or uni-, bi- or trifascicular block requires discontinuation of the drug unless an artificial pacemaker is used. Digitalization is indicated for borderline or suspected heart failure or for atrial flutter or fibrillation to avoid sudden acceleration of AV conduction. In pregnancy, disopyramide may stimulate uterine contractions; it is excreted in human milk.

DRUG INTERACTIONS. The concomitant use of **other Type 1 antiarrhythmic agents or beta-blockers** with disopyramide should be reserved for life-threatening arrhythmias that are demonstrably unresponsive to single agent antiarrhythmic agents (risk of negative inotropic effects, prolonged conduction). Cotherapy with Class III agents or diuretics or erythromycin increases the risk of torsades de pointes.[32] Phenytoin or other inducers of hepatic enzymes may lower disopyramide plasma levels. Tricyclic antidepressants have anticholinergic effects which could be additive to those of disopyramide.

BENEFICIAL DRUG INTERACTION. Pyridostigmine bromide (**Mestinon Timespan,** 90 to 180 mg 3 times daily) or bethanechol (**Urecholine**) may reduce anticholinergic side-effects of disopyramide by inhibition of cholinesterase activity.[12]

## Class IB: Lidocaine (Lignocaine) and Similar Compounds

As a group, Class IB agents inhibit the fast sodium current (typical Class I effect) while shortening the action potential duration in non-diseased tissue (Fig. 8–2). The former has the more powerful effect, while the latter might actually predispose to arrhythmias, but ensures that QT-prolongation does not occur. Class IB agents act selectively on diseased or ischemic tissue, where they are thought to promote conduction block, thereby interrupting re-entry circuits. They have a particular affinity for binding with inactivated sodium channels with rapid onset-offset kinetics, which may be why such drugs are ineffective in atrial arrhythmias, since the action potential duration is so short.[24]

## LIDOCAINE KINETICS

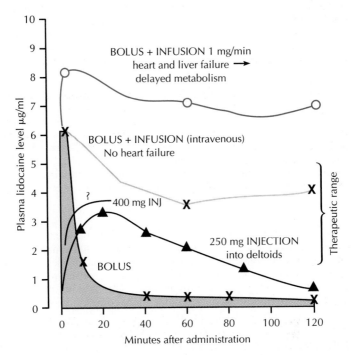

**FIGURE 8–5.** Lidocaine kinetics. To achieve and to maintain an adequate blood level of lidocaine requires an initial bolus or intramuscular injection followed by an infusion. For an intramuscular injection to give sustained high blood levels may require a dose of 400 mg. Note that in the presence of cardiac or liver failure, delayed metabolism increases the blood level with danger of toxic effects. Fig. copyright L.H. Opie. Modified from Fig. 23–12, L.H. Opie, The Heart: Physiology, Metabolism, Pharmacology and Therapy, Grune and Stratton, Orlando, 1984.

### Lidocaine (Lignocaine)

Lidocaine (**Xylocaine; Xylocard**) has become the standard intravenous agent for suppression of arrhythmias associated with AMI and with cardiac surgery. The concept of prophylactic lidocaine to prevent VT and VF in AMI is increasingly being abandoned.[84,87] The drug has no role in the control of chronic recurrent ventricular arrhythmias. Lidocaine acts preferentially on the ischemic myocardium[1] and is more effective in the presence of a high external potassium;[36] therefore hypokalemia must be corrected for maximum efficacy (also for other Class I agents).

PHARMACOKINETICS. The bulk of an intravenous dose of lidocaine is rapidly de-ethylated by liver microsomes. The two critical factors governing lidocaine metabolism and hence its efficacy are liver blood flow (decreased in old age and by heart failure, beta-blockade, and cimetidine) and liver microsomal activity (enzyme inducers). Since lidocaine is so rapidly distributed within minutes after an initial intravenous loading dose, there must be a subsequent infusion or repetitive doses to maintain therapeutic blood levels (Fig. 8–5). Lidocaine metabolites circulate in high concentrations and may contribute to toxic and therapeutic actions. The half-life increases with prolonged (> 24 hours) infusion.

DOSE. A constant infusion would take 5 to 9 hours to achieve therapeutic levels (1.4 to 5.0 μg/ml), so standard therapy includes a loading dose of 75 to 100 mg intravenously[87] or 400 mg intramuscularly.[1] Thereafter lidocaine is infused at 2 to 4 mg/min for 24 to 30 hours, aiming at 3 mg/min, which prevents VF but may cause serious side-effects in about 15% of patients, in half of whom the lidocaine dose may have to be reduced.[1] Poor liver blood flow (low cardiac output or beta-blockade), liver disease, or cimetidine or halothane therapy calls for halved dosage. The dose should also be decreased for elderly patients in whom toxicity develops more frequently and after 12 to 24 hours of infusion.

SIDE-EFFECTS. Lidocaine is generally free of hemodynamic depressive side-effects, even in patients with CHF, and it seldom impairs nodal function or conduction. The higher infusion rate of 3 to 4 mg/min may result in drowsiness, numbness, speech disturbances, and dizziness, especially in patients over 60 years of age. Minor adverse neural reactions can occur in about half the patients, even with 2 to 3 mg/min of lidocaine.[1] Occasionally there is SA arrest especially during coadministration of other drugs that potentially depress nodal function.

DRUG INTERACTIONS AND COMBINATIONS. In patients receiving cimetidine, propranolol, or halothane, the hepatic clearance of lidocaine is reduced and toxicity may occur more readily, so that the dose should be reduced. With hepatic enzyme inducers (barbiturates, phenytoin, and rifampin) the dose needs to be increased. Combination of lidocaine with early beta-blockade is not a contraindication, although there is no reported experience. The obvious precaution is that bradyarrhythmias may become more common because beta-blockade reduces liver blood flow. Hence a standard dose of lidocaine would have potentially more side-effects including sinus node inhibition.

LIDOCAINE FAILURE. If lidocaine apparently fails, is there hypokalemia? Are there technical errors? Is the drug really called for or should beta-blockade rather be used? If none of these factors is present, a blood level is taken (if available) and the infusion rate can be increased cautiously until development of the central nervous system effects (confusion, slurred speech). Alternatively or concomitantly, Class IA agents are tried (especially procainamide) before resorting to Class III agents, such as bretylium or amiodarone.

CLINICAL USE. *Should lidocaine be administered routinely to all patients with AMI?* The question has been asked for at least 16 years. Increasingly the answer is no.[87] It is "an idea whose time is all but gone."[84] At the present low rates of ventricular fibrillation, due to more frequent use of thrombolytic therapy and beta-blockade, about 400 patients with suspected AMI must be treated to save one from VF.[84] Thus it is uncertain whether prophylactic lidocaine is cost-effective, especially bearing in mind that its use might substantially increase mortality.[63]

*Should lidocaine be used routinely before attempted defibrillation of ventricular tachyarrhythmias?* The answer is no—any benefits are cancelled by the greater delays involved in achieving defibrillation.[89]

*When can it be used?* When tachyarrhythmias seriously interfere with hemodynamic status in patients with AMI (especially when already beta-blocked) and during cardiac surgery or general anesthesia.

*When should lidocaine not be used?* "Prophylactically" or when there is bradycardia or bradycardia plus ventricular tachyarrhythmias, when atropine (or pacing) and not lidocaine is required.

## Tocainide

Tocainide (**Tonocard**) is an oral analog of lidocaine. The major side-effects are neurologic; GI side-effects are also frequent. Neutropenia and agranulocytosis, though rare, limit its use. A major advantage is that there are few drug interactions.

The usual oral dose is 300 to 600 mg 3 times daily; twice-daily administration may be effective. The dose should be decreased in renal failure (renal excretion), as well as in the elderly (low glomerular filtration rate).

The approved indication in the USA is treatment of symptomatic ventricular arrhythmias. That includes those refractory to more conventional antiarrhythmics, such as quinidine, procainamide, and propranolol.[1] Hypersensitivity can cause second- or third-degree heart block in the absence of an artificial pacemaker. In the package insert, nondigitalized atrial flutter or fibrillation is mentioned as a relative contraindication because of the danger of ventricular acceleration (unexpected effect on atrial tissue).

Tocainide frequently causes dose-dependent nervous system (28%) and GI reactions (11%), including lightheadedness or dizziness, paresthesia or numbness in the extremities, tremor, nausea, vomiting, or diarrhea.[1] Such side-effects cause discontinuation in about one-fifth of patients. Serious immune-based side-effects, such as pulmonary fibrosis, may occur. Serious blood dyscrasias, such as leukopenia and thrombocytopenia, occur in about 0.2% of patients treated with this drug. Therefore, it should be limited for use in life-threatening ventricular arrhythmias or carefully selected patients with less severe arrhythmias. Proarrhythmic effects may occur. CHF may be aggravated.[16]

Weekly blood counts are required for the first 3 months, with periodic counts thereafter. Patients should report bruising or bleeding or symptoms of infection (throat, chest).

## Mexiletine

Mexiletine (**Mexitil**), like lidocaine, is used chiefly against ventricular arrhythmias. Unlike lidocaine, it can be given orally. There are several arguments favoring it as one of several reasonable choices as a first-line agent in ventricular arrhythmias requiring therapy: (1) its comparable efficacy to quinidine; (2) little or no hemodynamic depression; (3) no QT-prolongation; and (4) no vagolytic effects. However, frequent GI and central nervous side-effects limit the dose and possible therapeutic benefit. Like other Class 1B agents, it may fail to improve mortality.[87]

PHARMACOKINETICS. Mexiletine is well absorbed with a high bioavailability and reaches peak plasma levels in 2 to 4 hours. The therapeutic blood level is 1 to 2 μg/ml. Ninety percent is metabolized in the liver to inactive metabolites and the rest excreted in the urine as unchanged mexiletine.[1] The half-life is 10 to 17 hours in normals. Higher than normal plasma levels are found in chronic liver disease but not in renal failure. Mexiletine is lipophilic and enters the brain (central nervous side-effects).

DOSE. The oral loading dose is 400 mg if high initial levels are required, followed by 300 to 1200 mg (given with food or antacid) in three divided daily doses, starting 2 to 6 hours after the loading dose. In the USA, the highest approved dose is 900 mg daily. The intravenous dose (not in the USA) is 100 to 250 mg (2.5 mg/kg) at 12.5 mg/min, then 2.0 mg/kg/h for 3.5 hours, then 0.5 mg/kg/h as long as needed. In Europe, sustained-release capsules (**Perlongets**) have a usual dose of 360 mg twice daily. The dose of mexiletine should be reduced in severe liver disease and in CHF. In pregnant women, the drug seems safe although it crosses the placental barrier. In the elderly, the dose must be reduced because of possible central nervous system side-effects and because hepatic metabolism is decreased.

INDICATIONS. The major approved indication is treatment of life-threatening ventricular arrhythmias. In the chronic oral prophylaxis of ventricular arrhythmias postinfarction, mexiletine 300 mg 8-hourly is as effective as procainamide.[1] A similar dose of mexiletine can be combined with quinidine (about 1 g daily) with a lower incidence of side-effects and better antiarrhythmic action than with higher doses of either agent alone.[1] In VT resistant to more conventional drugs or in the suppression of induced VT,[64] mexiletine alone gives only modest benefit.[1] In a major clinical trial on postinfarct patients, mexiletine reduced Holter-monitored arrhythmias in the first 6 months without improved mortality over 1 year; in fact, mortality tended to increase.[1]

SIDE-EFFECTS. The major problem is a narrow therapeutic-toxic margin,[1] so that in patients with ventricular arrhythmias resistant to conventional agents, an adequate antiarrhythmic effect is only obtained in 25% or fewer of patients without significant side-effects. Dizziness and mild disorientation may result from a single oral dose of 400 mg. During chronic therapy, side-effects include indigestion in 40%, tremor or nystagmus (10%, higher in some series) and confusional states in less than 10%. Severe side-effects occur in about 35% of patients receiving 1 g or more per day.[1] Nausea may be decreased by giving the drug with food. In about 5% of patients, bradycardia and hypotension may occur.[1] While a proarrhythmic effect cannot be excluded,[87] torsades de pointes is rare. Liver damage occasionally occurs. Intravenous prochloroperazine 12.5 mg can be given 5 minutes before mexiletine injection to lessen dizziness and vomiting.

CONTRAINDICATIONS. Cardiogenic shock or second- or third-degree heart block without a pacemaker. Relative contraindications are bradycardia, conduction defects, hypotension, hepatic failure, and severe renal or myocardial failure. Caution in patients with liver damage or seizures.

DRUG INTERACTIONS AND COMBINATION THERAPY. Narcotics delay the GI absorption of mexiletine. Hepatic enzyme inducers decrease plasma levels of mexiletine. Concurrent disopyramide or beta-blocker therapy predisposes to a negative inotropic effect.[1] Mexiletine elevates plasma levels of theophylline.[38] The drug may be combined with quinidine and amiodarone,[1] provided contraindications are observed and appropriate dose regimens of the two drugs are chosen.

## Phenytoin (Diphenylhydantoin)

Phenytoin (**Dilantin, Epanutin**) has four specific uses. First, in digitalis-toxic arrhythmias, it maintains conduction or even enhances it, especially in the presence of hypokalemia; it also inhibits delayed afterdepolarizations.[1] Second, phenytoin is effective against the ventricular arrhythmias occurring after congenital heart surgery.[1] Third, phenytoin is used in the congenital prolonged QT-syndrome when beta-blockade alone has failed; here, reliable comparative studies have not been done. Why phenytoin is so effective in the ventricular arrhythmias of young children is not known. Fourth, occasionally in patients with epilepsy and arrhythmias this dual action comes to the fore.

The intravenous dose is 10 to 15 mg/kg over 1 hour followed by oral maintenance of 400 to 600 mg/day (2 to 4 mg/kg/day in children). The long half-life allows once daily dosage with, however, the risk of serious side-effects including dysarthria, pulmonary infiltrates, lupus, gingivitis, and macrocytic anemia.

Phenytoin is an inducer of hepatic enzymes and therefore alters the dose requirements of many other drugs used in cardiology, including quinidine, lidocaine and mexiletine.

## Moricizine

Moricizine (**Ethmozine**) is a phenothiazine derivative, originally from the USSR and approved in the USA for management of documented ventricular life-threatening arrhythmias. Electrophysiologically, it has both lidocaine-like Class IB properties and also prolongs the PR and QRS times, while leaving the QT-interval unchanged. Therefore *moricizine may represent a "mixed" Class IB/IC agent.* The phenothiazine-like structure (which could perhaps predispose to QT-prolongation) also suggests a third antiarrhythmic mechanism through a central nervous system effect. Clinically, it is effective for the treatment of both ventricular and supraventricular arrhythmias. In patients with AV nodal re-entrant tachycardia, the drug acts by slowing retrograde conduction. In patients with tachycardias complicating the WPW syndrome, the drug increases anterograde and retrograde refractoriness in the re-entry limbs.[1] Moricizine is rapidly and extensively metabolized in the liver with a half-life of approximately 2 to 5 hours. The usual dose for adults is 600 to 900 mg in 3 divided doses 8-hourly with dose reduction in the elderly. Neurologic side-effects, most evident during intravenous infusion (not available in USA), include nervousness, dizziness, and vertigo. During oral therapy, side-effects are slight and include dizziness, paresthesia, headache and nausea. In the CAST-II study,[44] 13% suffered dizziness. Moricizine has only mildly depressant effects on LV function. Moricizine was evaluated for possible benefit in postinfarct ventricular premature systoles in which the flecainide and encainide arms of the CAST study were stopped.[44] Moricizine was ineffective as well as harmful. It induced more cardiac arrests within the first 2 weeks of initiation of therapy.

## Class IC Agents

These agents have acquired a particularly bad reputation because of their proarrhythmic effects in the CAST study[7] (flecainide), as well as in the CASH study[43] (propafenone). As a group they have three major electrophysiological effects. First, they are powerful inhibitors of the fast sodium channel causing a marked depression of the upstroke of the cardiac action potential. Second, they have a marked inhibitory effect on His-Purkinje conduction with QRS widening. Third, they markedly shorten the action potential duration of only Purkinje fibers leaving unaltered that of the surrounding myocardium.[21] Class IC agents are all potent antiarrhythmics used largely in the control of ventricular tachyarrhythmias resistant to other drugs. Their markedly depressant effect on conduction may explain their significant proarrhythmic action, to which the discrepancies in the action potential duration between Purkinje and ventricular tissue may contribute by promoting inhomogeneity.[21] Proarrhythmic effects limit the use of these agents in supraventricular tachycardias, particularly in the case of recurrent atrial fibrillation or flutter in the presence of structural heart disease.[13]

### Flecainide

Flecainide (**Tambocor**) is effective for the treatment of both supraventricular and ventricular arrhythmias. Its proarrhythmic potential limits its use. The reason for the emphasis, especially in the presence of structural heart disease, is because poor LV function exaggerates the proarrhythmic effects.[55] The negative inotropic effect also limits its use in ischemic heart disease or dilated cardiomyopathy. The drug should only be started under careful observation in hospital, using a gradually increasing low oral dose with checks of serum levels. This procedure will not, however, avoid all the excess mortality as shown in the CAST study.[7]

**Pharmacokinetics** are as follows. Flecainide is well absorbed with a bioavailability as high as 95%, and peak plasma levels at 2 to 4 hours. When feasible, plasma trough levels should be monitored and kept below 1.0 µg/ml to avoid myocardial depression.[1] The plasma half-life is 12 to 27 hours (package insert). Flecainide is two-thirds metabolized by the liver to inactive metabolites, whereas one-third is excreted unchanged by the kidneys and a small amount in the feces.

The **initial dose** for sustained VT is 100 mg every 12 hours, increased every 4 days by 50 mg twice daily to a maximum of 400 mg/day. For paroxysmal supraventricular tachycardia or flutter or fibrillation, the initial dose is 50 mg every 12 hours up to 300 mg daily. Lower doses are required for patients with poor LV function or severe renal failure or those receiving amiodarone.

**Indications** are (1) life-threatening sustained ventricular tachycardia and (2) paroxysmal supraventricular tachycardia including WPW arrhythmias, and paroxysmal atrial flutter or fibrillation, in patients without structural heart disease.

Flecainide is **contraindicated** in the absence of life-threatening VT or SVT. It is contraindicated in patients with right bundle branch block and left anterior hemiblock unless a pacemaker is implanted. It is also contraindicated in the sick sinus syndrome,[1] when the left ventricle is depressed, and in the postinfarct state.

**Cardiac side-effects** include aggravation of ventricular arrhythmias in 5% to 12%[1] or possibly more in the presence of pre-existing LV failure, and threat of sudden death as in the CAST study.[7] The proarrhythmic effect is related to nonuniform slowing of conduction.[21,26] Monitoring the QRS-interval is logical[1] but "safe limits" are not established. Furthermore, as shown in the CAST study,[7] late proarrhythmic effects can occur. In patients with pre-existing sinus node or AV conduction problems, there may be worsening.

**Atrial proarrhythmic effects** are of two varieties. It will be recalled that when patients with rapid supraventricular arrhythmias are given quinidine, digitalis coadministration has been traditional to avoid the decrease in atrial rate being reflected in accelerated AV conduction and ventricular arrhythmias. A similar but more marked danger may occur during administration of flecainide,[65] so that as the atrial rate falls the ventricular rate might rise.[11] Therefore if prescribed for prevention of atrial flutter or fibrillation, they should probably be coadministered with digitalis, beta-blocker or verapamil to avoid accelerated AV conduction. Second, ventricular arrhythmias may be precipitated.[13]

**Extracardiac side-effects** are related to the central nervous system (blurred vision, dizziness, headache, nausea, paresthesias, fatigue, tremor, and nervousness). Yet in one trial they were uncommon and no different from placebo.[6]

**Drug interactions and combinations** are as follows. Additive inhibitory effects require great care when flecainide is combined with other agents inhibiting sinus or AV nodal function (beta-blockers, verapamil, diltiazem, digitalis), when there are additive negative inotropic effects (beta-blockers, verapamil, disopyramide) or when there may be combined effects on His-Purkinje conduction (quinidine, procainamide, and, to a lesser extent, disopyramide). Amiodarone increases flecainide plasma levels (decrease flecainide dose by half).[1] Concurrent beta-blockade reduces proarrthythmia (p 13).

## Propafenone

Propafenone (**Rythmol** in the USA, **Arythmol** in the UK, **Rytmonorm** in Europe) is a relatively new antiarrhythmic drug of predominant Class IC properties. Usually well tolerated, the spectrum of activity and some of the side-effects resemble those of other Class IC agents, including the proarrhythmic effect. In the CASH study,[43] propafenone was withdrawn from one arm because of increased total mortality and cardiac arrest recurrence. Propafenone is regarded as relatively safe in suppressing supraventricular arrhythmias including those of the WPW syndrome and recurrent atrial fibrillation.[80]

In keeping with its Class IC effects, propafenone blocks the fast inward sodium channel, has a potent membrane stabilizing activity and increases PR and QRS times without effect on the QT-interval. It also has mild beta-blocking and calcium antagonist properties.

Marked interindividual variations in its metabolism mean that the dose must be individualized. The variable plasma levels and plasma half-life (2 to 10 hours in normals, 12 to 32 hours in poor metabolizers) may be explained by genetic variations in hepatic metabolism; in 7% of whites, the hepatic cytochrome isoenzyme, P-450 2D6, is genetically absent, so that propafenone breakdown is much slower.[15]

The **dose** is 150 to 300 mg 3 times daily, up to 1200 mg daily with some patients needing 4 times daily dose and some only twice.

The approved **indications** in the USA are (1) life-threatening ventricular arrhythmias[15] and (2) suppression of supraventricular arrhythmias, including those of the WPW syndrome and recurrent atrial flutter or fibrillation.[80] These must be in the absence of structural heart disease.

**Relative contraindications** include pre-existing sinus, AV or bundle branch abnormalities, or depressed LV function. Asthma is also a relative contraindication, especially when the propafenone dose exceeds 450 mg daily,[19] probably from the mild beta-blocking qualities of the drug.

**Side-effects** are dose-related. Cardiac side-effects include PR and QRS-prolongation, and conduction block as well as sinus node inhibition. CHF may be precipitated by the modest negative inotropic effect.[33] These and other cardiac side-effects required discontinuation of the drug in 25% of patients in the ESVEM Trial.[51] Proarrhythmia manifests as incessant wide complex VT, typical of Class I agents, and presumably accounts for the increased total mortality in the CASH Study.[43]

**Drug interactions and combinations** are as follows. Like other Class IC agents, propafenone is likely to interact adversely with drugs depressing nodal function or intraventricular conduction, or the inotropic state. Propafenone has been combined with quinidine or procainamide at reduced doses of both drugs in the treatment of PVCs. Propafenone substantially increases serum digoxin levels and increases the anticoagulant effect of warfarin.[23]

## Class II Agents: Beta-Adrenergic Antagonists

Whereas Class I agents are increasingly suspect from the long-term point of view, beta-blockers have a good record in reducing post-MI mortality.[87] The general arguments for beta-blockade include (1) the role of tachycardia in precipitating some arrhythmias, especially those based on triggered activity; (2) the increased sympathetic activity in patients with sustained VT[67] and in patients with AMI; (3) the fundamental role of the second messenger of beta-adrenergic activity, cyclic AMP, in the causation of ischemia-related VF;[62] and (4) the associated antihypertensive and anti-ischemic effects of these drugs. The mechanism of benefit of beta-blockade in postinfarct patients is uncertain, but is likely to be multifactorial and probably antiarrhythmic in part.[62]

The **indications** for antiarrhythmic therapy by beta-blockade include the following (Fig. 8–6). It is used especially for inappropriate or unwanted sinus tachycardia, for paroxysmal atrial tachycardia provoked by emotion or exercise, for exercise-induced ventricular arrhythmias, in the arrhythmias of pheochromocytoma (combined with alpha-blockade to avoid hypertensive crises), in the hereditary prolonged QT-syndrome, and sometimes in the arrhythmias of mitral valve prolapse. In AMI, the cardiodepressant effects argue against the use of beta-blockers as antiarrhythmic agents of choice, but in appropriate dosage and in patients without manifest heart failure, beta-blockade may be used to prevent and control supraventricular and ventricular arrhythmias. A common denominator to most of these indications is increased sympathetic beta-adrenergic activity. Beta-blockers are also effective as monotherapy

β–BLOCKADE

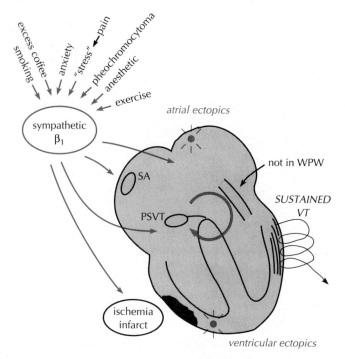

**FIGURE 8–6.** Principles of use of Class II agents (beta-blockers). Beta-blockade is antiarrhythmic therapy for a wide variety of arrhythmias. However, it does not prevent recurrences of atrial flutter or fibrillation, unless these are initiated by an atrial ectopic beat. Fig. copyright L.H. Opie.

in severe recurrent VT not obviously ischemic in origin,[5] and empirical beta-blocker therapy seems as good as electrophysiologic guided therapy with Class I or Class III agents.[85]

### Which Beta-blocker for Arrhythmias?

The antiarrhythmic activity of the various beta-blockers is reasonably uniform, the critical property being that of beta-adrenergic blockade, without any major role for associated properties such as membrane depression (local anesthetic action), cardioselectivity, and intrinsic sympathomimetic activity having no major influence on the antiarrhythmic potency. In the USA, the beta-blockers licensed for antiarrhythmic activity include propranolol, sotalol, and acebutolol. The latter is particularly attractive because of its cardioselectivity, its favorable or neutral effect on the blood lipid profile (Chapter 10), and its specific benefit in one large postinfarct survival trial. Metoprolol 25 to 100 mg twice daily was the agent chosen with empirical beta-blockade was compared with electrophysiologic guided antiarrhythmic therapy.[85] Sotalol uniquely combines Class II and III activity. The **drawback** to beta-blockade antiarrhythmic therapy continues to be the many patients with absolute or relative contraindications including pulmonary problems, conduction defects, or overt heart failure. Mild LV dysfunction no longer is an absolute contraindication (see Chapter 2). Despite these defects, beta-blockers are at present the closest to an ideal class of antiarrhythmic agents because of their broad spectrum of activity and because of their established safety record.

**TABLE 8–5**   COMPARISON OF PROPERTIES OF TWO MIXED CLASS III
AGENTS, SOTALOL AND AMIODARONE

|  | SOTALOL | AMIODARONE |
|---|---|---|
| Mechanism of action | Class II, III | Class I, III (II, IV) |
| Dose | Titrate upwards | Load then titrate downwards |
| SVT | + + | + + |
| Recurrent AF | + | + + |
| WPW arrhythmias | + | + + |
| Incessant VT | + + | + + |
| Early postinfarct | +, + /0 | + + |
| Late postinfarct | + + | + + |
| Proarrhythmia | torsades in 4%* | torsades or other proarrhythmias 2–5%* |
| Other adverse effects | fatigue, bradycardia, dyspnea | very common, up to 75% at doses of 400 mg or more* |

\* in VT/VF population, package inserts.

## Mixed Class III Agents: Amiodarone and Sotalol

As the evidence for the possible long-term harm of most Class I agents mounts, attention has shifted to Class II and especially Class III agents (Table 8–5). In the ESVEM trial[52] sotalol was better than six Class I antiarrhythmics. Amiodarone, in contrast to Class I agents, exerts a favorable effect on post-MI patients according to a meta-analysis.[70] Both are mixed, not pure, Class III agents, a quality that may be of crucial importance.

The **built-in problem** with Class III agents is as follows. These compounds act by lengthening the action potential duration and hence the effective refractory period, and must inevitably prolong the QT-interval to be effective. In the presence of added hypokalemia or other specific factors, QT-prolongation may predispose to torsades de pointes. This may especially occur with agents causing a simultaneous bradycardia, when agents such as sotalol become more effective in prolonging action potential duration—a "reverse use-dependency."[20] By acting only on the repolarization phase of the action potential, Class III agents should leave conduction unchanged. However, amiodarone, sotalol and bretylium all have additional properties that modify conduction—amiodarone being a significant sodium channel inhibitor, sotalol a beta-blocker, and bretylium initially releasing catecholamines.

Of the Class III agents, amiodarone makes the action potential pattern more uniform throughout the myocardium, thereby opposing electrophysiologic heterogeneity that underlies some serious ventricular arrhythmias. The efficacy of amiodarone is generally thought to exceed that of other antiarrhythmic compounds.

Despite several common electrophysiologic features, Class III agents are structurally, pharmacokinetically, and electrophysiologically dissimilar, so that neither the antiarrhythmic effects nor the clinical indications are interchangeable.

The two major Class III agents currently under further evaluation are sotalol and amiodarone. Although both are liable to cause torsades de pointes, the incidence of this serious proarrhythmia seems lower in amiodarone-treated patients than in sotalol-treated patients for reasons that are not clear. On the other hand, amiodarone has a host of multisystem potentially serious side-effects which sotalol does not.

## Amiodarone

Amiodarone (**Cordarone**) is a unique "wide spectrum" antiarrhythmic agent, chiefly Class III but with also powerful Class I activity and ancilliary Class II and Class III activity.[71] Its established antiarrhythmic benefits need to be balanced against, first, the slow onset of action of oral therapy that, in turn, may require large oral loading doses. Second, the serious side-effects, especially pulmonary infiltrates, mean that there must be a fine balance between the maximum antiarrhythmic effect of the drug and the potential for the side-effects. Third, there are a large number of potentially serious drug interactions, some of which predispose to torsades de pointes, which is nonetheless rare when amiodarone is used as a single agent. In recurrent supraventricular arrhythmias, low-dose amiodarone may be strikingly effective with little risk of side-effects. Otherwise, the use of amiodarone in as low a dose as possible should be restricted to selected patients with refractory ventricular arrhythmias especially in the post-MI group. In general, the status of this drug is changing from that of a "last ditch" agent to one that is increasingly used when life-threatening arrhythmias are being treated. It may not, however, be used without an adequate knowledge of its side-effect profile.

ELECTROPHYSIOLOGY. Amiodarone lengthens the effective refractory period by prolonging the action potential duration in all cardiac tissues, including the bypass tract. It also has a powerful Class I antiarrhythmic effect inhibiting inactivated sodium channels at high stimulation frequencies.[1] Amiodarone also noncompetitively blocks alpha- and beta-adrenergic receptors (Class II effect). A calcium antagonist (Class IV) effect might explain bradycardia and AV nodal inhibition and the relatively low incidence of torsades de pointes.[35] Furthermore, there are coronary and peripheral vasodilator actions.[54] Amiodarone is therefore a complex antiarrhythmic agent that shares at least some of the properties of each of the four electrophysiologic classes of antiarrhythmics.

PHARMACOKINETICS. After variable (30% to 50%) and slow GI absorption, amiodarone is very slowly eliminated with a half-life of about 25 to 110 days.[1] The onset of action after oral administration is delayed and a steady-state drug effect ("**amiodaronization**"[1]) may not be established for several months unless large loading doses are used. Even when given intravenously, its full electrophysiologic effect is delayed.[70] Amiodarone is lipid-soluble and extensively distributed in the body and highly concentrated in many tissues, especially in the liver and lungs. It undergoes extensive hepatic metabolism to the pharmacologically active metabolite, desethylamiodarone. A correlation between the clinical effects and serum concentrations of the drug or its metabolite has not been clearly shown, although there is a direct relation between the oral dose and the plasma concentration, and between metabolite concentration and some late effects, such as that on the ventricular functional refractory period.[29] The therapeutic level, not well defined, may be between 1.0 and 2.5 µg/ml, almost all of which (95%) is protein bound. Amiodarone is not excreted by the kidneys but rather by the lacrimal glands, the skin, and the biliary tract.

DOSE. When reasonably rapid control of an arrhythmia is needed, the initial **loading regime** (patient hospitalized) is 1,200 to 1,600 mg in 2 to 4 divided doses usually given for 7 to 14 days, which is then reduced to 400 to 800 mg/day for a further 1 to 3 weeks. More recently, the trend has been to omit the 800 mg stage, but there are no controlled data. Thereafter a maintenance dose that rarely needs to exceed 200 to 400 mg/day is given as a single dose. The loading dose is essential because of the slow onset of full action with a delay of about 10 days.[1] By using a loading dose, sustained ventricular tachycardia can be controlled after a mean interval of 5 days.[82] **Down-**

**ward dose adjustment** may be required during prolonged therapy to avoid development of side-effects while maintaining optimal anti-arrhythmic effect. Maintenance doses for supraventricular arrhythmias are generally lower (200 mg daily or less) than those needed for serious ventricular arrhythmias. **Intravenous administration** (not yet in the USA, approval being sought) may be used for intractable arrhythmias[83] or for atrial fibrillation in AMI [5 mg/kg over 20 minutes, 500 to 1,000 mg over 24 hours, then orally[34]]. Studies currently under way suggest that efficacy of intravenous amiodarone predicts subsequent success with oral amiodarone.

INDICATIONS.   In the prophylactic control of life-threatening ventricular tachyarrhythmias, especially post-MI, amiodarone is generally regarded as one of the most effective agents available, yet strict controlled studies are missing.[71] Amiodarone is highly effective in preventing recurrences of paroxysmal atrial fibrillation or flutter,[53,68] of paroxysmal supraventricular tachycardias and in WPW arrhythmias.[1] Amiodarone may be tried for variant angina complicated by severe ventricular arrhythmias.

CONTRAINDICATIONS.   In the USA, the drug should not be used unless adequate doses of other ventricular antiarrhythmics have been tested or are not tolerated. Contraindications to amiodarone are severe sinus node dysfunction with marked sinus bradycardia or syncope, second- and third-degree heart block, and known hypersensitivity.

CURRENT TRIALS.   Early results on several different trials suggest that amiodarone can reduce postinfarct mortality in patients with asymptomatic complex ventricular arrhythmias.[70,78] In another relatively small study, post-MI patients not eligible for beta-blockade received either amiodarone or placebo for one year with an improvement in cardiac mortality and a lessening of complex ventricular arrhythmias.[45] The results of the Canadian and European Myocardial Infarct Amiodarone Trials (CAMIAT and EMIAT) are still awaited. In the CASCADE study,[42] patients who were survivors of out-of-hospital ventricular fibrillation not associated with a Q-wave infarction were randomized to treatment by empiric amiodarone or conventional antiarrhythmic drug therapy guided by electrophysiological testing, Holter recording, or both. Of the total 228 patients enrolled in the study, 105 had automatic defibrillators implanted. Survival free of cardiac death, resuscitated ventricular fibrillation or syncopal defibrillator shock was better for the patients treated with amiodarone than with conventional therapy (chiefly quinidine, procainamide, flecainide, or drug combinations) (for GESICA study in CHF, see p 240).

SIDE-EFFECTS.   In higher doses, there is an unusual spectrum of toxicity, the most serious being pneumonitis, potentially leading to pulmonary fibrosis and occurring in up to 10% to 17% at doses of about 400 mg/day, and may be fatal in 10% (package insert).

PULMONARY SIDE-EFFECTS.   Pulmonary toxicity may be dose-related.[1] Pulmonary complications usually regress if recognized early and if amiodarone is discontinued, and the patient kept alive by symptomatic therapy, which may include steroids.

CARDIAC SIDE-EFFECTS AND TORSADES DE POINTES.   Amiodarone may inhibit the SA or AV node (about 2% to 5%). Although generally regarded as a safe drug from the hemodynamic point of view, two recent abstracts suggest that amiodarone might increase mortality in patients with markedly depressed LV function[69,72] in whom a negative inotropic effect might dominate over the vasodilator action especially during drug loading.[54] Although torsades is relatively rare with amiodarone,[35] special care needs to be taken in CHF to avoid hypokalemia and digoxin toxicity (Fig. 8–8).

CNS SIDE-EFFECTS.   Proximal muscle weakness, peripheral neuropathy, and neural symptoms (headache, ataxia, tremors, impaired memory, insomnia, dreams) occur with variable incidence.[3]

THYROID SIDE-EFFECTS. Amiodarone also has a complex effect on the metabolism of thyroid hormones (it contains iodine and shares a structural similarity to thyroxine), the main action being to inhibit the peripheral conversion of $T_4$ to $T_3$ with a rise in the serum level of $T_4$ and a small fall in the level of $T_3$; serum reverse $T_3$ is increased as a function of the dose and duration of amiodarone therapy. In most patients, thyroid function is not altered by amiodarone; in about 3% to 5% hypothyroidism or hyperthyroidism may develop; the exact incidence varies geographically. **Hyperthyroidism** may precipitate arrhythmia breakthrough and should be excluded if new arrhythmias appear during amiodarone therapy. At a low dose of amiodarone (200 to 400 mg daily), there may be biochemically documented but clinically silent alterations in thyroid function in 10% of patients.[1] We recommend biannual thyroid function tests of which the most useful is the TSH.

GI SIDE-EFFECTS. These were uncommon in the GESICA study.[52A] Yet nausea can occur in 25% of patients with CHF, even at a dose of only 200 mg daily.[17] Increased plasma levels of liver function enzymes may occur in 10% to 20% of all patients.[1] These effects usually resolve with dose reduction.

TESTICULAR DYSFUNCTION. This is a recently reported side-effect, detected by increased gonadotropin levels in patients on long-term amiodarone.[48]

LESS SERIOUS SIDE-EFFECTS. Corneal microdeposits develop in nearly all adult patients given prolonged amiodarone. Symptoms and impairment of visual acuity are rare and respond to reduced dosage. Macular degeneration rarely occurs. In over 10% of patients, a photosensitive slate-grey or bluish skin discoloration develops after prolonged therapy, usually exceeding 18 months. Avoid exposure to sun and use a sunscreen ointment with UVA and UVB protection. The pigmentation regresses slowly on drug withdrawal.

LONG-TERM USE. In one series, at 12 months of therapy the incidence of success against VT or VF was just over 50% which, however, fell to 30% at 2 years, while at 4 years the chances of a patient being alive and still on amiodarone were only about 20%.[2] On the other hand: (1) discontinuation of amiodarone leads to an even worse prognosis;[28] and (2) other investigators show that amiodarone is effective in nearly 60% of patients unresponsive to other antiarrhythmic drugs, even after 5 years.[18]

DRUG INTERACTIONS. The most serious interaction is an additive **proarrhythmic effect** with other drugs prolonging the QT-interval, such as Class IA antiarrhythmic agents, phenothiazines, tricyclic antidepressants, thiazide diuretics, and sotalol (Fig. 8–8). Amiodarone may increased quinidine and procainamide levels (these combinations are not advised). With **phenytoin,** there is a double drug interaction. Amiodarone increases phenytoin levels while at the same time phenytoin enhances the conversion of amiodarone to desethylamiodarone.[73] Amiodarone prolongs the prothrombin time and may cause bleeding in patients on **warfarin,** perhaps by a hepatic interaction;[1] decrease warfarin by about one-third and retest the INR (p 263). Amiodarone increases the plasma digoxin concentration,[1] predisposing to digitalis toxic effects (not arrhythmias because amiodarone protects); decrease **digoxin** by about half and remeasure digoxin levels. Amiodarone, by virtue of its weak beta-blocking and calcium antagonist effect, tends to inhibit nodal activity and may therefore interact adversely with beta-blocking agents and calcium antagonists.[1]

PRECAUTIONS. Check baseline pulmonary, thyroid, and liver func-

## CLASS III: SOTALOL & AMIODARONE
### possible indications

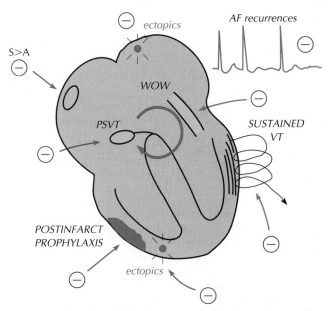

**FIGURE 8–7.** Principles of use of Class III agents (sotalol and amiodarone). One of the major differences lies in the side-effects. With sotalol, torsades de pointes is a greater risk, whereas with amiodarone there are many multisystem side-effects. Fig. copyright L.H. Opie.

tions and plasma electrolytes. To initiate therapy, the patient requires hospitalization, especially for life-threatening VT/VF. For recurrences of atrial fibrillation (not licensed in the USA), therapy can be initiated on an outpatient basis. Drug interactions must be considered. During chronic therapy the ECG and Holter recordings are monitored and periodic chest x-rays and thyroid tests are required. Keep the dose as low as possible. Intravenous amiodarone and bretylium have equal efficacy for the treatment of hemodynamically severe VT, incessant VT or VF, but there is more hypotension over 48 hours with bretylium.[60]

**COMPARATIVE STUDIES.** Postinfarct, amiodarone 400 mg daily was better than propranolol 160 mg daily.[14] In refractory VT or VF, in noninfarct patients, amiodarone seemed similar to sotalol although initially with less dropouts;[2] this study needs confirmation.

**DRUG DISCONTINUATION.** Due to adverse reactions up to 20% of patients may require drug discontinuation. The risk is reappearance of the life-threatening ventricular arrhythmia after a variable period. Similar problems apply to dose reduction. Extended hospitalization may be needed during this drug washout period, the duration of which depends on the variable but extremely prolonged half-life of amiodarone. The possibility of an adverse post-withdrawal interaction with a new antiarrhythmic must be considered.

### Sotalol

Sotalol (**Betapace** in the USA, **Sotacor** in Europe) has long been used outside the USA for control of severe ventricular arrhythmias when amiodarone toxicity is feared. Recently sotalol has been licensed in the USA for documented life-threatening ventricular arrhythmias, including sustained ventricular tachycardia. As a Class III agent, it has additional antiarrhythmic qualities by prolonging the refractory period of atrial, AV nodal, bypass tract, and ventricular tissue (Fig. 8–7). As a mixed Class II and Class III agent, it also has all the beneficial actions of the beta-blocker (Fig. 8–6). Inevitably, it is also susceptible to the Achilles heel of all Class III agents, namely torsades de pointes.

The pure Class III investigational agent **d-sotalol**, without the beta-blocking qualities of standard sotalol, increased mortality in postinfarct patients with a low ejection fraction (SWORD study). Another study comparing d-sotalol with amiodarone in serious ventricular tachycardia continues.

ELECTROPHYSIOLOGY. When added to isolated tissue in high concentrations, sotalol prolongs the action potential duration (APD) and causes aftercontractions,[59] the latter presumably mediated by excess cytosolic calcium that may possibly result from the prolonged APD. Excess cytosolic calcium is also the hypothetical basis of early afterdepolarizations associated with torsade de pointes. In man, Class II effects are sinus and AV node depression. Class III effects are prolongation of the action potential in atrial and ventricular tissue and prolonged atrial and ventricular refractory periods, as well as inhibition of conduction along any bypass tract in both directions. APD prolongation with, possibly, enhanced calcium entry may explain why the negative inotropic effect is less than expected.[57A]

PHARMACOKINETICS. It is a noncardioselective, water-soluble (hydrophilic), non-protein-bound agent, excreted solely by the kidneys, with a plasma high-life of 12 hours. Dosing every 12 hours gives trough concentrations half of those of the peak values.

INDICATIONS. Due to the combined Class II and Class III properties, sotalol is theoretically active against a wide variety of arrhythmias, including sinus tachycardia, paroxysmal supraventricular tachycardia, WPW arrhythmias with either anterograde or retrograde conduction, recurrence of atrial fibrillation,[58] ischemic ventricular arrhythmias, and recurrent sustained ventricular tachycardia or fibrillation.[81] For postinfarct prevention, the data are favorable[74] but not as convincing as for propranolol. Furthermore, high-dose therapy in the early postinfarct period is not advised (package insert). Possibly the benefit of beta-blockade in these conditions is balanced by an increased incidence of torsades de pointes.[81]

MAJOR TRIAL. The major outcome study with sotalol was the ESVEM Trial[52] in which this drug in a mean dose of about 400 mg daily was better at decreasing death and ventricular arrhythmias than any of six Class I agents. The major indication was sustained monomorphic ventricular tachycardia (or ventricular fibrillation) induced in an electrophysiologic study. None of the drugs, however, was compared with controls. Nor should it be forgotten that the patients were highly selected.[57A]

DOSE. The dose range is 160 to 640 mg/day given in two divided doses. Keeping the dose at 320 mg or less per day lessens side-effects, including torsades de pointes. Yet doses of 320 to 480 mg may be needed to prevent recurrent VT or VF. In the early postinfarct period (see Indications), the drug should be used cautiously and titrated upwards with care. When given in two divided doses, steady-state plasma concentrations are reached in 2 to 3 days. In patients with renal impairment or in the elderly, or when there are risk factors for proarrhythmia, the dose should be reduced and the dosing interval increased. The IV dose (not in USA) is 100 mg over 5 minutes.[56A]

SIDE-EFFECTS. These are those of beta-blockade added to which is the risk of torsades de pointes. Aggravation of heart failure might be less than with standard beta-blockers.[57A]

PRECAUTIONS AND CONTRAINDICATIONS. The drug should be avoided in patients with serious conduction defects, including sick sinus syndrome, in bronchospastic disease, in diabetics, in overt CHF, and when there are evident risks of proarrhythmia. In pregnancy, the

## LONG QT WITH RISK OF TORSADES

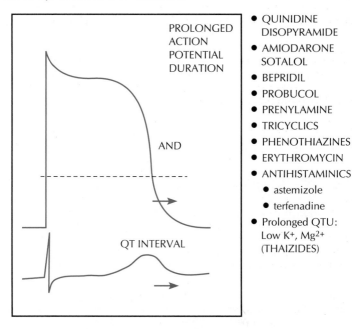

PROLONGED
ACTION
POTENTIAL
DURATION

AND

QT INTERVAL

- QUINIDINE
  DISOPYRAMIDE
- AMIODARONE
  SOTALOL
- BEPRIDIL
- PROBUCOL
- PRENYLAMINE
- TRICYCLICS
- PHENOTHIAZINES
- ERYTHROMYCIN
- ANTIHISTAMINICS
  - astemizole
  - terfenadine
- Prolonged QTU:
  Low K+, Mg2+
  (THAIZIDES)

FIGURE 8–8.  Therapeutic agents, including antiarrhythmics, that may cause QT-prolongation. Hypokalemia causes QTU not QT-prolongation. Some antiarrhythmic agents act at least in part chiefly by prolonging the action potential duration, such as amiodarone and sotalol. QT-prolongation is therefore an integral part of their therapeutic benefit. On the other hand, QT- or QTU-prolongation, especially in the presence of hypokalemia and other electrolyte disturbances or when there is cotherapy with one of the other agents prolonging the QT-interval, may precipitate torsades de pointes. Fig. copyright L.H. Opie and modified from Reference 1.

drug is category B. It is not tetragenic but does cross the placenta and may depress fetal vital functions. Sotalol is also excreted in mother's milk.

RISK FACTORS FOR PROARRHYTHMIA.  Torsades de pointes is more likely if there is a low plasma potassium, when there is a high sotalol dose, when there is bradycardia, when the corrected QT-interval is prolonged, in patients with LV failure, and in the female gender. Risk of torsades de pointes is increased whenever there is cotherapy with Class IA drugs, amiodarone or other drugs prolonging the QT-interval. There is risk of torsades de pointes whenever the drug is started or whenever the dose is increased and the QT-interval should be monitored (not to exceed 500 msec, QTc). The plasma potassium and magnesium should also be checked before starting therapy and intermittently during diuretic cotherapy.

DRUG INTERACTIONS.  As a beta-blocker, sotalol interacts adversely with other drugs depressing LV mechanical function, the SA node, or AV node, including calcium channel blockers and disopyramide. There is no pharmacokinetic interaction with digoxin. Catecholamine depletion by reserpine predisposes to sinus node depression. Cotherapy with other drugs predisposing to torsades de pointes (Fig. 8–8) should be avoided, including diuretics, Class IA antiarrhythmics, amiodarone, phenothiazine, and probucol. Such reservations are not absolute restrictions. Low-dose sotalol (up to 360 mg daily) has been carefully combined with Class IA agents with apparent improvement in control of sustained VT. The dropout rate was, however, 26%.[49]

COMPARATIVE STUDIES.  Compared with lidocaine,[56A] both given intravenously as 100 mg over 5 minutes, **sotalol** was better at terminating sustained VT. In *recurrent atrial fibrillation*, sotalol was as effective as quinidine[58] or propafenone.[80] Sotalol has the advantage of controlling the ventricular response rate. In the only direct comparison between sotalol and amiodarone,[2] these two drugs gave similar results over one year in patients with sustained VT not responding to a Class I drug. The initial amiodarone dose was 1,600 mg daily working down to mean maintenance dose of 400 mg daily. For sotalol, on the other hand, the dose was titrated upwards from an initial dose in the range of 160 to 320 mg daily to 160 to 640 mg daily (mean 491 mg). The authors believe that amiodarone would have been more toxic over a longer period, and that its excessively long half-life (25 days or more) could lead to problems when the drug had to be withdrawn because of adverse or toxic effects. Hence the authors recommend sotalol rather than amiodarone as the first choice Class III agent.

### Bretylium Tosylate

Bretylium (**Bretylol**) is generally limited to recurrent VF or VT after lidocaine and DC cardioversion have failed in the setting of AMI. It differs from all other antiarrhythmics in being concentrated in the terminal sympathetic neurons, where it accumulates initially to release stored norepinephrine (NE) and then to inhibit further release of NE with a "chemical" sympathectomy.[1] Bretylium also has Class III activity in Purkinje fibers, but less in ventricular muscle and none in atrial tissue. There is little inhibitory effect on nodal or conduction tissue.

**Pharmacokinetically,** bretylium is widely distributed after intravenous administration to various tissues and then excreted almost entirely by the kidneys by active tubular secretion. There is no liver metabolism and the elimination half-life is 7 to 9 hours (much prolonged in renal failure).

The initial **dose** of 5 mg/kg can be increased to 10 mg/kg in the absence of hypotension (major problem). It should be diluted 1:4 to a minimum of 50 ml with 5% dextrose or sodium chloride and infused over 10 to 30 minutes to minimize nausea and vomiting.[1] In emergencies, however, it is given undiluted by rapid intravenous injection. After loading, a constant infusion of 1 to 2 mg/min may be given, or the loading dose may be repeated at 1 to 2 hour intervals.

Regarding **indications,** bretylium may have a special use in patients subject to defibrillation and external cardiac massage. In seven patients with VF after AMI,[1] bretylium 5 to 10 mg/kg was given intravenously with the patient's arm raised above the heart, and resuscitation was continued. In five patients, defibrillation ensued without DC shock. In a series of 27 patients treated by a hospital cardiac arrest team, VF was resistant to 30 minutes of conventional electric and pharmacologic procedures (lidocaine plus one or more of the following: procainamide, propranolol, and phenytoin),[1] yet after a single intravenous bolus of bretylium tosylate (5 mg/kg), 20 patients were successfully defibrillated by DC shock. A randomized clinical trial of 147 patients compared bretylium and lidocaine in VF occurring outside the hospital; the two drugs were equieffective.[1] Similarly, intravenous bretylium and intravenous amiodarone are equieffective for incessant VT or VF, though half of the bretylium-treated patients had hypotension.

Thus the major **side-effect** is drug-induced hypotension, which can be treated by vasopressor catecholamines or by protriptyline (5 mg every 6 hours) which pharmacologically antagonizes the hypotensive effect.[1] With bretylium, initial sympathomimetic effects (transient hypertension and increased arrhythmias) probably result from transient discharge of NE from the terminal neurons. Nausea and vomiting are common after rapid intravenous bolus injection.

## Class IV Agents: Verapamil, Diltiazem and Adenosine

**Verapamil and diltiazem** inhibit slow channel dependent conduction through the AV node. Verapamil has been a major advance in the acute therapy of supraventricular arrhythmias (see Chapter 3). Diltiazem is of similar value to verapamil, and the intravenous form is now licensed in the USA for (1) control of rapid ventricular rate in atrial fibrillation or flutter (but not in WPW arrhythmias) and (2) in AV nodal re-entrant tachycardia for rapid conversion to sinus rhythm; this indication includes narrow QRS-complex supraventricular arrhythmias associated with the WPW syndrome. The dose is 0.05 to 0.45 mg/kg given intravenously over 2 minutes and the major adverse effect is hypotension.[50]

The **potassium channel openers** are indirect calcium antagonists. These agents hyperpolarize the cell membrane thereby moving the polarity away from that required for "opening" of the slow calcium channel, so that they are particularly useful in supraventricular tachycardias with re-entrant circuits utilizing the AV node. Adenosine given intravenously is increasingly used to inhibit the AV node in supraventricular re-entrant tachycardias with the same locus of action in the middle of the AV node as has verapamil. Because of its extremely short half-life, serious hemodynamic side-effects are rare.

## Adenosine

Adenosine (**Adenocard**), has multiple cellular effects, including potassium channel opening, and inhibition of the sinus and especially the AV node.[41] It is now the first-line agent for terminating narrow complex paroxysmal SVT in many countries.

PHARMACOKINETICS. Adenosine has an extremely short half-life of 10 to 30 seconds. However, the effect in precipitating bronchoconstriction in asthmatic patients is of unknown mechanism and can last for 30 minutes.[41]

DOSE. The drug is given as an initial rapid intravenous bolus of 6 mg followed by a saline flush to obtain high concentrations in the heart. If it does not work within 1 to 2 minutes, a 12 mg bolus is given that may be repeated once. At the appropriate dose, the antiarrhythmic effect occurs as soon as the drug reaches the AV node.[9] The initial dose needs to be reduced to 3 mg or less in patients taking calcium antagonists or beta-blockers or dipyridamole (see Drug Interactions), or in the elderly who are at risk of sick sinus syndrome.

INDICATIONS. The chief indication is narrow complex SVT (AV nodal re-entrant tachycardia, AV tachycardia in WPW). Adenosine has no effect on the basic atrial arrhythmia, such as an ectopic focus or flutter. Whereas it terminates AV nodal tachycardias, it may unmask atrial activity in atrial flutter or atrial tachycardia. In **wide complex tachycardia** of uncertain origin, adenosine can help the management. This tachycardia can either be VT or SVT (with aberrant conduction). In the latter case, adenosine is likely to stop the tachycardia, whereas in the case of VT there is unlikely to be any major adverse hemodynamic effect and the tachycardia continues. There is therefore a combined therapeutic-diagnostic test.[41] Very occasionally adenosine is effective in certain types of VT, such as those induced by exercise in an anatomically normal heart (right ventricular outflow tachycardia).

SIDE-EFFECTS. Those ascribed to the effect of adenosine on the potassium channel are short-lived, such as headache, provocation of chest pain, flushing, and excess sinus or AV nodal inhibition. Bronchoconstriction can last for longer and precipitate dyspnea especially in asthmatics. Transient new arrhythmias at the time of chemical cardioversion occur in about 65%.

CONTRAINDICATIONS. Asthma or history thereof, second- or third-degree AV block, sick sinus syndrome.

DRUG INTERACTIONS. Dipyridamole inhibits the breakdown of adenosine and therefore the dose of adenosine must be markedly reduced in patients receiving dipyridamole.[25,39] Methylxanthines (caffeine, theophylline) competitively antagonize the interaction of adenosine with its receptors, so that it becomes less effective.

ADENOSINE VS. VERAPAMIL OR DILTIAZEM. In patients pretreated with beta-blocking drugs or with myocardial failure, adenosine is preferred to verapamil or diltiazem in the treatment of SVT to avoid combined depressant effects on the SA and AV nodes. Therefore adenosine is replacing intravenous verapamil or diltiazem for the rapid termination of narrow QRS complex SVT.[41] Verapamil by its myocardial depression and peripheral vasodilation can be fatal when given to patients with VT, adenosine with its very transient effects leaves true VT virtually unchanged. When the wide complex tachycardia is in fact SVT with aberrant conduction, adenosine should also be effective.

### ATP (adenosine triphosphate)

ATP probably acts by conversion to adenosine and is likewise used in supraventricular arrhythmias. Intravenous ATP 10 to 20 mg was somewhat more effective than intravenous verapamil 5 to 10 mg in terminating SVT[4] at the cost of more side-effects (AV block, new arrhythmias, noncardiac side-effects of adenosine). **Striadyne** is a mixture of ATP, adenosine, and other nucleosides often used in Europe.

## Metabolic Agents

**Hypokalemia** predisposes to ventricular arrhythmias especially in the context of AMI and during the use of agents prolonging the action potential duration when torsades becomes a risk. In such situations, **potassium infusions** may be required. It is prudent always to check plasma potassium during antiarrhythmic therapy or during digoxin therapy or at the start of AMI.[1]

**Magnesium salts** given intravenously are reported to be of benefit in the therapy of torsades[37] and also in the arrhythmias of early AMI. The routine use of magnesium in AMI has become unpopular since the negative results of the large ISIS-4 study (Chapter 9).

## Combination Therapy

A combination of antiarrhythmic agents may be used when single drug treatment fails or when the dose must be reduced because of side-effects. There are no outcome studies on combination therapy. Some logical "rules" are, first, not to combine agents of the same class or subclasses, or agents with potentially additive side-effects, such as the extra risk arrhythmias with Class IA and Class IC agents,[1] or the added QT-prolongation with Class IA agents and sotalol or amiodarone.[1] Second, a logical combination is that of a Class I drug that preferentially binds to inactivated sodium channels (Class IB), with a drug binding preferentially to activated channels such as a Class IA drug,[40] thus explaining the benefits of mexiletine combined with quinidine[10] or mexiletine with procainamide.[1] Third, there is some hope that combining propranolol with flecainide might diminish the proarrhythmic effects of the latter, yet the obvious problem is the combined negative inotropic effects of these two drugs. When sotalol followed by amiodarone has failed as maximal therapy, combination of amiodarone with a beta-blocker is not logical, because even amiodarone has mild beta-blocking properties. Thus, addition of mexiletine or procainamide to sotalol or amiodarone becomes logical. The latter drugs may have little or no proarrhythmic effects.[87] When oral antiarrhythmics are exhausted, increasing use is made of an AICD (Automatic Implanted Cardioverter-Defibrillator). Alternatively, the time might come to break the rules, for example by

## CLASS 1A & III AGENTS: TORSADES DE POINTES

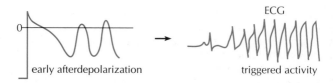

## CLASS 1C AGENTS: WIDE COMPLEX VT

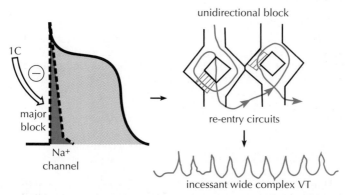

**FIGURE 8–9.**   Major proarrhythmic mechanisms.[26] Class IA and Class III agents widen the action potential duration and in the presence of an early afterdepolarization through complex mechanisms can give rise to triggered activity of the variety known as torsades de pointes. Note major role of QT-prolongation (Fig. 8–8). Class IC agents have as their major proarrhythmic mechanism a powerful inhibition of the sodium channel particularly in conduction tissue. Increasing heterogeneity together with unidirectional block sets the stage for re-entry circuits and monomorphic wide complex ventricular tachycardia. Fig. copyright L.H. Opie.

combining Class IA agents with sotalol,[49] although stringent data on safety and efficacy of this combination are lacking.

## Proarrhythmic Effects of Antiarrhythmic Compounds

The concept that proarrhythmia can offset the benefits of an antiarrhythmic agent has been established by the CAST study,[7] in which an initial "test period" of flecainide was used to show antiarrhythmic benefit without any early proarrhythmic effect; and yet during the actual prolonged study period there was an increased mortality. Moricizine, in contrast, had an early proarrhythmic effect within 2 weeks. Meta-analysis shows that of the Class I agents, quinidine is most suspect, with disopyramide and especially procainamide less so.[87] It is only the proarrhythmic effect of the Class I agents that has been established in a proper prospective study. There are two basic mechanisms for proarrhythmia:[26] prolongation of the action potential duration and QT-interval, particularly when combined with diuretic-induced hypokalemia or when there is bradycardia (next section), and, second, incessant wide complex tachycardia often terminating in VF (Fig. 8–9). The former typically occurs with Class IA and Class III agents, the latter with Class IC agents. In addition, incessant VT can complicate therapy with any Class I agent when conduction is sufficiently severely depressed. Of the Class III agents, sotalol may be particularly prone to cause torsades de pointes because of its reverse use dependency,[20] so that the action potential duration is prolonged more in the presence of bradycardia. A third type of proarrhythmia is when the patient's own tachycardia, previously paroxysmal, becomes incessant—the result of either Class IA or IC agents.[22] Not only early vigilance is required with the institution of therapy with antiarrhythmics of the Class IA, IC and III types, but continuous vigilance is required throughout therapy. Furthermore, the CAST study[7] shows that proarrhythmic sudden death can occur even when ventricular premature complexes are apparently eliminated. Solutions to this problem include (1) avoiding the use of Class I, and especially Class IC, agents, (2) not treating unless the overall effect will clearly be beneficial, and (3) ultimately defining better those subjects at high risk for proarrhythmia and arrhythmic death.[22]

Measurement of **QT-dispersion** in the precordial chest leads is a simple, noninvasive measure of the risk of torsades de pointes.[56,57] Whereas Class IA drugs increased the QT-dispersion, amiodarone decreased this measure. Much more simply, markedly increased PVCs during titration of Class I drugs heralds increased risk of proarrhythmic death.[91]

## QT-Prolongation and Torsades de Pointes

Delayed repolarization is a mechanism for controlling arrhythmias (Class IA and III agents) that at the same time predisposes to potentially life-threatening arrhythmias. It is clinically recognized by a prolonged QT or QTc (corrected for heart rate exceeding 440 msec) or QTU-interval.[1] The prolonged QT-syndrome may either be acquired or be a congenital abnormality (Romano-Ward and related conditions). The realization that quinidine, disopyramide, procainamide and related Class IA agents, Class III agents, and others (Fig. 8–8) can all prolong the QT-interval has led to a reassessment of the mode of use of such agents in antiarrhythmic therapy. Serious problems may arise when antiarrhythmic QT-prolongation is combined with any other factor increasing the QT-interval or QTU, such as bradycardia, hypokalemia, hypomagnesemia, hypocalcemia, intense or prolonged diuretic therapy, or combined Class IA and Class III therapy. A number of noncardiac drugs prolong the QT-interval (mechanism unclear), including tricyclic antidepressants, phenothiazines, erythromycin, and some antihistaminics, such as terfenadine and astemizole. When amiodarone is given to patients not receiving diuretics or other drugs who are not hypokalemic and without pre-existing QT-prolongation, torsades de pointes is very rare, possibly because it has mixed class effects.

PREVENTION. Probably the most effective way to avoid the drug-induced QT-syndrome is by regular monitoring of the ECG for the appearance of ventricular pauses, post-pause T-wave changes, and late cycle PVCs,[1] as well as QT-prolongation, while checking blood potassium and magnesium, and using a potassium-sparing diuretic whenever possible. Measurement of QT-dispersion should be considered.

TREATMENT. Torsades de pointes is best treated by agents that shorten the QT-interval such as isoproterenol or temporary cardiac pacing. Isoproterenol is contraindicated in ischemic heart disease and the congenital prolonged QT-syndrome. Alternatively, use intravenous magnesium sulfate.[37] If the QT-interval is not markedly prolonged, torsades de pointes is excluded and therapy with conventional ventricular antiarrhythmic agents is acceptable.[1]

For **congenital QT-prolongation,** the underlying cause may be an imbalance of the sympathetic drive coming from the left and right sympathetic chains. The therapy now becomes full dose beta-blockade, with added phenytoin if needed,[1] and/or left stellate ganglionectomy.

## Arrhythmias in Congestive Heart Failure

"Prophylactic" antiarrhythmic therapy is contraindicated in CHF, especially in view of the high incidence of bradyarrhythmic deaths.[27] The incidence of sudden death seems to be falling since the widespread introduction of ACE inhibitors.[77] Is there a special place for the use of amiodarone in patients with "high density" PVCs? The current VA Co-operative study (CHF-STAT) suggests not.[84A] In contrast, in the Argentinian study over 2 years, amiodarone added to standard triple therapy reduced mortality by 28%, but arrhythmias were not an entry criteria.[52A,75] In **significantly symptomatic arrhythmias,** it is first essential to pinpoint precipitating factors such as hypokalemia, hypomagnesemia, or use of sympathomimetics, phosphodiesterase inhibitors, or digoxin. The hemodynamic status of the myocardium must be made optimal because LV wall stress per se is arrhythmogenic. ACE inhibitors should help to limit LV size. Antiarrhythmics are only given after documentation of benefit by electrophysiological studies or by ambulatory monitoring.[52] Logically, beta-blockers in initial low doses could be expected to improve LV function and to help prevent the arrhythmias.

A PARADOX: ANTIARRHYTHMICS MAY WORSEN CHF. Here is the paradox: Ventricular arrhythmias can be a fatal event in CHF, yet antiarrhythmic agents can precipitate CHF. Besides beta-blockers and calcium antagonists, Class I agents[16,33] and sotalol may all precipitate CHF. In the Argentinian trial, amiodarone was well tolerated.[75] In the European trial, amiodarone 400 mg daily was as likely as sotalol to precipitate CHF.[2] Paradoxically, when a lower dose of amiodarone (200 mg) was used, the ejection fraction increased from 19% to 29%, possibly through the peripheral vasodilator and mild beta-blocking effects of the drug.[54]

PHARMACOKINETICS OF ANTIARRHYTHMICS IN CHF. In CHF, diverse factors can influence antiarrhythmic drug kinetics. For example, the volume of distribution is decreased by about 50% so that the loading dose should be lower. In addition, liver blood flow and hepatic metabolism are decreased so that the maintenance dose needs to be lower. The elimination half-life is prolonged which tends to decrease the dose. Because antiarrhythmics may increase the severity of CHF,[16] therapy needs to be started at low doses in hospitalized patients, and side-effects as well as the hemodynamic and metabolic status of the patients need to be carefully monitored.

## Principles of Treatment of Ventricular Tachycardia

First, a full work-up and optimal cardiac and electrolyte status are required. There is no unanimity of cardiologic opinion on the principles and indications for antiarrhythmic therapy, nor on the relative merits of noninvasive or invasive monitoring in drug selection.[30] Nonetheless, in the EVSEM study,[52] **empiric therapy** by sotalol, guided by Holter monitoring, appeared to be an effective procedure. Enthusiasm for drug choice by serial electrophysiologic testing must also be dampened by the finding that this complex procedure was no better than empiric metoprolol.[85] The experience of many cardiologists not specializing in arrhythmia therapy is likely to be limited to a small number of drugs and to Holter monitoring. For the specialist, the additional information achieved by at least one invasive electrophysiologic study is probably worth it. For each category of agent, the profile of electrophysiologic and hemodynamic side-effects needs to be matched against the clinical situation in the individual patient. The potential for proarrhythmic events and the lack of firm evidence for prevention of sudden death by antiarrhythmics needs stressing. Exceptions to these reservations appear to be (1) postinfarct beta-blockade that prolongs life and reduces sudden death; (2) postinfarct amiodarone, apparently favorable but still under evaluation;[70] and (3) acute therapy of truly life-threatening, serious symptomatic ventricular arrhythmias where any drug stopping the VT will save from sudden death (but not necessarily improve total mortality).

The practice of treating **recurrent VT** or **cardiac arrest** has changed in the following ways. First, the drug of choice is more likely to be a Class III than a Class I agent. Second, one or two antiarrhythmic drugs may be used, but if not effective, an **automatic implanted cardioverter defibrillator (AICD)** is used rather than trying three or more antiarrhythmic drugs in succession. The choice of an AICD is particularly made in patients with a left ventricular LV ejection fraction of below 30% to 35%, in whom the likelihood of finding a successful antiarrhythmic drug is decreased and the risk of sudden death is increased.

Limitation of AICDs should also be mentioned. They reduce sudden death but not total mortality.[93] AICD and the best medical therapy (sotalol and amiodarone) are being compared in the NIH-sponsored AVID trial [Antiarrhythmics Versus Implantable Defibrillators, see Zipes[93]].

(For ventricular arrhythmias in AMI, see Table 11–5.)

## Ablation for Supraventricular Arrhythmias

Pharmacologic management of supraventricular arrhythmias, including atrial fibrillation, is discussed in Chapter 11 (Tables 11–3 and 11–4). For refractory cases, ablation of the AV node or the bypass tract is increasingly used as appropriate. When this "map and zap" approach fails, surgical intervention is the next option.

For **atrial flutter,** a new and promising procedure with about 85% to 90% success is ablation of the isthmus between the tricuspid valve and the inferior vena cava and/or the coronary sinus.[92] In severe refractory **atrial fibrillation** not responding to AV nodal inhibition by drugs, ablation of the AV node is now an option.[90]

## Antiarrhythmics and Implantable Devices

Antiarrhythmic drugs may affect the defibrillation threshold of an AICD, or the pacing stimulation threshold. In general, Class IC drugs and amiodarone (animal data) increase these thresholds. Conversely, beta-blockers and sotalol do not alter the VF or pacing threshold. If a patient has an AICD and antiarrhythmic therapy is changed, VT may have to be induced to properly reset the device since the VT rate may be different. If the VT rate is slower than the AICD setting, the device will not be activated.[88]

## Summary

The complexity of the numerous agents available and the ever-increasing problems with side-effects and proarrhythmic events underline the requirement for careful cardiological evaluation and monitoring in patients receiving such drugs. In terms of drug effects, the therapy of supraventricular arrhythmias is assuming an increasingly rational basis with a prominent role for verapamil or diltiazem and adenosine in supraventricular tachycardia with AV nodal re-entry. Sodium blockers can inhibit the bypass tract or retrograde fast AV nodal fibers, as can Class III agents, such as sotalol or amiodarone. Ablation is preferentially used for difficult cases.

The therapy of ventricular arrhythmias remains a controversial and constantly evolving area of development, and antiarrhythmic drug therapy may be only one avenue of overall management. A distinction must be made between suppression of premature ventricular complexes and the control of VT/VF. In AMI, lidocaine is no longer given prophylactically. In postinfarct patients, beta-blockers remain the drugs of choice, while amiodarone is under evaluation. In CHF, optimal management of the hemodynamic and neurohumoral status, including the use of ACE inhibitors, takes preference over the prophylactic use of antiarrhythmic drugs. Amiodarone looks promising.

In other patients, whether or not ventricular arrhythmias should be treated largely depends on the nature and severity of the underlying heart disease and the nature of the arrhythmia. All seriously symptomatic arrhythmias need therapy; whether asymptomatic arrhythmias should be treated is a moot point, even if they look "premalignant" and "life-threatening." Not only has there been no definite proof that treatment of asymptomatic arrhythmias improves mortality, but the CAST study[7] showed a definite proarrhythmic risk for the use of flecainide or encainide in post-myocardial infarction patients. This risk may apply to varying degrees, to most Class I agents, especially quinidine. Therefore, the choice of drug has now shifted to Class III agents, such as sotalol or amiodarone; the former has a greater risk of torsades de pointes, while the latter has complex multisystem side-effects which though unpleasant can be lessened by using the lowest feasible dose. Therefore, automatic implantable cardioverter defibrillators are increasingly used in really high risk patients with serious ventricular tachyarrhythmias. Nonetheless, it is not known whether, besides reducing sudden death, the implantable devices also reduce total mortality.

# Acknowledgement

We thank Bramah Singh MD for review of this chapter.

# References

*For references from Second Edition, see Singh et al. (1991)*

1. Singh BN, Opie LH, Marcus FI. Antiarrhythmic agents. In: Opie LH (ed), Drugs for the Heart, Third Edition. WB Saunders Company, Philadelphia,1991, pp 180–216.

*References from Third Edition*

2. Amiodarone vs Sotalol Study Group. Eur Heart J 1989; 10:685–694.
3. Anastasiou-Nana MI, Anderson JL, Gilbert EM, et al. Circulation 1989; 80 (Suppl II):II–651.
4. Belhassen B, Glick A, Laniado S. Circulation 1988; 77:795–805.
5. Brodsky MA, Allen BJ, Luckett CR, et al. Am Heart J 1989; 118:272–280.
6. CAPS (Cardiac Arrhythmia Pilot Study) Investigators. Am J Cardiol 1988; 61:501–509.
7. CAST Investigators (Cardiac Arrhythmia Suppression Trial). N Engl J Med 1989; 321:406–412.
8. CAST Study—Akhtar M, Breithardt G, Camm AJ, et al. Circulation 1990; 81:1123–1127.
9. DiMarco JP, Sellers TD, Lerman BB, et al. J Am Coll Cardiol 1985; 6:417–425.
10. Dorian P, Berman ND. Circulation 1989; 80 (Suppl II):II–651.
11. Epstein M, Jardine RM, Obel IWP. SA Med J 1988; 74:559–562.
12. Euler DE, Wedel VA, Scanlon PJ. J Cardiovasc Pharmacol 1989; 14:430–437.
13. Falk RH. Ann Intern Med 1989; 111:107–111.
14. Fournier C, Brunet M, Bah M, et al. Eur Heart J 1989; 10:1090–1100.
15. Funck-Brentano C, Kroemer HK, Lee JT, Roden DM. N Engl J Med 1990; 322:518–525.

16. Gottlieb SS, Kukin ML, Medina N, et al. Circulation 1990; 81:860–864.
17. Hamer AWF, Arkles B, Johns JA. J Am Coll Cardiol 1989; 14:1768–1774.
18. Herre JM, Sauve MJ, Malone P, et al. J Am Coll Cardiol 1989; 13:442–449.
19. Hill MR, Gotz VP, Harman E, et al. Chest 1986; 90:698–702.
20. Hondeghem LM, Snyders DJ. Circulation 1990; 81:686–690.
21. Ikeda N, Singh BN, Davis LD, Hauswirth O. J Am Coll Cardiol 1985; 5:303–310.
22. Josephson ME. Ann Intern Med 1989; 111:101–103.
23. Kates RE, Yee Y-G, Kirsten EB. Clin Pharmacol Ther 1987; 42:305–311.
24. Langenfeld H, Weirich J, Kohler C, Kochsiek K. J Cardiovasc Pharmacol 1990; 15:338–345.
25. Lerman BB, Wesley RC, Belardinelli L. Circulation 1989; 80:1536–1543.
26. Levine JH, Morganroth J, Kadish AH. Circulation 1989; 80:1063–1069.
27. Luu M, Stevenson WG, Stevenson LW, et al. Circulation 1989; 80:1675–1680.
28. Marks ML, Graham EL, Powell JL, et al. Circulation 1989; 80 (Suppl II):II–651.
29. Mitchell LB, Wyse G, Gillis AM, Duff HJ. Circulation 1989; 80:34–42.
30. Podrid J. Ann Rev Med 1987; 38:1–17.
31. Pollick C. Am J Cardiol 1988; 62:1252–1255.
32. Ragosta M, Weihl AC, Rosenfeld LE. Am J Med 1989; 86:465–466.
33. Ravid S, Podrid PJ, Lampert S, Lown B. J Am Coll Cardiol 1989; 14:1326–1330.
34. Schutzenberger W, Leisch F, Kerschner K, et al. Br Heart J 1989; 62:367–371.
35. Singh BN. Am J Cardiol 1989; 63:867–869.
36. Singh BN, Nademanee K. Am Heart J 1985; 109:421–430.
37. Tzivoni D, Banai S, Schuger C, et al. Circulation 1988; 77:392–397.
38. Vacek JL, Sztern MI, Botteron GW, et al. J Am Coll Cardiol 1990; 15:39A.
39. Watt AH, Bernard MS, Webster J, et al. Br J Clin Pharmacol 1986; 21:227–230.
40. Woosley RL. In: Hurst JW, Schlant RC, et al. (eds) The Heart, 7th Edition. McGraw-Hill Information Services Company, New York, 1990, pp 1682–1711.

## New References

41. Camm AJ, Garratt CJ. Adenosine and supraventricular tachycardia. N Engl J Med 1991; 325:1621–1629.
42. CASCADE study—The CASCADE Investigators. Randomized antiarrhythmic drug therapy in survivors of cardiac arrest (the CASCADE Study). Am J Cardiol 1993; 72:280–287.
43. CASH Study—Siebels J, Cappato R, Ruppel R, et al. Preliminary results of the Cardiac Arrest Study Hamburg (CASH). Am J Cardiol 1993; 72:109F–113F.
44. CAST-II Study—The Cardiac Arrhythmia Suppression Trial II (CAST-II) Investigators. Effect of the antiarrhythmic drug moricizine on survival after myocardial infarction. N Engl J Med 1992; 327:227–233.
45. Ceremuzynski L, Kleczar E, Krzeminska-Pakula M, et al. Effect of amiodarone on mortality after myocardial infarction: A double-blind, placebo-controlled, pilot study. J Am Coll Cardiol 1992; 20:1056–1062.
46. Clyne CA, Estes III NAM, Wang PJ. Moricizine. N Engl J Med 1992; 327:255–260.
47. Coplen SE, Antman EM, Berlin JA, et al. Efficacy and safety of quinidine therapy for maintenance of sinus rhythm after cardioversion. A meta-analysis of randomized control trials. Circulation 1990; 82:1106–1116.
48. Dobs AS, Sarma S, Guarnieri T, Griffith L. Testicular dysfunction with amiodarone uses. J Am Coll Cardiol 1991; 18:1328–1331.
49. Dorian P, Newman D, Berman N, et al. Sotalol and Type IA drugs in combination prevent recurrence of sustained ventricular tachycardia. J Am Coll Cardiol 1993; 22:106–113.
50. Dougherty AH, Jackman WM, Naccarelli GV, et al. Acute conversion of paroxysmal supraventricular tachycardia with intravenous diltiazem. Am J Cardiol 1992; 70:587–592.
51. ESVEM Investigators. The ESVEM trial. Electrophysiologic Study Versus Electrocardiographic Monitoring for selection of antiarrhythmic therapy of ventricular tachycardia. Circulation 1989; 70:1354–1360.
52. ESVEM Investigators—Mason JW, for the Electrophysiologic Study Versus Electrocardiographic Monitoring (ESVEM) Investigators. A comparison of seven antiarrhythmic drugs in patients with ventricular tachyarrhythmias. N Engl J Med 1993; 329:452–458.
52A. GESICA study—Doval HC, Nul DR, Grancelli HO, et al. for Grupo de Estudio de la Sobrevida en la insuficiencia Cardiaca en Argentina (GESICA). Randomised trial of low-dose amiodarone in severe congestive heart failure. Lancet 1994; 344:493–498.
53. Gosselink ATM, Crijns HJGM, van Gelder IC, et al. Low-dose amiodarone for maintenance of sinus rhythm after cardioversion of atrial fibrillation or flutter. JAMA 1992; 267:3289–3293.
54. Gottlieb SS, Riggio DW, Lauria S, et al. High dose oral amiodarone loading exerts important hemodynamic actions in patients with congestive heart failure. J Am Coll Cardiol 1994; 23:560–564.
55. Herre JM, Titus C, Oeff M, et al. Inefficacy and proarrhythmic effects of flecainide

and encainide for sustained ventricular tachycardia and ventricular fibrillation. Ann Intern Med 1990; 113:671–676.

56. Hii JTY, Wyse G, Gillis AM, et al. Precordial QT-interval dispersion as a marker of torsade de pointes. Disparate effects of Class IA antiarrhythmic drugs and amiodarone. Circulation 1992; 86:1376–1382.

56A. Ho DSW, Zecchin RP, Richards DAB, et al. Double-blind trial of lignocaine versus sotalol for acute termination of spontaneous sustained ventricular tachycardia. Lancet 1994; 344:18–23.

57. Hohnloser SH, van de Loo A, Kalusche D, et al. Does sotalol-induced alteration of QT-dispersion predict drug effectiveness or proarrhythmic hazards? (abstr). Circulation 1993; 88:I–397.

57A. Hohnloser SH, Woosley RL. Sotalol. N Engl J Med 1994; 331:31–38.

58. Juul-Moller S, Edvardsson N, Rehnqvist-Ahlberg N. Sotalol versus quinidine for the maintenance of sinus rhythm after direct current conversion of atrial fibrillation. Circulation 1990; 82:1932–1939.

59. Kaumann AJ, Olson CB. Temporal relation between long-lasting aftercontractions and action potentials in cat papillary muscles. Science 1968; 161:293–295.

60. Kowey PR, for the IV Amiodarone Investigators. A multicenter randomized double-blind comparison of intravenous bretylium with amiodarone in patients with frequent malignant ventricular arrhythmias (abstr). Circulation 1993; 88:I–396.

61. Leon AR, Merlino JD. Quinidine: its value and danger. Heart Disease and Stroke 1993; 2:407–413.

62. Lubbe WF, Podzuweit T, Opie LH. Potential arrhythmogenic role of cyclic AMP and cytosolic calcium overload: Implications for prophylactic effect of beta-blockers in myocardial infarction and proarrhythmic effects of phosphodiesterase inhibitors. J Am Coll Cardiol 1992; 19:1622–1633.

63. MacMahon S, Collins R, Peto R, et al. Effects of prophylactic lidocaine in suspected acute myocardial infarction. JAMA 1988; 260:1910–1916.

64. Manolis AS, Deering TF, Cameron J, Estes III NAM. Mexiletine: Pharmacology and therapeutic use. Clin Cardiol 1990; 13:349–359.

65. Marcus FI. The hazards of using type IC antiarrhythmic drugs for the treatment of paroxysmal atrial fibrillation (editorial). Am J Cardiol 1990; 66:366–367.

66. Mariano DJ, Schomer SJ, Rea RF. Effects of quinidine on vascular resistance and sympathetic nerve activity in humans. J Am Coll Cardiol 1992; 20:1411–1416.

67. Meredith IT, Broughton A, Jennings GL, Esler MD. Evidence of a selective increase in cardiac sympathetic activity in patients with sustained ventricular arrhythmias. N Engl J Med 1991; 325:618–624.

68. Middlekauff HR, Wiener I, Savon LA, Stevenson WG. Low-dose amiodarone for atrial fibrillation: Time for a prospective study? Ann Intern Med 1992; 116:1017–1020.

69. Middlekauff HR, Stevenson WG, Saxon LA. Amiodarone is not safe for advanced heart failure patients with a history of torsades de pointes (abstr). J Am Coll Cardiol 1993; 21:243A.

70. Nademanee K, Singh BN, Stevenson WG, Weiss JN. Amiodarone and post-MI patients. Circulation 1993; 88:764–774.

71. Nattel S, Talajic M, Fermini B, Roy D. Amiodarone: Pharmacology, clinical actions, and relationships between them. J Cardiovasc Electrophysiol 1992; 3:266–280.

72. Navarro-Lopez F, Cosin J, Guindo J, et al. A controlled trial of amiodarone vs metoprolol in post-myocardial infarction patients with ventricular ectopic activity: Three year follow-up (abstr). J Am Coll Cardiol 1993; 21:243A.

73. Nolan PE, Erstad BL, Hoyer GL, et al. Steady-state interaction between amiodarone and phenytoin in normal subjects. Am J Cardiol 1990; 65:1252–1257.

74. Nora M, Zipes DP. Empiric use of amiodarone and sotalol. Am J Cardiol 1993; 72:62F–69F.

75. Nul DR, Doval H, Grancelli H, et al. Amiodarone reduces mortality in severe heart failure (abstr). Circulation 1993; 88 (Suppl I):I–603. (See Reference 52A.)

76. Opie LH. In: Schlant RC, Alexander RW (eds). Adverse cardiovascular drug interactions. The Heart, 8th edition. McGraw-Hill, New York, 1994, pp 1971–1985.

77. Pahor M, Gambassi G, Carbonin P. Antiarrhythmic effects of ACE inhibitors: A matter of faith or reality? Cardiovasc Res 1994; 28:173–182.

78. Pfisterer ME, Kiowski W, Brunner H, et al. Long-term benefit of 1-year amiodarone treatment for persistent complex ventricular arrhythmias after myocardial infarction. Circulation 1993; 87:309–311.

79. Rea RF, Hamdan M, Schomer SJ, Geraets DR. Inhibitory effects of procainamide on sympathetic nerve activity in humans. Circ Res 1991; 69:501–508.

80. Reimold SC, Cantillon CO, Friedman PL, Antman EM. Propafenone versus sotalol for suppression of recurrent symptomatic atrial fibrillation. Am J Cardiol 1993; 71:558–563.

81. Ruffy R. Sotalol. J Cardiovasc Electrophysiol 1993; 4:81–98.

82. Russo AM, Beauregard LA, Waxman HL. Oral amiodarone loading for the rapid treatment of frequent, refractory, sustained ventricular arrhythmias associated with coronary artery disease. Am J Cardiol 1993; 72:1395–1399.

83. Scheinman MM, for the IV Amiodarone Study Group. Multicenter study of the

dose response to intravenous amiodarone in patients with refractory ventricular tachycardia/fibrillation (abstr). Circulation 1993; 88:I–396.

84. Singh BN. Routine prophylactic lidocaine administration in acute myocardial infarction. An idea whose time is all but gone? Circulation 1992; 26:1033–1035.

84A. Singh SN, Fletcher RD, Fisher SG, et al. Results of the congestive heart failure survival trial of antiarrhythmic therapy (Veterans Affairs Cooperative Study Program 320)(abstr). Circulation 1994; 90:2939.

85. Steinbeck G, Andresen D, Bach P, et al. A comparison of electrophysiologically guided antiarrhythmic drug therapy with beta-blocker therapy in patients with symptomatic, sustained ventricular tachyarrhythmias. N Engl J Med 1992; 327:987–992.

86. Task Force of the Working Group on Arrhythmias of the European Society of Cardiology. The Sicilian Gambit. A new approach to the classification of antiarrhythmic drugs based on their actions on arrhythmogenic mechanisms. Circulation 1991; 84:1831–1851.

87. Teo KK, Yusuf S, Furberg D. Effects of prophylactic antiarrhythmic drug therapy in acute myocardial infarction. An overview of results from randomized controlled trials. JAMA 1993; 270:1589–1595.

88. Tworek DA, Nazari J, Ezri M, Bauman JL. Interference by antiarrhythmic agents with function of electrical cardiac devices. Clin Pharm 1992; 11:48–56.

89. Weaver WD, Fahrenbruch CE, Johnson DD, et al. Effect of epinephrine and lidocaine therapy on outcome after cardiac arrest due to ventricular fibrillation. Circulation 1990; 82:2027–2034.

90. Windecker S, Plumb VJ, Epstein AE, Kay GN. Does AV nodal ablation impair long-term survival compared with medical treatment of atrial fibrillation (abstr)? J Am Coll Cardiol 1994; 23:84A.

91. Wyse DG, Morganroth J, Ledingham R, et al, for the CAST and CAPS Investigators. New insights into the definition and meaning of proarrhythmia during initiation of antiarrhythmic drug therapy from the Cardiac Arrhythmia Suppression Trial and its pilot study. J Am Coll Cardiol 1994; 23:1130–1140.

92. Xie B, Murgatroyd FD, Heald SC, et al. Catheter ablation for atrial flutter substrate using low energy direct current: Results of long-term follow-up (abstr). J Am Coll Cardiol 1994; 23:84A.

93. Zipes DP. Implantable cardioverter-defibrillator. Lifesaver or a device looking for a disease? Circulation 1994; 89:2934–2936.

# Notes

# 9 Antithrombotic Agents: Platelet Inhibitors, Anticoagulants, and Fibrinolytics

B.J. Gersh • L.H. Opie

The Emperor said: "I wonder whether breathlessness results in death or life?"

Chi'i P answered: "When there are blockages in the circulation between the viscera, then death follows. . . ."

The Emperor said: "What can be done with regard to treatment?"

Chi'i P replied: "The method of curing is to establish communication between the viscera and the vascular system. . . ."

The Yellow Emperor's Classic of Internal Medicine (ca. 2000 BC)

## Mechanisms of Thrombosis

### Pro- and Anti-Aggregatory Factors

These opposing factors are normally finely balanced. To protect against vascular damage and the risk of bleeding to death, the pro-aggregatory system is poised rapidly to form a thrombus to limit any potential hemorrhage. As long as the **vascular endothelium** is intact, at least four anti-aggregatory mechanisms keep the blood flowing (Fig. 9–1). As coronary endothelial damage appears to be a prominent feature of ischemic heart disease, there is a constant risk that pro-aggregatory forces will dominate with the risk of further vascular damage, and sometimes thrombosis.

To **form a thrombus,** the three steps are (1) exposure of the circulating blood to a thrombogenic surface, such as a damaged vascular endothelium, resulting from a ruptured atherosclerotic plaque; (2) a sequence of platelet-related events, involving platelet adhesion, platelet activation, and platelet aggregation, with release of agents further promoting aggregation and causing vasoconstriction; and (3) triggering of the clotting mechanism with an important role for thrombin in the formation of fibrin, the latter cross-linking to form the backbone of the thrombus. Thrombin is in itself a very powerful stimulator of platelet adhesion and aggregation. Once formed, the thrombus may be broken down by plasmin-stimulated fibrinolysis. Current antithrombotic medications include those inhibiting platelets (antiplatelet agents), those preventing coagulation (anticoagulants) and fibrinolytics. The typical arterial thrombus at the site of a coronary stenosis has a white head due to platelet aggregation, and a red tail due to stasis beyond the lesion.

The above sequence relates to the three main types of agents considered in this chapter. First, **platelet inhibitors** may be expected to act on arterial thrombi and to help prevent their consequences such as myocardial infarction and transient ischemic attacks (TIAs). Second, **anticoagulants** given acutely (heparin) should limit further formation of fibrin, and when given chronically (warfarin) should prevent thromboembolism derived from veins such as those in the legs, or from a dilated left atrium. Third, **fibrinolytics** will be most useful in clinical syndromes of acute arterial thrombosis and occlu-

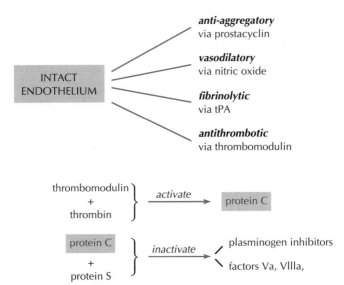

FIGURE 9–1. Factors protecting against coagulation directly or indirectly depend on an intact endothelium. Fig. copyright L.H. Opie.

sion, typified by acute myocardial infarction (AMI), but also including peripheral arterial thrombosis. Different sites of action of these three types of agents mean that combination therapy can be logical, for example adding together thrombolytic agents with antiplatelet agents and anticoagulants in the management of AMI.

PLATELET FUNCTION. In addition to their potential for acting against arterial thrombosis, it may be predicted that platelet inhibitors should also protect against other proposed consequences of platelet malfunction such as excessive vasoconstriction. Platelets, perhaps by release of platelet-derived growth factor (PDGF), may also stimulate smooth muscle cell proliferation and migration into the subintimal layer with subsequent synthesis of connective tissue and intimal hyperplasia, thereby promoting the development of atheroma.

PLATELET ADHESION TO THE INJURED VESSEL WALL (Fig. 9–2). This is the first of the three steps involving platelets in the development of an arterial thrombus. Endothelial injury promotes platelet adhesion in two ways. First, there is release from the endothelium of von Willebrand factor to which platelets adhere. Second, microfibrils of collagen from the deeper layers of the vessel become exposed as a result of endothelial injury, thereby promoting platelet adhesion.

PLATELET RECEPTORS AND ACTIVATION. Superficial injury to the platelets activates **platelet receptors,** which are membrane glycoproteins (GP). Activated receptors bind more readily to the von Willebrand factor (receptor GP Ib) or subendothelial collagen (receptor GP Ia) or fibrinogen (**receptor GP IIb/IIIa**). These receptors have a twofold function. They help to activate platelets by releasing calcium from the endoplasmic reticulum (Fig. 9–3) and they allow macromolecules such the circulating von Willebrand factor (a high molecular weight protein) to "chain" receptors together and thereby to promote platelet adhesion. Thrombin, although a protease in the coagulation process, can act as a classic ligand that activates platelet receptors by cleaving a specific extracellular amino acid domain of the platelet receptor, thereby exposing the active ligand.[57] The activated receptor raises platelet calcium both by inhibiting adenylcyclase and by stimulating phospholipase C.[57]

PLATELET AGGREGATION (aggregation means a mass brought together). The critical event is a rise in intracellular platelet calcium level (Fig. 9–3). Several mediators including collagen from endothelial injury,

## PLATELET ADHESION AND AGGREGATION

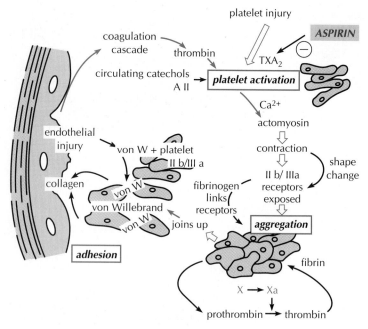

FIGURE 9–2. The three basic processes of (1) platelet adhesion; (2) platelet activation; and (3) platelet aggregation set in motion by endothelial and platelet injury. The bottom sequence indicates activation of coagulation by the intrinsic (platelet) pathway. $TXA_2$ = thromboxane $A_2$; EPI = epinephrine; ADP = adenosine diphosphate; von Willebrand = von Willebrand factor. Fig. copyright L.H. Opie.

thrombin, ADP released from injured platelets, and serotonin from hemolyzed red cells, act by stimulating the formation of inositol trisphosphate ($IP_3$). The thromboxane $A_2$ synthesized in the damaged vessel wall inhibits the formation of cyclic AMP, thereby removing a brake on the production of $IP_3$. $IP_3$ mobilizes calcium from the endoplasmic reticulum. An enhanced platelet calcium has several consequences, including (1) stimulation of the pathways breaking down the platelet phospholipids eventually to form thromboxane $A_2$ (Fig. 9–3) and (2) activation of platelet actin and myosin to cause contraction. Contraction of the platelets or mechanical shear stress[93] exposes the glycoprotein receptor GP IIb/IIIa which mediates the final common path in platelet aggregation by allowing a greater rate of interaction with various macromolecules including the von Willebrand factor, fibrinogen and thrombin. These macromolecules bind the platelets to each other and to those platelets already adhering to the vessel wall.

ACTIVATION OF CLOTTING MECHANISMS. The **intrinsic coagulation pathway** involves the generation of thrombin during activation of the platelet membrane (Fig. 9–2). The **extrinsic coagulation pathway** involves thromboplastin generated by the vessel wall, which then converts prothrombin to thrombin. Prothrombin is one of several vitamin-K-dependent clotting factors; the oral anticoagulants such as warfarin are vitamin-K-antagonists. Thrombin from either source enhances platelet membrane activation further to promote platelet aggregation and to convert fibrinogen to fibrin, which adheres to platelet surfaces to stabilize and fix the arterial thrombus. The end result is a platelet- and fibrin-rich thrombus, adherent to the vessel wall. This whole process may be dynamic and repetitive.[74] Fibrinolytic mechanisms, involving the conversion of plasminogen to plasmin, act to limit the size of the clot and eventually to dissolve it at least in part.

## Platelet Receptors

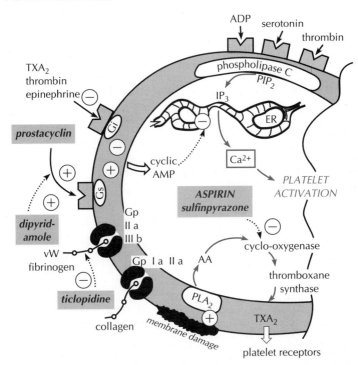

**FIGURE 9–3.**   Role of intracellular platelet calcium control systems and site for therapeutic agents. Crucial is the role of $IP_3$ in mobilizing calcium from the endoplasmic reticulum (ER). Note role of ADP, serotonin, collagen and thrombin in promoting formation of $IP_3$ and different mechanism of action of thromboxane $A_2$ ($TXA_2$). $IP_3$ = inositol trisphosphate; $PIP_2$ = phosphatidylinositol diphosphate; PDE = phosphodiesterase; AA = arachidonic acid. Fig. copyright L.H. Opie.

**Platelets and Vascular Contraction.**   During and after platelet aggregation, platelets release 5-hydroxytryptamine (serotonin) and other potentially important products such as platelet factor 4 and beta-thromboglobulin that may help in the formation of the hemostatic plug. Serotonin normally causes vasodilation in the presence of an intact vascular endothelium. In contrast, when the endothelium is damaged, serotonin causes vasoconstriction that may promote vascular stasis and thrombosis. Hence platelets are suspected of a role in vasoconstrictive diseases such as coronary spasm or Raynaud's disease.

## Platelet Inhibition by Aspirin

Aspirin (acetylsalicylic acid) irreversibly acetylates cyclo-oxygenase, and activity is not restored until new platelets are formed. Platelets, being very primitive cells, cannot synthesize new proteins so that aspirin removes all the platelet cyclo-oxygenase activity for the lifespan of the platelet. Therefore, aspirin stops the production of the pro-aggregatory thromboxane $A_2$ (Fig. 9–4) and eventually acts as an indirect antithrombotic agent.[1] On the other hand, aspirin also has important nonplatelet effects and in the vascular endothelium likewise inactivates cyclo-oxygenase that could diminish formation of anti-aggregatory prostacyclin. The difference is that vascular cyclo-oxygenase can be resynthesized within hours. Despite potentially conflicting effects that aspirin has by lessening synthesis of both thromboxane $A_2$ and prostacyclin, the overwhelming clinical message is that the antithrombotic effects predominate.[74]

## ASPIRIN ACTION

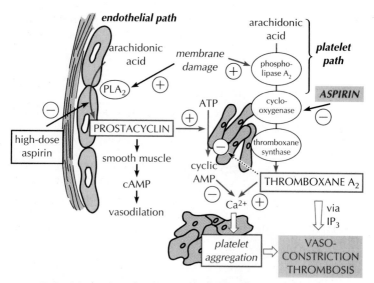

**FIGURE 9–4.** Mechanism of aspirin action. The critical event in platelet aggregation is an increase of platelet calcium that can be inhibited by prostacyclin (PGI₂) and promoted by thromboxane A₂ (see Fig 9–3). Aspirin inactivates cyclooxygenase to inhibit formation of thromboxane A₂ and in high doses inhibits prostacyclin formation in the vascular endothelium. Fig. copyright L.H. Opie.

ASPIRIN KINETICS. Aspirin undergoes substantial presystemic hydrolysis to form salicylic acid, which is only a weak inactivator of cyclooxygenase with a longer half-life of 2 to 3 hours versus 15 to 20 minutes for aspirin.[1] Although even very low doses of aspirin, such as 20 mg, have a documented platelet inhibitory effect, and may selectively inhibit the formation of thromboxane A₂ rather than prostacyclin,[74] the problem with such doses is that the full antithrombotic effect takes up to 48 hours to be manifest. In contrast, with standard doses, the effect comes on within hours. Thus full-dose aspirin should be given at the start of symptoms of acute myocardial infarction.[109]

### Clinical Indications for Aspirin

The clinical indications for this remarkable drug keep expanding. A recent mega-meta-analysis on 140,000 patients in 300 studies confirmed prophylactic benefit after previous myocardial infarction, in angina, after stroke, or after bypass surgery, and established efficacy for women as well as men.[43] Aspirin works in hypertensives and in diabetics.

STABLE ANGINA. In stable angina, aspirin 75 mg daily (when compared with placebo) caused a 34% reduction in acute myocardial infarction and sudden death in the Swedish SAPAT study[114] which was on about 2,000 patients, half being male. Both aspirin and placebo were added to the beta-blocker sotalol, given at an average dose of 160 mg per day. In the smaller study of Ridker et al.[108] on 333 men, aspirin (325 mg on alterate days) given for an average of 60 months, reduced first myocardial infarction by 87%.

UNSTABLE ANGINA. There is general agreement that aspirin should be given both in the acute and follow-up phases.[47,74] Although aspirin in its own right reduces AMI and death, even in doses as low as 75 mg daily[110] it does not consistently decrease anginal pain.[22,33] A meta-analysis of seven trials on the follow-up after unstable angina also show benefits for aspirin in reducing AMI, stroke and vascular death.[43] In two studies, doses of 75 or 325 mg daily were effective.[1,111]

Aspirin was started during hospitalization and continued for up to 2 years. It is now standard practice to combine heparin and aspirin, starting the two together for two reasons. First, the differential diagnosis from AMI may not be clear and, second, aspirin should be on board when heparin is discontinued to prevent recurrences of unstable angina.[123]

NON-Q-WAVE MYOCARDIAL INFARCTION. The principles of treatment by aspirin are similar to those used for unstable angina.[47]

ACUTE MYOCARDIAL INFARCTION. In view of the ISIS-2 trial[18] in which 160 mg aspirin was started as soon as possible and continued for 1 month, the use of oral aspirin as soon as possible after the onset of symptoms is now standard. Theoretically, an initial dose of 325 mg is preferable.[135] Self-administration of aspirin on suspicion of AMI would appear to be a simple and potentially effective procedure.[109]

POSTINFARCT FOLLOW-UP. By 1988 there had been nine randomized trials.[2] Pooled data show that vascular mortality decreased by 13%, nonfatal myocardial infarction by 31%, nonfatal stroke by 42%, and all vascular events by 25%. Aspirin 300 to 325 mg daily given indefinitely is a reasonable recommendation accepting that absolutely definitive data on doses are not available and that lower doses are now often used. No additional benefit is derived from cotherapy with dipyridamole.

POST-THROMBOLYTIC FOLLOW-UP. In ISIS-2,[18] aspirin continued for 1 month had added benefit to that achieved by streptokinase. In the APRICOT study,[44] standard dose aspirin (325 mg per day) given for 3 months after thrombolytic therapy reduced reinfarction, revascularization rate, and increased left ventricular ejection fraction.[44]

POST-CORONARY BYPASS SURGERY. This is another firm indication for aspirin, with the aim of avoiding thrombotic graft closure and also in the hope of lessening long-term graft arteriosclerosis. Aspirin should be started immediately after surgery and continued for at least 1 year and probably indefinitely.[74] In a large series, aspirin 325 mg given 12 hours before surgery and thereafter daily was as good as aspirin 1,000 mg daily plus dipyridamole or sulfinpyrazone.[12] Very low-dose aspirin (50 mg daily) combined with dipyridamole helped to prevent graft closure in a prospective randomized trial[27] and could be recommended for 1 year. In view of the small increase in risk of bleeding with **preoperative aspirin,**[12,76] preoperative dipyridamole is started and then stopped soon after the operation while continuing aspirin started 6 to 12 hours postoperatively and continued for at least 1 year.[74] In patients already on aspirin, the risk of bleeding is not sufficiently serious to delay surgery.

CORONARY ANGIOPLASTY. Pretreatment with aspirin together with acute heparin is strongly recommended to prevent acute thrombotic closure.[74] To prevent **restenosis, aspirin 500 mg daily is better than 100 mg daily.**[58A]

TRANSIENT ISCHEMIC ATTACKS (TIAs). For TIAs, the huge doses initially used (1,300 mg daily) have dwindled first to 300 mg daily[37] then to 75 mg daily[112] and even down to 30 mg daily.[62] In the recent Swedish trial,[112] aspirin 75 mg daily reduced stroke or death by 18% over 32 months in 1,360 patients, one-third being female. Hence, aspirin is now the standard recommendation for both genders, usually in a dose of 325 mg daily.[69] Some experts still prefer higher doses.[69]

PREVENTION OF STROKE (NONCARDIOGENIC). For primary prevention, the data for aspirin are not convincing and there may be an increased hazard.[14] In secondary prevention, aspirin forms part of a comprehensive preventative program[74] including control of blood pressure.[69]

PREVENTION OF STROKE IN ATRIAL FIBRILLATION. When warfarin is contraindicated or the patient is not at high risk of stroke, aspirin provides at least some protection (see Atrial Fibrillation, under section on Warfarin).

OTHER INDICATIONS. Less firm indications for aspirin are: (1) **artificial heart valves** to prevent emboli (recently, the combination of warfarin and low-dose aspirin has been validated,[129] although in the past the combination warfarin-dipyridamole was preferred to warfarin plus standard-dose aspirin because of the increased risk of bleeding); (2) **arteriovenous shunts,** aspirin 160 mg daily decreases thrombosis; (3) **peripheral vascular disease**—prophylactic aspirin prevents angiographic progression especially in smokers and hypertensives;[1] (4) **renovascular hypertension**—a little-known study shows that aspirin reduces the blood pressure in this specific type of hypertension, presumably by inhibiting formation of those prostaglandins involved in renin release;[17] and (5) in **diabetic retinopathy,** to stop the rate of evolution of microaneurysms.[58] In **pregnancy-induced hypertension,** aspirin 50 mg daily does not work[90] contrary to previous information.

## Aspirin Side-effects

High-dose aspirin causes GI side-effects in many patients, whereas the standard dose (150 to 300 mg daily) lessens the incidence to about 40% compared with about 30% in placebo.[37] GI side-effects (dyspepsia, nausea, vomiting) may be dose-limiting in about 10 to 20% of patients. Such side-effects may be reduced by **buffered** or **enteric-coated aspirin** or by taking aspirin with food. GI bleeding may occur in about 5%, of patients with frank melena in only about 1% per year and hematemesis in about 0.1% per year. A really low dose of aspirin (30 mg daily) substantially reduces the incidence of bleeding, but leaves gastric side-effects virtually unchanged.[62] In some studies, **hemorrhagic stroke** has been a side-effect.[108] Even though not confirmed in larger studies,[112,114] the FDA warns against self-administration of aspirin because of the slight risk of stroke.[72] Uncommonly, gout may be aggravated because aspirin impairs urate secretion.

## Contraindications

Aspirin intolerance, hemophilia, history of GI bleeds or of peptic ulcer or other potential sources of GI or genito-urinary bleeding. Congestive heart failure (CHF) is a contraindication to **Alka-Seltzer** (sodium content) as are renal failure or stones or hepatic cirrhosis. *Relative contraindications* include dyspepsia, iron deficiency anemia, gout, and the possibility of enhanced peri-operative bleeding unless the dose is only 20 mg daily.[1] Aspirin, especially in high doses, may exaggerate a bleeding tendency. Common sense says that retinal hemorrhages are a contraindication unless very low-dose or controlled-release aspirin is used, yet data are lacking. Periodic hemoglobin checks may detect occult GI bleeding. Because it decreases the urinary excretion of uric acid, it is contraindicated in gout.

## Drug Interactions

Concurrent **warfarin** and aspirin predispose to bleeding especially if doses are high. For low-dose combination, see Reference 55A. Generally, nonsteroidal anti-inflammatory drugs (NSAIDs) attenuate the efficacy of **antihypertensive therapy** by complex mechanisms; aspirin appears not to share this interaction. Nonetheless, aspirin may lessen the efficacy of the **ACE inhibitor** enalapril, so that a low aspirin dose is required (p 125). Aspirin may decrease the efficacy of **uricosuric drugs** such as sulfinpyrazone and probenecid. The **risk of aspirin-induced GI bleeding** is increased by alcohol, corticosteroid therapy, and other NSAIDs. Concurrent warfarin and aspirin predispose to bleeding especially if doses are high. Enteric-coated preparations may have their efficacy reduced by antacids by altering the pH of the stomach. Phenobarbital, phenytoin, and rifampin decrease aspirin efficacy by induction of the hepatic enzymes metabolising aspirin. The effect of **oral hypoglycemic agents** and insulin might be enhanced. Both **thiazides** and aspirin decrease excretion of uric acid with increased risk of gout.

### Standard- versus Low-dose Aspirin

Knowledge that aspirin 300 mg daily is as good as 1,200 mg for TIA prevention[37] meant that a dose of approximately 300 mg became standard. Since then, the beneficial use of 160 mg daily for 1 month in the ISIS-2 trial[18] means that this lower dose is now widely accepted as having prophylactic efficacy. Meta-analysis suggests a dose range of 75 to 325 mg daily.[43] The present trend is to make the standard tablet strength 100 to 160 mg. Even lower doses of aspirin (75 mg daily) have beneficial effects in stable angina[114] or in the follow-up of unstable angina[110] or in the prevention of TIAs.[112] Minute doses of aspirin such as 30 mg daily can still theoretically achieve cyclo-oxygenase inhibition and may be as good as higher doses in prevention of TIAs.[62] Possibly a controlled release aspirin may allow a greater platelet (thromboxane $A_2$) than vascular (prostacyclin) inhibitory effect.[56]

### Primary Prevention by Aspirin—Is it Worth It?

Our recommendation, supported by a meta-analysis of three trials on about 30,000 subjects,[43] is that aspirin should not be used prophylactically in the general apparently healthy population, especially not in the elderly.[25] The FDA warn against a slightly increased risk of hemorrhagic stroke.[72] When a comprehensive attack on risk factors is being mounted, however, low-dose aspirin appears a useful adjunct to other measures.[14] Thus in patients with established coronary artery disease or peripheral vascular disease, 75 to 325 mg aspirin daily is reasonable.[6,11,43,114]

### Aspirin—Summary

Aspirin is now of proven value both in stable and unstable angina to prevent myocardial infarction. In acute myocardial infarction, aspirin should be given right at the start of symptoms. In postinfarct patients, 325 mg daily is recommended by the FDA, but 160 mg seems equally reasonable. In patients with TIAs, aspirin reduces recurrent attacks. Aspirin reduces the incidence of early graft closure following bypass surgery. Aspirin is also used in selected patients with artificial heart valves or arteriovenous shunts. Aspirin may reduce thromboembolism in some patients with atrial fibrillation. The optimal dose of aspirin remains uncertain, but about 160 to 325 mg daily has become standard. Most trials showing beneficial outcome have used 160 to 325 mg daily with a few trials on TIAs using 1,300 mg daily. In other trials on TIAs, 75 mg or even 30 mg daily also seem effective. In the rare case of clear contraindications to aspirin, such as definite allergy or gastric intolerance even with enteric coated low-dose preparations, alternate antiplatelet regimes are required.

## Alternate Antiplatelet Regimes

In general, platelet inhibition by sulfinpyrazone or dipyridamole or aspirin combined with either of these or by ticlodipine has results very similar to those of aspirin alone.[43]

### Dipyridamole

Dipyridamole (**Persantine**) is one of several agents that can be used instead of aspirin. Dipyridamole has five effects. First, there are the well-known coronary vasodilator effects mediated by the inhibition of adenosine transport, which is the basis of the dipyridamole-thallium stress test. Second, it inhibits platelet adhesion to the damaged vessel. Third, dipyridamole may potentiate the anti-aggregatory effect of prostacyclin.[1] Fourth, at high and supraclinical doses,[1] dipyridamole enhances cyclic AMP formation and lowers platelet calcium, thereby inhibiting platelet aggregation (Fig. 9–3). In comparison with aspirin, dipyridamole has far more inhibitory effects on platelet adhesion to the vessel wall and much less on platelet aggregation. There have been few clinical trials using dipyridamole alone; usually combination with aspirin is undertaken, and in almost all trials there is no convincing evidence that dipyridamole adds anything to the benefits obtained by aspirin alone.

DOSE. Most trials have used 75 mg three times daily. The manufacturers recommend 50 mg three times daily, taken at least 1 hour before meals.

SIDE-EFFECTS. GI irritation (common); vasodilatory and hypotensive effects such as intractable headache, dizziness, flushing, syncope, occasional angina pectoris ("coronary steal").

INDICATIONS. In **patients with prosthetic valves,** therapy by dipyridamole plus anticoagulation by warfarin is the only licensed indication on the basis of five trials showing that the combination is superior to placebo.[26] Dipyridamole dramatically increases the antithrombotic effect of aspirin on artificial surfaces,[1] hence the **combination of aspirin plus dipyridamole** makes most sense when dealing with prosthetic valves or prosthetic bypasses. The success of low-dose aspirin combined with warfarin[129] and the general results of meta-analysis[43] do, however, argue against combining of aspirin plus dipyradimole plus warfarin.

In **saphenous vein bypass grafts,** the large Goldman study[12] showed no better patency for the combination dipyridamole-aspirin than for aspirin.

In **peripheral vascular disease,** dipyridamole 75 mg plus aspirin 330 mg each three times daily limited the angiographic progress of the disease.[1] Aspirin alone was also effective but less so.

In **renal disease** (type 1 membranoproliferative glomerulonephritis), dipyridamole helps to prevent deterioration.[1]

In **threatened strokes** and **TIAs,** dipyridamole 75 mg three times daily with aspirin 325 mg three times daily improved survival and decreased both nonfatal and fatal strokes,[9] yet meta-analysis shows that the results are no better than those of aspirin alone.[43]

In **ischemic syndromes** such as angina pectoris, acute myocardial infarction, postinfarct follow-up, or TIAs or stroke, aspirin alone is appropriate for almost all these conditions. This conclusion is based on a comprehensive review of 145 trials on 70,000 "high-risk" patients.[43]

The only **specific indication** for dipyridamole is aspirin intolerance. In patients with prosthetic mechanical valves, dipyridamole may be added to aspirin and warfarin if thromboembolism persists.

DRUG INTERACTIONS. Because dipyradimole leads to accumulation of adenosine, the potential hypotensive effects of **adenosine** given intravenously for supraventricular tachycardia may become serious and the dose of adenosine must be reduced.

## Ticlopidine

This agent (**Ticlid**) irreversibly inhibits the transformation of the GPIIa/IIIb receptor to its active form. Hence it prevents fibrinogen-induced platelet-platelet interaction (Fig. 9–3).

PHARMACOKINETICS. Its kinetics are nonlinear, with a markedly decreased clearance with repeated dosing. Thus maximum inhibition of platelet aggregation takes 8 to 11 days of dosing (manufacturer's data).

CLINICAL STUDIES.  In the Canadian-American ticlopidine study[5] on 1,072 patients with recent thromboembolic stroke (74% with carotid or vertebrobasilar disease), ticlopidine in a dose of 250 mg twice daily reduced stroke, myocardial infarction, and vascular death, although disappointingly the overall death rate was unchanged.[5] In another large study,[122] ticlopidine was better than aspirin (650 mg twice daily) in TIA prevention. However, over 3 years of treatment plasma cholesterol increased by 9%. Ticlopidine can also be used to manage unstable angina,[1] to prevent vascular complications in intermittent claudication and to control diabetic retinopathy.[94]

INDICATIONS.  Ticlopidine is licensed as follows. It is indicated to reduce the risk of thrombotic stroke (fatal or nonfatal) in patients who have experienced stroke precursors, and in patients who have had a completed thrombotic stroke. Because ticlopidine is associated with a risk of neutropenia/agranulocytosis, which may be life-threatening, it should be reserved for patients who are intolerant of aspirin therapy where indicated to prevent stroke.[69] A standard dose is 250 mg twice daily taken with food.

SIDE-EFFECTS.  The major problem with ticlopidine lies in neutropenia (2.4%), the subject of a boxed warning in the package insert. There may also be minor bleeding (up to 10%), skin rash (up to 15%), liver toxicity (4%) and diarrhea (ticlopidine 22%, placebo 0%)—which are all, however, reversible.[94] The neutropenia occurs within the first 3 months of treatment.

ESSENTIAL PRECAUTION.  It is, therefore, essential that a complete blood count and white cell differential be performed every 2 weeks till the end of the third month (manufacturer's information).

META-ANALYSIS.  In the recent overview,[43] ticlopidine was not better than aspirin in the prevention of myocardial infarction, stroke, or vascular death. In a large primary prevention trial in women, aspirin failed to reduce the incidence of stroke.[98] Because of the severe side-effects of ticlopidine and the meta-analysis referred to, aspirin is still chosen even in females.

## Sulfinpyrazone

This agent (**Anturane**) also inhibits cyclo-oxygenase and has similar ultimate effects to those of aspirin, decreasing the production of prostacyclin and thromboxane $A_2$. In addition, it is a uricosuric agent. The mechanism of action on the cyclo-oxygenase is different from that of aspirin in that sulfinpyrazone competitively and reversibly *inhibits* the enzyme, whereas aspirin *inactivates* it, so that sulfinpyrazone is much weaker.[1] The critical questions are (1) whether sulfinpyrazone, which is more expensive and needs multiple daily doses, gives any added protection to patients already taking aspirin; and (2) whether sulfinpyrazone might be used as an alternative to aspirin. The answer to the first question is no, and to the second, yes.[43]

INDICATIONS.  In the USA, the only licensed **indication** is gouty arthritis, chronic or intermittent. In mitral stenosis, however, a prospective blinded study over 4 years showed that sulfinpyrazone (200 mg 4 times daily) decreased thromboembolism and reverted the shortened platelet survival time toward normal.[1]

DOSE.  That most commonly used, 800 mg/day in 4 doses, is "at the lower end of the dose-response curve and close to the maximum tolerable level."[1]

CONTRAINDICATIONS. These include peptic ulcer, renal impairment, and renal stones.[1] Early after AMI, sulfinpyrazone may cause temporary renal failure, so that the dose must be kept low.[1]

DRUG INTERACTIONS. Sulfinpyrazone, being highly bound (98% to 99%) to plasma proteins, may displace warfarin to precipitate bleeding. Sulfinpyrazone may potentiate the effects of sulfa drugs, sulfonylureas, and insulin.

COMMENT. Except in gout, when aspirin impairs urate excretion, aspirin is the preferred platelet-inhibitor, being effective in only one daily dose and having been much better tested.[43]

## Other Platelet Inhibitors

INDOMETHACIN. Besides inhibiting cyclo-oxygenase, indomethacin is an anti-inflammatory. Indomethacin is seldom used as a specific antiplatelet agent in patients with cardiovascular diseases, because it also inhibits the formation of vasodilatory prostaglandins. The vasoconstrictive action is likely to be worse in the presence of endothelial damage.[1] Thus indomethacin may (1) promote coronary vasoconstriction;[1] (2) attenuate the effects of antihypertensive agents such as beta-blockers and diuretics; and (3) cause clinical deterioration in patients with CHF and hyponatremia.[1]

THROMBOXANE SYNTHETASE INHIBITORS. These agents, under evaluation, have two important theoretical advantages: (1) they might divert precursors from formation of thromboxane to that of prostacyclin by the so-called "endoperoxide steal"; and (2) they specifically inhibit the formation of thromboxane yet not that of prostacyclin. The major problem is the short half-life of the effect on the synthetase.

THROMBOXANE RECEPTOR ANTAGONISTS. Also under evaluation, these agents should block the vasoconstrictory and pro-aggregatory effects of thromboxane.

NONSPECIFIC PLATELET INHIBITORS. These include beta-blockers, calcium antagonists, alpha-receptor antagonists, ketanserin, and nafazatrom.

ENDOTHELIAL INTEGRITY AND ACE INHIBITORS. Agents maintaining endothelial integrity have indirect antiplatelet effects. For example, during ACE inhibition increased formation of bradykinin is potentially protective. Such mechanisms may explain reduced reinfarction after prolonged therapy with ACE inhibitors. Heparin and aspirin, by their indirect platelet protective effects, can also be expected to maintain endothelial integrity.

ANTIBODY c7E3 AGAINST PLATELET IIb/IIIa RECEPTOR. This monoclonal antibody fragment is directed against the receptor mediating the final common pathway of platelet aggregation (Fig. 9–2). It helps to inhibit restenosis after revascularization[127] and is under test in unstable angina. The FDA has now approved c7E3 Fab for use in angioplasty in patients thought to be at high risk of ischemic complications.

## Acute Anticoagulation: Heparin

Anticoagulation, when given for an acute indication such as myocardial infarction, or acute venous thrombosis, or acute pulmonary embolism, is usually initiated by intravenous heparin given for 4 to 5 days while awaiting the effect of oral warfarin. Alternatively, in uncomplicated AMI, only heparin may be used till the patient is mobile.[1] Either heparin sodium or heparin calcium may be used. Heparin may be given by infusion, intermittent injection, or subcutaneously but not orally. In patients with bleeding disorders or in whom the effects of bleeding could be serious (subacute bacterial endocarditis, GI or genito-urinary lesions), ultralow-dose heparin should be considered.

## THROMBOSIS AND LYSIS

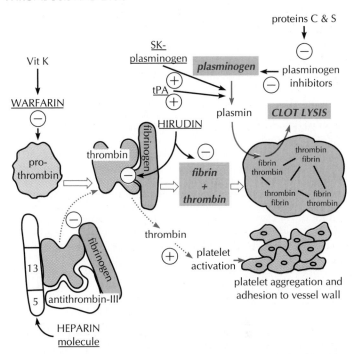

**FIGURE 9–5.** The coagulation cascade with sites of therapeutic attack. Crucial to the formation of the clot is the conversion of fibrinogen into fibrin and the binding of fibrin to thrombin, followed by crossbinding of fibrin. Antithrombin-III prevents the binding of Fibrinogen to thrombin, hence is an anticoagulant. Heparin promotes the activity of antithrombin-III. Once fibrin is thrombin-bound, heparin is not active, because antithrombin-III no longer interacts with thrombin. Thus, to break down the fibrin-thrombin combination requires fibrin-olytics such as tPA or streptokinase (SK). Warfarin works by inhibiting the production of prothrombin. PAI = plasminogen activator inhibitor; FDP = fibrin disintegration products. Fig. copyright L.H. Opie.

### Mechanism of Action of Heparin

Heparin is a heterogeneous mucopolysaccharide with extremely complex effects on the coagulation mechanism, and on blood vessels. Heparin also exerts direct antiplatelet effects by binding to and inhibiting the von Willebrand factor. Furthermore, chronic heparin administration has ill-understood effects in lessening experimental atheroma and in promoting angiogenesis.[115] *The major effect of heparin is interaction with antithrombin-III and thrombin.* Inhibition of thrombin by heparin requires (1) binding of heparin to antithrombin-III by a unique pentasaccharide segment of the heparin molecule, and (2) simultaneous binding of heparin to thrombin by thirteen additional saccharide units.[135] Heparin-antithrombin-III also inhibits factor Xa and a number of other clotting factors. Only about one-third of all the heparin molecules exert this important action. Heparin, therefore, inhibits the thrombin-induced platelet aggregation that initiates un-stable angina and venous thrombosis (Fig. 9–5). The dose-effect relationship is difficult to predict because heparin is a heterogeneous group of molecules extracted by a variety of procedures and having variable strength from batch to batch. Heparin also variably binds to plasma proteins, endothelial cells, and macrophages. The binding to these cells inactivates some of the heparin, the rest leaving the circulation by the renal route. These complexities, added to the difficulty of controlling the dose, mean that heparin is far from ideal as an intravenous anticoagulant and explain why fixed dose regimes are not optimal for serious disease.

## Administration

INTRAVENOUS HEPARIN.   The **standard intravenous schedule** for AMI or unstable angina is usually a 5,000 unit intravenous bolus, followed by 1,000 units/hour for 48 hours or more[80] with control of the dose by the activated partial thromboplastin time (next section). According to GUSTO-II, there must be no dose increase in patients over 80 kg. United States Pharmacopeia units may be about 10% to 15% more potent than the international units used in other countries. The heparin may be diluted either in isotonic saline or in dextrose water (which may be better in AMI). **Intermittent injection** may be preferred in AMI when it is crucial to avoid fluid overload; the schedule is 10,000 units given as an initial dose, followed by 5,000 to 10,000 units every 4 to 6 hours. **Ultralow-dose intravenous heparin** (1 unit/kg/h for 3 to 5 days, about 17,000 units/day) seems as effective as other methods in preventing postoperative deep vein thrombosis.

CONTROL OF THE DOSE OF INTRAVENOUS HEPARIN.   When heparin is given in AMI or unstable angina, meticulous laboratory control of the heparin dose is required (activated partial thromboplastin time or APTT of 1.5 to 2.5 times normal, up to 60 to 85 seconds with monitoring at 6, 12 and 24 hours).[80] Higher values incur the risk of cerebral bleeding.[81A] Patients with optimal heparinization and an APTT of twice normal have greater coronary artery patency than others.[45] As already emphasized, this method is far from ideal perhaps because of prolonged laboratory turn-around time. A new development is a bedside device that gives APTT within 3 minutes.[49] The APTT has an inherent limitation in that different commercial reagents give different APTT values.[135]

SUBCUTANEOUS HEPARIN.   This route is as good as others for the treatment of deep vein thrombosis unless it is proximal.[135] After the initial intravenous loading dose, heparin may be given as a deep subcutaneous injection 10,000 units 8-hourly or 15,000 12-hourly, using a different site at each rotation. The dose required is about 10% higher than with the intravenous route. Low-dose subcutaneous heparin is adequate in the **prophylaxis of surgical thromboembolism** where the schedule is 5,000 units subcutaneously 2 to 8 hours preoperation and every 12 hours for 7 days.[135]

## Heparin: Precautions and Side-effects

An increased danger of **heparin-induced hemorrhage** exists in patients with subacute bacterial endocarditis, hematological disorders including hemophilia, hepatic disease, and GI or genito-urinary ulcerative lesions. GUSTO-IIA and TIMI-9A found a *narrow therapeutic window* for heparin plus thrombolytic therapy.[81A,125A] To avoid intracerebral hemorrhage, the recommended doses of heparin should not be exceeded. Platelet plugs are the main hemostatic defence of heparinized patients, and the coadministration of aspirin, sulfinpyrazone, dipyridamole or indomethacin may predispose to bleeding, as may **heparin-induced thrombocytopenia,** which occurs in about 10% of patients after heparin for 5 days or more[1] and is usually reversible upon heparin withdrawal. Usually the thrombocytopenia is asymptomatic. If not, and if acute anticoagulation is essential, a heparinoid (p 262) may be used. Platelet abnormalities may also, paradoxically, predispose to **heparin thrombosis** characterized by a "white clot."[86] **Heparin hemorrhage** may occur in clinically inapparent sites such as the adrenal glands, which is potentially life-threatening and demands immediate cortisol replacement. Some patients have **heparin resistance,** and high-dose heparin with APTT monitoring every 4 hours is advised. Heparin is derived from animal tissue and occasionally causes **allergy;** a trial dose of 100 to 1,000 units is required in allergic patients.

**Heparin overdosage** is treated by stopping the drug and, if clinically required, giving **protamine sulfate** (1% solution) as a very slow infusion at no more than 50 mg in any 10-minute period.

## Indications for Heparin

ACUTE MYOCARDIAL INFARCTION. The urgent use of prophylactic heparin as an **intravenous bolus** (5,000 units) followed by an infusion (1,000 units/hour) is logical during thrombolysis by tPA. Heparin is often used to initiate protection against venous thrombosis, possibly to help prevent further coronary artery thrombosis, and to prevent mural thrombosis and systemic embolism. Heparin, continued for at least 48 hours, is essential with tPA to prevent reocclusion.[80] Intravenous heparin is required in a lower dose when thus used than in unstable angina for which thrombolysis is not recommended. *With streptokinase, concurrent heparin seems not to be necessary for the effects of this fibrinolytic agent.*[135] When tPA is not used and when heparin is chosen, the dose schedules are not clear. In uncomplicated infarcts, where heparin is given chiefly against the development of deep vein thrombosis, there is no need for repetitive checks of the APTT and a fixed dose regime could be considered.

In patients with borderline heart failure, sodium loading can be avoided by the use of **calcium heparin (Calciparine,** 5,000 to 20,000 USP units/ampoule) and by diluting heparin in dextrose water rather than in saline. Heparin is usually given until the patient is mobile, or until oral anticoagulants take effect. In uncomplicated AMI, the present trend is to give only heparin.

HEPARIN IN UNSTABLE ANGINA. Dose-adjusted heparin is highly effective (and better than aspirin) in preventing myocardial infarction[124] and in decreasing anginal pain and electrocardiographic features of ischemia.[22] An intravenous bolus of 5,000 units is followed by an infusion of 1,000 units per hour[124] and after 6 hours the dose is adjusted to an APTT of 1.5 to 2.5 times baseline.[124] An average dose is 32,000 units per 24 hours.[135] Fixed bolus injections of heparin are ineffective.[22] The heparin is continued for 5 to 6 days. Stopping heparin without aspirin exposes the patient to risk of rebound of unstable angina.[123] Aspirin 160 to 325 mg is started at the onset in nonprior users.[47]

Logically, because heparin and aspirin have different and additive antithrombotic mechanisms, the combination should be better than either agent alone in unstable angina. This simple supposition has been difficult to prove and more trials are needed.[74]

HEPARIN IN CORONARY ANGIOPLASTY. High doses of heparin may prevent acute thrombotic closure; the combination with aspirin is often used.

PROXIMAL VENOUS THROMBOSIS. High-dose continuous intravenous heparin, adjusted to the APTT is required for 5 to 6 days while oral warfarin is started.[85] Thrombolytic therapy is not needed.[102A]

TREATMENT OF VENOUS THROMBOEMBOLISM. Three routines are possible: intravenous infusion, intermittent intravenous infusion, and the subcutaneous route. These all seem comparable.[135] Doses are, after an initial intravenous bolus of 5,000 units, (1) 32,000 units per 24 hours by continuous infusion or (2) 17,500 units subcutaneously every 12 hours, both adjusted by APTT.

PREVENTION OF VENOUS THROMBOEMBOLISM. Subcutaneous heparin is adequate.

PREGNANCY ANTICOAGULATION. Heparin is the anticoagulant of choice in pregnancy (Table 11–8). Yet if given in doses greater than 20,000 units daily for more than 5 months, it can cause osteoporosis.[135]

## Low Molecular Weight Heparins (LMW)

These constitute about one-third of the molecular weight of heparin and are also heterogeneous in size. Approximately 25% to 30%

of the molecules of various preparations contain the crucial 18 or more saccharide units to bind to both antithrombin-III and thrombin (Fig. 9–5). The remaining molecules of LMW heparin bind only to factor Xa. LMW heparins, still under evaluation, have better bioavailability and a longer plasma half-life than standard heparin. They need only be given subcutaneously in a fixed dose and once daily. They are as effective as standard APTT-monitored heparin when given intravenously.[85] At present they are the agents of choice when heparin is contraindicated, but the disadvantage is expense.[113] Yet, time of skilled personnel is saved by having to avoid APTT tests, dose adjustments, and an intravenous infusion. In future, the convenience and simplicity of administration will probably make these popular agents, especially if the price decreases.

**Heparinoids** are similar in properties to LMW heparin but consist chiefly (80%) of **heparan** sulfate. One preparation, **Organan,** does not immunologically cross-react with heparin. It can, therefore, be used for **heparin-induced thrombocytopenia.**

### Specific Antithrombins

Under test are several agents of which the prototype is **hirudin,** which is a leech peptide now synthesized as recombinant hirudin, with a molecular sequence similar to that of the catalytic site of the thrombin receptor on platlets and on smooth muscle cells. *Hirudin binds directly with high affinity to several sites on thrombin and can inactivate thrombin already bound to fibrin (clot-bound thrombin) which heparin cannot do.*[73] Hirudin does not require endogenous cofactors such as antithrombin III for its activity. Also, unlike heparin, hirudin can inhibit thrombin-induced platelet aggregation.[128] Finally, again unlike heparin, hirudin does not interact with platelets nor the vascular endothelium to cause hemorrhage in that way. Intracranial or other hemorrhage has been a serious side-effect in three trials,[81A,84,125A] so that the hirudin dose has been reduced to 0.1 mg/kg bolus followed by 0.1 mg/kg/h. Related compounds are **hirulog,**[126] **hirugen,** and **argatroban.**[132] New molecular techniques have led to agents that inhibit activated factor X. Another approach is to activate **protein-C** (Fig. 9–1). The latter when activated is a powerful antithrombotic which destroys activated factors V and VIII; the possibility of infusing activated protein-C is now being explored.

## Oral Anticoagulation: Warfarin

Warfarin ( = **Coumarin; Coumadin; Panwarfin**) is the most commonly used oral anticoagulant, because a single dose causes a stable anticoagulation as a result of the excellent oral absorption and a circulating half-life of about 37 hours; warfarin also has remarkably few side-effects apart from bleeding. Drug interactions are many.

MECHANISM OF ACTION.   As a group, the oral anticoagulants inactivate vitamin-K in hepatic microsomes, thereby interfering with the formation of vitamin-K-dependent clotting factors including prothrombin (Fig. 9–5). There is a delay in onset of action of 2 to 7 days.[135]

PHARMACOKINETICS.   Oral warfarin, after rapid and complete absorption, is almost totally bound to plasma albumin with a half-life of 37 hours. It is metabolized in the hepatic microsomes to inactive metabolites excreted in urine and stool.

DOSE.   A standard procedure is to give warfarin 5 mg/day for 5 days, checking the prothrombin time daily until it is in the therapeutic range, and then to check it at three times weekly for up to 2 weeks. Avoiding a large primary dose may avoid an excess fall of prothrombin and may decrease the risk of skin necrosis. When an urgent effect is required, an initial loading dose of warfarin 10 to 15 mg daily is used. Patients with heart failure or liver disease require lower doses. The maintenance dose, although often 4 to 5 mg daily, may vary from 1 to 20 mg daily. This wide range means that doses must be individualized according to the INR (next section).

INR VERSUS PROTHROMBIN TIME. The effect of warfarin is monitored by reporting the INR (International Normalized Ratio) which is the prothrombin time that would be obtained if international reference thromboplastin, as approved by the World Health Organization, were used. This thromboplastin has an International Sensitivity Index (ISI) of 1. Although the INR is far more accurate than the prothrombin ratio,[65] in the USA the INR is not yet used as widely as it should. Up to one-third of laboratories cannot give data on the standardization of thromboplastin. Yet to interpret the prothrombin time accurately requires a knowledge of the ISI (see Table 4, Hirsh and Fuster[136]). *The results of these inaccuracies can be a major loss of the efficacy of warfarin.*[65] Currently, two levels of intensity of warfarin therapy are recommended: a medium dose with an INR of 2.0 to 3.0 and a higher dose with an INR of 2.5 to 3.5.[136] Prosthetic heart valves require the greatest possible intensity of safe anticoagulation and the INR is at the top end of the medium range, i.e., about 3.0 (corresponding roughly to a prothrombin ratio of 1.5). Less intense anticoagulation is appropriate with an INR of 2.0 to 3.0 or a prothrombin ratio of about 1.3 to 1.5 for for deep vein thrombosis with pulmonary embolism, AMI in the early stages or with risk of thromboembolism, and for patients with thromboembolism thought to be at high risk of stroke. In patients with atrial fibrillation without valvular heart disease, the lower limits are an INR of only 1.5 and a prothrombin ratio of about 1.2.[119] These are only approximate rules, but the current tendency is to reduce the intensity of anticoagulation required. The modest loss of efficacy is balanced by the lesser risk of serious bleeding. Once the steady-state warfarin requirement is known, the INR is checked only once every 4 to 6 weeks.

DOSE REDUCTION. This is required in the presence of CHF, liver damage from any source (alcohol, malnutrition), and renal impairment (which increases the fraction of free drug in the plasma). Thyrotoxicosis enhances the catabolism of vitamin-K to decrease the dose of warfarin needed, whereas myxedema has the opposite effect. In the elderly, the dose is decreased because the response to warfarin becomes better as age increases. A high intake of dietary **vitamin-K** (green salads) reduces warfarin effectiveness. Some fad diets alternate high and low salad periods which causes INR control to vascillate.

DRUG INTERACTIONS WITH WARFARIN. Warfarin may be subject to approximately 80 drug interactions.[1] **Inhibitory interactions** include drugs such as cholestyramine that reduce absorption of vitamin-K or of warfarin, and drugs such as barbiturates or phenytoin that accelerate warfarin degradation in the liver. **Potentiating drugs** include the cardiovascular agents allopurinol, quinidine,[1] and amiodarone.[1] Drugs that decrease warfarin degradation and increase the anticoagulant effect include a variety of antibiotics such as metronidazole (**Flagyl**), co-trimoxazole (**Bactrim**), and also the antiulcer agent, cimetidine.

Antiplatelet drugs such as aspirin may potentiate the risk of bleeding with a big interindividual variation. Very high doses of aspirin (6 to 8 tablets/day) impair the synthesis of clotting factors. In contrast, a low-dose combination (aspirin 80 mg and warfarin 3 mg daily) is often safe.[55A] Sulfinpyrazone powerfully displaces warfarin from blood proteins, to reduce the dose of warfarin required down to 1 mg in some patients.[1] *The safest rule is to tell patients on oral anticoagulation not to take any over-the-counter drugs without consultation, and for the physician to checklist any new drug used.* If in doubt, more frequent measurements of the INR are required.

CONTRAINDICATIONS. These include recent stroke, uncontrolled hypertension, hepatic cirrhosis, and potential GI and genito-urinary bleeding points such as hiatus hernia, peptic ulcer, gastritis, colitis, proctitis, and cystitis.[1] If anticoagulation is deemed essential, the risk-to-benefit ratio must be evaluated carefully. Old age is not in itself a contraindication to anticoagulation, although the elderly are more likely to bleed.[13] In **pregnancy,** warfarin is contraindicated in the first trimester (tetragenic) and also in the last (risk of fetal bleeding); category X; consider chronic subcutaneous heparin for valve prophylaxis.[1]

ELDERLY PATIENTS. Age in itself is not a contraindication to warfarin,[1] but brings with it a greater risk of various conditions predisposing to bleeding. For example, there is a higher INR for the same warfarin dose.[71] Because of potential compliance problems and the risk of accidental falling or cerebrovascular accident or other co-morbid conditions, warfarin is often not given in the elderly.

WARFARIN-ASSOCIATED SKIN NECROSIS. The cause of this rare but potentially serious skin condition is ill-understood. It may occur on the third to eighth day of therapy.[136] A **protein-C deficiency** may predispose[1] especially when high-dose warfarin is initiated after cardiopulmonary bypass (which lowers protein-C).

PRO-COAGULATORY EFFECT AFTER CARDIAC SURGERY. Occasionally warfarin promotes thrombosis supposedly by inhibiting protein-C, which is also the proposed explanation for skin necrosis. Hence, warfarin should be started in very low doses under heparin cover after cardiac surgery.

WARFARIN OVERDOSE. Excess hypoprothrombinemia without bleeding or with only minor bleeding can be remedied by dose reduction or discontinuation. The risk of bleeding is decreased dramatically by lowering the intended INR from 3.0 to 4.5 down to 2.0 to 3.0, which generally can be achieved by reducing warfarin by only 1 mg daily.[136] If bleeding becomes significant, oral or subcutaneous **vitamin-K$_1$** 2 to 5 mg may be required. In patients with prosthetic valves, vitamin-K should be strictly avoided because of the risk of valve thrombosis, unless there is a life-threatening intracranial bleed. In patients unresponsive to vitamin-K, the order of choice is: (1) a concentrate of the prothrombin group of coagulation factors including II, IX and X; (2) fresh frozen plasma 15 ml/kg; and (3) fresh, whole blood transfusion.

## AMI and Pulmonary Embolism: Indications for Warfarin

ACUTE MYOCARDIAL INFARCTION. The use of full-dose intravenous heparin followed by oral anticoagulant therapy has become standard during the hospital phase of myocardial infarction, provided that relative or absolute contraindications are absent. Nonetheless, in uncomplicated or smaller infarcts, warfarin is often omitted. Oral anticoagulation should be started 4 to 5 days before heparin therapy is discontinued.

EARLY POSTINFARCT ANTICOAGULATION. Accumulating evidence[136] suggests that within the first 3 to 6 months, mural thrombosis and the subsequent incidence of systemic thromboembolism is more frequent in patients with large anterior Q-wave infarctions, apical dyskinetic areas identifiable echocardiographically (even before any intraventricular thrombus is present), severe left ventricular (LV) dysfunction, congestive heart failure, and atrial fibrillation. Furthermore, the likelihood of systemic thromboembolism is greatest in the first 3 months post-discharge. Good evidence supports the use of oral warfarin for a 3 to 6 month period in these specific postinfarct patients, especially those with mural thrombosis,[130] aiming at an INR of 2.0 to 3.0.

PROLONGED ORAL ANTICOAGULATION. Chronic postinfarct therapy, previously given for years, has now lost its popularity. Three separate studies in patients with mean ages of 61 to 68 years[1,40,46] show that warfarin can reduce recurrent MI and cerebral vascular events, the risk of cerebral hemorrhage being outweighed by the benefit of reduced ischemic stroke.[52] Conceivably the benefit of an equal advantage would have been found with aspirin alone.[74]

POSTINFARCT ANTICOAGULATION VERSUS ASPIRIN. Aspirin and oral anticoagulation are associated with an almost identical total mortality with, however, different side-effects.[1] The incidence of bleeding was 6 times higher in the anticoagulant group and the GI problems 5 times higher in the aspirin group (500 mg three times daily). For a prolonged antithrombotic effect postinfarct, aspirin is much simpler and is recommended by the FDA. A standard dose would now be 160 to 325 mg daily[52] or even lower, down to 75 mg daily.[43] Two ongoing trials are assessing the effects of long-term low-dose warfarin.[52] The CARS study compares aspirin 160 mg daily with aspirin 80 mg plus warfarin 3 mg daily and with aspirin 80 mg plus warfarin 1 mg daily.[55A] The CHAMP study compared low-intensity warfarin (INR 1.5 to 2.5) plus aspirin 80 mg daily with aspirin 160 mg daily, using as end-points the incidence of reinfarction. *At present we do not advise routine postinfarct oral anticoagulation, but rather a careful evaluation of the needs of each individual patient,* with preference for aspirin started as soon as possible after the onset of myocardial ischemia and continued indefinitely unless there are clear contraindications. Warfarin is chosen for patients at high risk of systemic embolization because of atrial fibrillation, CHF, or mobile mural thrombus.

UNSTABLE ANGINA AT REST. *Oral anticoagulation is generally not undertaken* especially because such patients may come to coronary artery surgery or balloon angioplasty. In patients with severe repetitive attacks of **variant angina,** there is a risk of secondary coronary thrombosis following coronary spasm, and oral anticoagulation is logical although unproven. In others, low-dose aspirin remains the pragmatic albeit unproven approach to the prevention of spasm-induced platelet stasis and thrombosis.

WARFARIN FOR VENOUS THROMBOEMBOLISM. In deep venous thrombosis, warfarin is initiated concurrently with intravenous heparin, the latter for 4 to 5 days as standard therapy for acute episodes. Thereafter, oral anticoagulation alone is continued for at least 3 months.[16] A less intense regime (INR 2 to 3) is effective and safer than a more intense regime (INR 3.0 to 4.5).[135] In patients with recurrent venous thrombosis or with risk factors such as antithrombin-III deficiency, protein-C or S deficiency, or malignancy, indefinite treatment should be considered.

For objectively documented **pulmonary embolism,** heparin followed by oral warfarin is used as for deep vein thrombosis. Warfarin is continued for approximately 6 months in the absence of recurrences; when the latter occur, indefinite therapy is considered.

## Atrial Fibrillation: Indications for Warfarin

Atrial fibrillation in the presence of heart disease is strongly associated with thromboembolism.[1] The two logical steps are cardioversion (if possible) and anticoagulation. In general, the benefits of warfarin far exceed the risk of hemorrhage.[55] The only clear indications for withholding warfarin are (1) lone atrial fibrillation in younger patients and (2) a bleeding diathesis. **Cardioversion** in patients with atrial fibrillation increases the risk of an embolus. After 3 days of atrial fibrillation, anticoagulation for 3 weeks is strongly recommended (if feasible) prior to elective cardioversion, followed by another 2 to 4 weeks thereafter.[106] Postcardioversion quinidine has been replaced by amiodarone or sotalol (Chapter 8). For urgent cardioversion, intravenous heparin is used as cover followed by warfarin (exception: not for atrial flutter.[60] For policy thereafter, see Table 11–3.

MITRAL STENOSIS OR REGURGITATION. In patients with mitral valve disease, the risk of thromboembolism is greatest in those with atrial fibrillation, marked left atrial enlargement, and previous embolic episodes. Anticoagulation is strongly indicated in this setting. In contrast, in patients with mitral stenosis with sinus rhythm, anticoagulation is usually reserved for secondary prevention after the first episode of systemic embolism.[1] An argument can be made for earlier anticoagulation if the left atrium is dilated.

HYPERTENSIVE HEART DISEASE. This condition is a suggested indication for anticoagulation only if there is marked left atrial or LV enlargement, or in the presence of atrial fibrillation. Uncontrolled hypertension (systolic blood pressure greater than 160 mmHg) is usually a contraindication, although there are no good data defining the "safe" blood pressure levels.

ISCHEMIC HEART DISEASE. In the presence of good LV function, atrial fibrillation is an unsettled indication for anticoagulation. LV failure strengthens the argument for anticoagulation.[1] Chronic LV aneurysm of itself with sinus rhythm is not an indication for oral anticoagulation.[1]

DILATED CARDIOMYOPATHY. There is a substantial risk of systemic embolism, particularly if there is atrial fibrillation; anticoagulants effectively reduce thromboembolism.[1]

THE TACHYCARDIA/BRADYCARDIA SYNDROME. This condition may be complicated by atrial fibrillation and thromboembolism. Anticoagulation may require consideration, especially if there is underlying organic heart disease (ischemic heart disease, hypertension, cardiomyopathy). Yet the evidence is unproven.

ATRIAL SEPTAL DEFECTS. In older patients with atrial septal defects and pulmonary hypertension, anticoagulation is strongly recommended as prophylaxis against in situ pulmonary arterial thromboses or, rarely, paradoxical emboli. Anticoagulation is also required for those with repaired septal defects who later develop atrial fibrillation.

THYROTOXIC HEART DISEASE. In patients with atrial fibrillation and thyrotoxicosis, the first aim is to render the patient euthyroid which reverts the atrial fibrillation in the majority.[8] In the others, cardioversion should be performed at about the 16th week after the patient becomes euthyroid. Anticoagulation cover is required and should be maintained for 4 weeks after the conversion.[8]

INTERMITTENT ATRIAL FIBRILLATION. When this lasts a few hours, the choices vary from no treatment in lone atrial fibrillation (next paragraph) to warfarin in elderly patients thought to be at higher risk.

"LONE" ATRIAL FIBRILLATION. In the absence of any other cardiac or precipitating condition, including thyrotoxicosis, atrial fibrillation may be rare.[1] In patients younger than 60 years and without hypertension, the risk of thromboembolism is no greater than that in any age- and sex-matched population, so that the morbidity of anticoagulant therapy outweighs the potential advantages.[19] Elderly patients with "lone" atrial fibrillation have a somewhat increased risk of TIAs or stroke without any increased mortality or risk of AMI, so that anticoagulation or aspirin needs consideration.[20]

PATIENTS PRESENTING WITH ATRIAL FIBRILLATION AND ACUTE EMBOLIC STROKE. Although anticoagulation is required, cerebral hemorrhage must first be excluded by computed tomography which, in the case of large strokes, must be delayed for about 1 week for full evolution to occur.[53]

ATRIAL FIBRILLATION—CONCLUSIONS. Of the above groups, those with a history of hypertension, ischemic heart disease, or CHF make up the vast majority of patients with chronic **nonvalvular atrial fibrillation.** There are now strong arguments especially in "high-risk patients" favoring low-intensity anticoagulation based on six controlled studies.[48,55,64] Risk stratification allows triage with warfarin for high-risk and aspirin for low-risk patients. Besides age (> 65 years), there are four other risk factors: a history of hypertension, diabetes, CHF, and previous stroke or TIA.[48] Patients with a recent TIA or minor stroke are at particularly high risk of recurrence.[64] Warfarin is much better than aspirin in reducing stroke in high risk patients. Only when the risk of bleeding is six times greater than average is anticoagulation justifiably withheld in such patients.

## Prosthetic Heart Valves: Use of Warfarin

In patients with **mechanical prosthetic heart valves,** warfarin is standard and the recommended INR is 2.5 to 3.5.[136] This is lower than the previously proposed range and it is given in the hope that benefit may be retained with less risk of bleeding.[30] Adding an antiplatelet agent to warfarin is logical. Thus, good results have been obtained with added aspirin 100 mg and an INR of close to 3.0.[129] Dipyridamole 400 mg daily may be chosen if aspirin is contraindicated or if further therapy is required, for example with continued emboli despite aspirin plus warfarin. In children or in others in whom warfarin is difficult to manage, aspirin is a reasonable alternative.[1] In patients with **bioprosthetic mitral valves,** the risk of thromboembolism is highest in the first three postoperative months when warfarin is required. Thereafter aspirin may be a reasonable alternative to warfarin.[136] Arguments for continued warfarin are strong when mitral bioprosthetic valves are combined with atrial fibrillation or a large left atrium or LV failure (Table 9–1). In patients with relative contraindications to warfarin or platelet inhibitors, those with a history of thromboembolism, marked left atrial enlargement, or atrial fibrillation are most in need of treatment. In **bioprosthetic aortic valves,** the risk is particularly low, so that aspirin for only 3 months is appropriate.[136]

## Marginal or Possible Indications for Warfarin

CEREBROVASCULAR ACCIDENT AND TRANSIENT ISCHEMIC ATTACKS (TIAs). Anticoagulation remains a source of fierce debate. Certainly in patients who have had a complete stroke, there is no evidence to support anticoagulation. When atrial fibrillation presents with an acute stroke, warfarin is indicated if cerebral hemorrhage is excluded by computed tomography.[53] In patients with recent TIAs (who do not undergo carotid surgery), aspirin 325 mg daily is recommended rather than anticoagulation.[69] In those intolerant of aspirin, ticlopidine is the next choice, with no evidence for dipyridamole or sulfinpyrazone.[69] Warfarin is only recommended when symptoms persist despite aspirin or when there is a major cardiac source for embolism.[69] **Suloctidil** is hepatotoxic.

PRIMARY PULMONARY HYPERTENSION. This entity includes a variety of histologic appearances and, probably, pathogenic mechanisms. Diffuse pulmonary thromboembolism or pulmonary arteriolar thrombosis call for anticoagulation. When the pathogenesis cannot be established, long-term anticoagulation is usually chosen.

MITRAL VALVE PROLAPSE. In patients with marked mitral valve prolapse and suggestive evidence of thrombotic or thromboembolic events, there might be an indication for warfarin or platelet inhibitors but this remains a moot issue.

## Oral Anticoagulants—Summary

In AMI, anticoagulants during the hospital phase are now standard, although many centers give only heparin, limited to the dura-

**TABLE 9–1**    **ANTITHROMBOTIC THERAPY FOR PROSTHETIC HEART VALVES: CURRENT RECOMMENDATIONS**

| VALVE | SITUATION | THERAPY |
|---|---|---|
| Mechanical | Routine | Warfarin* medium intensity + ASA |
| | ASA contraindicated | Warfarin + D 400 mg/day |
| | Problems such as bleeding | 1. Low-dose warfarin + ASA 80 mg/day or D 400 mg/day<br>2. D + ASA |
| | Recurrent embolism | Consider reoperation |
| Bioprosthetic | AVR routine | SC heparin for 7–10 days, then ASA for 3 months or longer |
| | MVR routine | SC heparin, then warfarin (INR 2.0–3.0) + ASA for 3 months, thereafter only ASA |
| | AF, LA thrombus, thromboembolism | Warfarin (INR 2.0–3.0) long-term |
| | Previous thromboembolism | High intensity warfarin + ASA |

AF = atrial fibrillation; ASA = aspirin 80 to 160 mg daily; AVR = aortic valve replacement; MVR = mitral valve replacement; D = dipyridamole; LA = left atrium; Sulf = sulfinpyrazone; SC = subcutaneous

Based on Turpie et al.,[129] Israel et al.[89] and Hirsh and Fuster.[136]

* Cannegieter et al.[54] suggest no ASA but only warfarin; Turpie et al.[129] suggest added ASA.

tion of bed rest, for uncomplicated AMI. Only a minority of patients qualify for limited anticoagulation for 3 to 6 months. Only a very few require prolonged anticoagulation, although this may change when the results of present trials with low-intensity postinfarct anticoagulation become available. Oral anticoagulants are frequently used to prevent systemic embolism especially in selected patients with atrial fibrillation and those with prosthetic heart valves or dilated cardiomyopathy. They are used both in the treatment and prevention of venous thrombosis and pulmonary embolism. Long-term anticoagulation requires a careful consideration of the risk-to-benefit ratio for the individual patient. For example, while benefit could well be achieved in a patient with chronic atrial fibrillation by meticulous anticoagulation, in a relatively noncompliant patient or in a patient with a vigorous physical lifestyle, it may be safer to use aspirin.

## Fibrinolytic (Thrombolytic) Therapy

*"The focus of the debate should shift toward the more rapid administration of a thrombolytic agent and away from the relative merits of one agent over another."*[134]

The present goal is "early patency, increased myocardial salvage, preserved LV function and lower mortality."[134] Besides better salvage, a patent infarct-related artery also improves remodeling and enhances electrical stability. Increased patency at 90 minutes can be translated into a mortality reduction at 30 days.[81] From these facts it follows that *the major aim is to achieve early reperfusion with a short "symptom-to-needle" and "door-to-needle" time in patients with suspected*

TABLE 9–2    COMPARATIVE DRUGS IN ISCHEMIC SYNDROMES

| DRUG THERAPY | EFFORT ANGINA | UNSTABLE ANGINA | AMI (EARLY) | AMI FOLLOW-UP |
|---|---|---|---|---|
| *Antithrombotics* | | | | |
| Aspirin | + + | + + | + + | + + |
| Heparin | 0 | + + | with tPA | 0 |
| Thrombolytics | 0 | 0 | + + | 0 |
| Warfarin | 0 | 0 | some | some |
| *Anti-ischemics* | | | | |
| Beta-blockers | + + | + + | + + | + + |
| Calcium antagonists | + + | ( + )* | 0 | ( + )* |
| Nitrates, IV | 0 | + + | + | 0 |
| Nitrates, oral | + + | + | + | 0 |

+ + = strongly indicated in view of editor (LH Opie); + = indicated; 0 = not indicated; * = non-DHPs; if no LV failure for follow-up; IV = intravenous.

*AMI and ST-elevation or bundle branch block.*[42,70] The principle of modern fibrinolytic therapy is the use of agents such as tPA and streptokinase which convert plasminogen into active plasmin (Fig. 9–6). Because thrombolytic agents simultaneously exert clot-dissolving and procoagulant actions and have significant serious side-effects, they must not be used in unstable angina where there is no benefit (Table 9–2).[125]

ULTRA-EARLY REPERFUSION (0 TO 1 HOUR OR SOON THEREAFTER). During the "golden" first hour, dramatic reductions in mortality can be obtained (Fig. 9–7). In two studies, such early reperfusion was achieved either by rushing the paramedical team to the patient or by streamlining the admission to hospital. In the MITI trial,[100] tPA and aspirin were started as soon as possible either at home or in hospital. Reperfusion within 70 minutes decreased the early death rate from 8.7% to 1.2%, while infarct size fell from 11.2% to 4.9%, when compared with a longer delay time up to 180 minutes. In the second study, similar mortality data were obtained with anistreplase given at a mean time of 60 minutes from onset of symptoms.[96]

EARLY REPERFUSION (2 TO 3 HOURS FROM ONSET). In the GUSTO trial,[80] there was no placebo group, but comparison with the expected mortality shows a 50% reduction in mortality for tPA plus aspirin plus heparin, with a mean start of reperfusion at 165 minutes.[81] There was nearly as good a result for streptokinase plus aspirin plus subcutaneous heparin. In those given tPA within 90 minutes, patency of the occluded artery was achieved in 81%, and the mortality was lowest in those with complete patency.[81] Improvements in indices of LV function also paralleled the degree of patency achieved.

INTERMEDIATE DELAY (4 TO 6 HOURS). Here the only data are on the early GISSI-1 and ISIS-2 studies when streptokinase was given without aspirin, and the reduction in mortality was about 22%.[134] Streptokinase plus aspirin or tPA plus aspirin plus heparin would presumably have done even better.

LATE INTERVENTION (7 TO 12 HOURS). Several studies with streptokinase show a modest reduction in mortality of about 12% and one study with tPA shows a reduction of about twice that of streptokinase. As there are no strict comparative studies over this timespan, all that can be said with confidence is that the benefit is less than when the agents are given earlier (Fig. 9–7).

VERY LATE REPERFUSION (13 TO 24 HOURS). Several large studies have failed to show any significant benefit on early mortality from reperfu-

THROMBOLYTICS AND PLASMIN

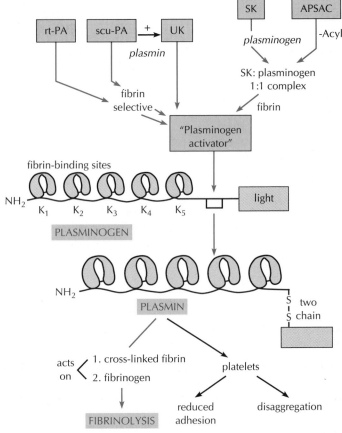

**FIGURE 9–6.** Basically thrombolytics act by promoting the conversion of plasminogen to plasmin, the latter being fibrinolytic. "Plasminogen activator" refers to the effects of tPA or streptokinase—plasminogen complex in catalyzing the conversion of plasminogen to plasmin. For abbreviations of fibrinolytics, see Table 9–3. Fig. modified from Reference 1.

sion at this time interval.[67,95] In a meta-analysis of 58,600 patients, late reperfusion appeared to be slightly beneficial without reaching statistical significance.[70] Yet, even later reperfusion could have other benefits according to the "open artery" hypothesis.

THE "OPEN ARTERY" HYPOTHESIS. The evidence for the benefits of early patency is now overwhelming.[50] The further proposal is that a patent reperfused artery, even if achieved days or possibly even weeks after AMI, confers protection of a different nature from that achieved by early thrombolytic salvage of the ischemic myocardium.[92] The benefits may include improved LV remodeling with a smaller LV cavity[84] and less electrical instability. Because patency by thrombolytic therapy becomes unlikely after 12 to 24 hours, revascularization by angioplasty or surgery theoretically becomes more appropriate. This hypothesis should now be tested by a prospective randomized trial.

## Which Thrombolytic?

Using early patency of the infarct-related artery as an end-point, randomized trials have shown that tPA was distinctly superior to streptokinase.[34,38] Likewise, pro-urokinase led to more rapid reperfusion and fewer bleeding complications than did intravenous streptokinase.[28] Such differences in early arterial patency have now been

**TABLE 9–3**     CHARACTERISTICS OF THROMBOLYTIC AGENTS

|  | RTPA | SK | APSAC | SCU-PA | UK |
|---|---|---|---|---|---|
| Fibrin selective | Yes | No | No | Yes | No |
| Plasminogen binding | Direct | Indirect | Indirect | Direct | Direct |
| Duration of infusion (min) | 180 | 60 | 2–5 | 90–180 | 5–15 |
| Half-life (min) | 8 | 23 | 90 | 7 | 16 |
| Fibrinogen breakdown | 1–2+ | 4+ | 3+ | 2+ | 3+ |
| Early heparin | Yes | No | No | ?No | ?No |
| Hypotension | No | Yes | Yes | No | No |
| Allergic reactions | No | Yes | Yes | No | No |
| Approximate cost/dose | $2300/ 100 mg | $300/ 1.5 MU | $1200/ 30 mg | High | $2200/ 3 MU |
| Patency at 90 min | 81[1]–88[2] (75)[7] | 53[3]–65[4] (53)[7] | 55[3]–65[5] | 71[4] | 66[6] |
| Patency at 2–3 hours | 73[8]–76[1] | 70[8]–73[1] | | | |
| Patency at 24 hours | 78[6]–85 | 81[3]–88[4] | 88[3]–92[5] | 85[4] | 73[6] |

Abbreviations: APSAC = anisoylated plasminogen streptokinase activator complex = anistreplase; MU = million units; scu-PA = single chain urokinase (prourokinase) plasminogen activator; SK = streptokinase; tPA = tissue plasminogen activator; UK = urokinase.

1 = GUSTO Angiographic Investigators[81]
2 = Purvis et al.[107]
3 = Hogg et al.[15]
4 = PRIMI Trial Study Group[28]
5 = Pacouret et al.[24]
6 = Neuhaus et al.[23]
7 = Mean value of 11 trials for streptokinase and 13 for tPA[7]
8 = Granger et al.[77]
For other data sources, see Marder and Sherry[1]

translated into a reduction of mortality in the GUSTO trial.[81] Now it is only the far greater expense of tPA (Table 9–3), the consistently greater risk of hemorrhagic stroke, and the need for dose-adjusted heparin that restrain the widespread preferential use of tPA. Hence, there are still situations when streptokinase is preferred,[73] such as hypertensive females in whom cerebral hemorrhage is less with streptokinase.[118]

Because tPA can reperfuse nearly 30 minutes earlier than streptokinase, the shorter the "symptom-to-needle" time, the more likely tPA will show a benefit above streptokinase. Long-term follow-up of GUSTO patients shows that the benefits of tPA became especially evident in non-anterior infarcts, showing a very delayed benefit of early reperfusion in this group.

### Tissue-Type Plasminogen Activator (tPA) = alteplase (Activase)

Tissue plasminogen activator (tPA) is a naturally occurring enzyme that binds to fibrin with a greater affinity than does streptokinase or urokinase; once bound it starts to convert plasminogen to plasmin on the fibrin surface. Hence, it is "clot-selective," though in clinical doses some systemic effects do occur. The dose of tPA required to produce nearly complete clot lysis (85%) can also produce some delayed bleeding. The very short half-life (Table 9–3) mandates cotherapy with intravenous heparin to avoid reocclusion.

INDICATIONS. Besides AMI, indications are pulmonary embolism, thrombosed arteriovenous shunts, and thrombosed St Jude valves.[117] Unstable angina is clearly not an indication.[22,125] Thrombolysis is not needed for deep vein thrombosis.[102A]

DOSE. Standard IV doses are 80 to 100 mg tPA spread over 3 hours. "Front-loading," as used in the GUSTO trial,[80] gives two-thirds of the total dose of 100 mg over the first 30 minutes, starting with an initial bolus of 15 mg, then 50 mg over 30 minutes, then 35 mg over 1 hour. Correcting for body weight, the doses used in the GUSTO trial[80] were 0.75 mg/kg over 30 minutes after the initial bolus, and then 0.5 mg/kg over 1 hour. *Splitting the standard dose of 100 mg into two bolus injections spaced by 30 minutes seems simpler and gives a 90 minute arterial patency of 88%.*[107] A higher total dose (150 mg) leads to no greater benefit and more cerebral hemorrhage.[34] Although an initial heparin bolus of 5,000 units is standard, the heparin can be delayed for at least 20 minutes after the start of tPA.[35] Thereafter intravenous heparin is continued for at least 48 hours, when subcutaneous heparin is substituted until hospital discharge. Chewable aspirin is started as soon as possible.

CONTRAINDICATIONS. These relate chiefly to hemorrhage. For example, any recent hemorrhage or cerebrovascular accident, advancing age with fear of intracranial hemorrhage, coagulation defects, recent surgical operations, hemorrhagic retinopathy, and high risk of left atrial thrombus as in mitral stenosis with fibrillation or subacute bacterial endocarditis are all contraindications. Prompt correction of hypertension before thrombolysis is required to lessen the risk of cerebral hemorrhage.[118] Potential sources of microemboli such as enlarged left atrium and ventricular or aortic aneurysms are also contraindications. Furthermore, recent peptic ulcer or pregnancy are also contraindications. Menstruation is not a contraindication provided that increased vaginal bleeding is acceptable.[91] Gentamicin sensitivity is a specific exclusion, because gentamicin is used in the preparation of tPA. Previous streptokinase is an indication, not a contraindication (because of the antigenicity of streptokinase).

COMPARISONS WITH PLACEBO. In the European Cooperative Study,[38] control patients were given 250 mg aspirin and a bolus injection of 5,000 units of heparin before the start of the trial while patients in the treatment group were also given 100 mg tPA over 3 hours. The 3 month mortality rate of patients treated by tPA was 59% lower.

COMPARISONS WITH STREPTOKINASE. Despite the much higher early patency rates with tPA, it has been difficult to achieve a corresponding fall in mortality. The major comparison between tPA and streptokinase has been in the large GUSTO trial,[80] in which tPA was marginally but decisively better than streptokinase. The benefit of tPA versus streptokinase on early mortality (30 days) is about 1 life saved per 100 treated[73] at risk of 0.2% to 0.3% increase in hemorrhagic stroke.[118] One year after treatment there is still a small mortality decrease of 11% in the tPA group.[53A]

COST-EFFECTIVENESS. The major disadvantage of tPA remains the greatly increased cost compared with streptokinase; both the cost of the agent and the cost of repeated heparin dose monitoring by the activated partial thromboplastin time (time of personnel, laboratory costs) must be taken into account. Dose-adjusted heparin gives no advantage in the case of streptokinase.[81]

COTHERAPY WITH HEPARIN. It is often thought that the GUSTO trial[80] settled the question of whether or not early intravenous heparin is required. In fact this trial[80] showed that in patients treated with tPA, intravenous heparin and chewable aspirin (160 to 320 mg) had the lowest 30-day mortality yet (6.3%). There is no decisive evidence that intravenous heparin was the crucial component in the therapy mix, although its use is logical to prevent reocclusion. Besides aspirin, about half of the patients were given intravenous atenolol 5 mg, and an unexpected 77% were given intravenous nitrates. In centers where the intravenous heparin component is deemed to be too expensive (time-consuming) or too difficult to regulate, it should be considered that a small European trial[59] showed that early patency with aspirin and tPA alone was 75%, whereas with heparin and tPA it was 83%. Thus, the apparent benefits of added heparin must be weighed against the increased expense, the probability that it contributes to the increased incidence of hemorrhagic stroke, and the general imprecision of heparin therapy (see section on Heparin). Probably, in time, low molecular weight heparin or new specific antithrombin agents will come to replace heparin.

SIDE-EFFECTS. The GUSTO trial[80] showed that the incidence of hemorrhagic stroke was slightly higher ($p < 0.03$) with tPA than with streptokinase yet the overall rate for all strokes was similar. In the streptokinase group, there were more allergic reactions and hypotension was more common. The overall incidence of bleeding was similar with both regimes, as judged by the requirement for infusion of whole blood. Coadministration of intravenous beta-blockade may reduce stroke as a complication of tPA.[36] Major bleeding requires cessation of the fibrinolytic agent and administration of fresh frozen plasma or whole blood. A present ethical problem is that infusion of whole blood is perceived among patients as being dangerous (risk of AIDS). Although some adverse reaction is quite common, serious complications, such as cytomegalovirus infection, are in fact very rare.[120]

UNEXPLAINED PROBLEMS WITH THE GUSTO TRIAL.[80] In the case of 30-day mortality, patients treated in Europe had some unexpected differences from those in the USA. One year mortality was, however, similarly decreased by tPA by 11% both in the USA and non-USA groups.[53A] It remains true that very early thrombolytic therapy is more important than the agent used (Fig. 9–7).

NEW TYPES OF tPA. The standard tPA consists predominantly of two chain molecules. In development are mutant or chimeric tPAs which may have longer half-lives, be resistant to the effects of plasminogen activator inhibition, and may have increased thrombolytic efficacy.

## Streptokinase

Streptokinase itself has no direct effect on plasminogen. It works by binding with plasminogen to form a 1:1 complex which becomes an active enzyme to convert plasminogen to plasmin.[42] In addition, streptokinase may increase circulating levels of activated protein-C which enhances clot lysis.[79]

DOSE AND RATE OF INFUSION OF STREPTOKINASE. In several mega-trials, the rate has been 1.5 million units of streptokinase in 100 ml of physiological saline in 1 hour. A higher dose (3 million units) can achieve a patency rate of 82% at 2.8 hours after the start, but is seldom used.[32]

COTHERAPY WITH HEPARIN IN AMI. Added subcutaneous heparin tends to give a greater incidence of stroke with no improvement in mortality.[109] Intravenous heparin is no better than the subcutaneous route.[80] Therefore, subcutaneous heparin is not essential cotherapy, whereas aspirin is.[88] Rather, heparin may be given for general reasons such as prevention of venous thrombosis or LV thrombus.

THROMBOLYTIC THERAPY

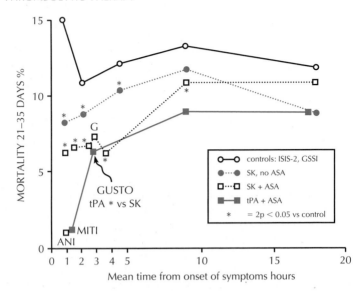

**FIGURE 9–7.** Approximate mortality figures for patients with acute myocardial infarction, according to the time from onset of symptoms and the treatment given. Mortality = 21 days for GISSI-I, 35 days for ISIS-2, 30 days for GUSTO. Data points are as follows. *Controls* for 0–6 hours pooled from GISSI and ISIS-2, plotting 2–4 hours as a mean time of 3 hours and 3–6 hours as a mean time of 4.5 hours. Controls for 7–24 hours pooled from ISIS-2, GISSI, EMERAS and LATE studies, taking 9 hours as the mean of 7–12 hours and 18 hours as the mean of 13–24 hours. SK no ASA (aspirin) from GISSI and ISIS-2. SK plus ASA from ISIS-2 and (for 6–24 hours) EMERAS. tPA plus ASA from GUSTO and for 6–24 hours from LATE. Significance points versus corresponding controls (not pooled controls) from each study, eg., Fig. 3 of ISIS-2 for SK and ASA up to 4 hours. Significance for SK and ASA at 9 hours from chi-squared data (SK plus ASA: 312/2869 vs. control 404/2854, p = 0.0011). For tPA plus ASA at 2.75 hours, see GUSTO; note corresponding SK and ASA data from GUSTO shown as G in open block. Fig. copyright L.H. Opie.

**INDICATIONS OTHER THAN AMI.** These are the same as for tPA. Infusion dose of streptokinase: 250,000 to 600,000 units over 30 minutes, then 100,000 units every hour for up to 1 week.

**CONTRAINDICATIONS.** These are similar to those for tPA, excluding gentamicin sensitivity. In addition, (1) recent streptococcal infections because bacterial toxins induce resistance to streptokinase, and (2) previous treatment by streptokinase because the antibodies diminish efficacy and there is an increased risk of allergy.[51] Hypertension may be less of a contraindication to streptokinase than to alteplase.[118] For hypotension, see next section.

**PRECAUTIONS** (not used in most mega-trials). Ideally check blood count and clotting factors before use. Discontinue heparin. Sometimes **intravenous hydrocortisone** 100 to 250 mg is given before streptokinase to prevent allergic reactions (not in most mega-trials). **Hypotension** occurs particularly in those with low pretreatment systolic blood pressure and the mortality is high.[83]

**SIDE-EFFECTS AND COMPLICATIONS.** Allergic reactions (Table 9–4) include fever and rashes, and rarely (0.1%) anaphylactoid reactions. Minor bleeding requires local measures, not cessation of lytic therapy (danger of rebound excess lytic state). Poststreptokinase bleeding diathesis is a risk especially with combined heparin therapy, but at present this combination is used less and less. For control of major bleeding, see tPA.

TABLE 9–4    SIDE-EFFECTS OF STREPTOKINASE AND tPA IN THE GUSTO
TRIAL

|  | STREPTOKINASE | tPA |
|---|---|---|
| Mortality, at 30 days | 7.4% | 6.3%* |
| Overall stroke | 1.40% | 1.55% |
| Hemorrhagic stroke† | 0.5% | 0.7%* |
| Major bleeds | 0.5% | 0.4% |
| Allergic reactions | 5.8%* | 1.6% |
| Hypotension | 12.5% | 10.1% |

Both agents with intravenous heparin

* Significant difference

† For risk factors, see Simoons et al.[118] In patients with streptokinase and no risk factors, the probability of stroke is 0.3%.

In patients with alteplase (tPA) and three risk factors, the probability is over 3%.

## Urokinase

This agent has similar indications, contraindications, and effects to streptokinase. However, being prepared from cultured human renal cells, allergic effects are minimal. Furthermore, a shorter half-life than streptokinase causes less sustained systemic fibrinolysis, and is a safer drug if early coronary bypass is the aim. A specific indication is for intraocular clot lysis (chosen because of absence of allergic properties). The defect of urokinase is its great expense. The **dose** for intracoronary use is 3 times that of streptokinase. For intravenous use high-dose urokinase (3 million units over 45 to 60 minutes) gives a low incidence of bleeding and reocclusion.[39]

## Anistreplase = APSAC (anisoylated plasminogen streptokinase activator complex), Eminase

Anistreplase is a stoichiometric combination of streptokinase and plasminogen, stabilized by the addition of the anisoyl group which is bound to the catalytic center of plasminogen. This modification ensures that the catalytic properties are stabilized. Once injected, anistreplase is deacylated at a controlled rate, so that it releases the streptokinase-plasminogen complex relatively slowly. Thus the drug can be given as a single intravenous dose. The latter point is its major advantage, so that prehospital use is feasible, although this advantage seems not to have been fully exploited. Prehospital administration of anistreplase, simpler than that of tPA, could lead to more patients being treated within the "golden" first 70 minutes.[100]

DOMICILIARY THROMBOLYSIS WITH ANISTREPLASE. In Europe a number of important trials have utilized anistreplase for initiating domiciliary thrombolysis. For example, in the GREAT trial,[78] early administration of anistreplase within 2 hours of the onset of symptoms led to a 50% reduction in the 3-month mortality, compared with the "standard" delay of 4 hours. Linderer et al.[96] showed a striking reduction in 21 day mortality down to only 1% when comparing those treated within 1.5 hours to those treated later (Fig. 9–7).

In the EMIP study,[68] about 1 hour to the onset of thrombolytic treatment was saved by "in-field" management. Nonetheless, to achieve significance in 30 day overall mortality needed pooling of data from five studies.

These advantages of domiciliary thrombolysis must be balanced against the complications of early reperfusion which might have to be managed at home, such as ventricular fibrillation and symptomatic bradycardia. Also the added delay in reaching hospital means that some of the complications of early AMI, such as shock, might have to be managed at home.

DOSE.   In the EMIP study,[68] anistreplase was given as a single intravenous injection of 30 units over 4 to 5 minutes. Linderer et al.[96] preceded this injection with 100 mg methylprednisolone to avoid allergy.

SIDE-EFFECTS.   Most common is hypotension, with some fall in blood pressure in about 60% of patients, with a severe fall in 7%.[78] This effect was treated as an allergic reaction and hydrocortisone and an antihistaminic were given. In ISIS-3, this agent gave more allergy and also more hemorrhagic stroke than did streptokinase.[88] The other side-effects noted in the EMIP study[68] were those of early reperfusion.

CONTRAINDICATIONS.   These are similar to those for streptokinase.

COTHERAPY WITH HEPARIN.   In the study with the best results on mortality,[96] anistreplase given at home was followed by aspirin upon hospital arrival and dose-adjusted heparin starting 6 hours after the anistreplase and continued for 3 days or more. Nonetheless, heparin does not add to the benefits of anistreplase, as shown by the DUCCS-1 study[61] in which withholding heparin reduced bleeding complications by 46% without changing the outcome.

## Combination of Fibrinolytic Agents

In the GUSTO trial,[80] tPA 90 mg with 1 million units of streptokinase, and with intravenous heparin, fared worse than tPA alone and was similar to streptokinase alone.

## Combination Fibrinolytic Therapy and Other Drugs

BETA-BLOCKADE.   In view of the benefits of early beta-blockade in myocardial infarction, and also of early thrombolysis, it is logical to consider a combination. In the TIMI-II trial,[101] there were less reinfarctions and recurrent ischemic episodes in patients receiving intravenous metoprolol, although there were few long-term benefits.[34] Logically, beta-blockade by reducing blood pressures should reduce intracerebral bleeding.[36] Thus, in **AMI with hypertension** (SBP > 165 mmHg and/or DBP > 95 mmHg[118]), intravenous esmolol (p 26) becomes an option for rapid control of blood pressure before thrombolytic therapy. Controlled studies, however, are lacking. In the GUSTO trial,[80] intravenous atenolol (5 mg) was used whenever possible, which was in about half the patients.

CALCIUM ANTAGONISTS.   Although no formal trial has been carried out, several mega-trials including ISIS-4 show that there is no negative interaction between fibrinolysis and the use of calcium antagonists.

NITRATES.   An oral mononitrate was combined with streptokinase in ISIS-4, whereas an intravenous followed by transdermal nitroglycerin was used in GISSI-3 (Chapter 5, Reference 61). Neither gave any added benefit beyond that achieved by the fibrinolytic. Intravenous nitroglycerin is one of several options to control blood pressure in hypertensives with AMI.

ACE INHIBITORS.   The benefit achieved by added oral captopril in ISIS-4 was slight and without statistical significance, and at the cost of excess hypotension and renal impairment (Table 9–5). In GISSI-3, lisinopril reduced mortality by 11% yet again at the cost of increased hypotension.

ACE INHIBITORS AND INTRAVENOUS NITRATES.   This combination actually reduced mortality by 17% in streptokinase-treated patients in GISSI-3 without further hypotension. It is impossible to ignore this large improvement in mortality, greater than that achieved in the GUSTO trial[80] for tPA versus streptokinase. Judging by the AIRE Study,[41] it

TABLE 9–5     ROLE OF ACE INHIBITORS IN FIBRINOLYTIC TRIALS

| TRIAL | AGENT | DOSE AND TIMING | EFFECT |
|---|---|---|---|
| ISIS-4 | Captopril | 6.25 mg initially up to 25 mg b.d. Start within 24 hours | 6% fall in mortality, NS. Hypotension doubled |
| CONSENSUS-II | Enalaprilat; then enalapril | 1 mg IV over 2 hours within 24 hours; then enalapril up to 20 mg 2× daily | Increased mortality in those with hypotension |
| GISSI-3 | Lisinopril | 2.5–5 mg initially up to 10 mg once daily. Start within 24 hours | 11% fall in mortality (p < 0.04). Hypotension doubled. |
| GISSI-3 | Lisinopril (L) and IV NG followed by transdermal NG (TN) | L as above TN mg/24 hours, left on for 14 hours per 24 hours | 17% fall in mortality (p = 0.02). Hypotension doubled. |
| AIRE | Ramipril | 2.5 mg 2× daily initially up to 5 mg 2× daily. Within 2–9 days of onset of AMI; only in clinical heart failure | 27% fall (p = 0.002) in 15 month mortality. No severe problems with hypotension although incidence doubled. |

For references, see Chapter 5.

is likely that the ACE inhibitor was particularly effective in a subgroup of patients with LV failure. In addition, it could have made the nitrate more effective by preventing nitrate tolerance.[99] It is recommended that the *combination ACE inhibitor plus intravenous nitroglycerin be used in patients with clinical signs of heart failure on the first day*. On the second day and thereafter, an ACE inhibitor on its own should be adequate as judged by the AIRE Study.[41] The routine use of vigorous ACE inhibition at the start of AMI is argued against by the negative results of CONSENSUS-II[121] in which intravenous enalaprilat caused frequent hypotension and excess mortality in that group. In the rather small PRACTICAL study,[105] enalapril started 9 to 10 hours after the onset of symptoms at a dose of only 1.25 mg (3 doses at 2-hourly intervals, then 5 mg three times daily) avoided initial hypotension, reduced postinfarct LV dilation, and improved mortality over 1 year. Hypotension (with associated renal failure) is the "Achilles heel" of the use of ACE inhibitors in acute infarction.

MAGNESIUM. Despite the positive results of several small earlier studies, ISIS-4 (Table 5–6) decisively showed that intravenous magnesium started after fibrinolysis gave no added benefit. Yet theoretically magnesium should be "on board" at the time of reperfusion to protect against reperfusion damage (see next section).

## Specific Thrombolytic Problems

DOMICILIARY TREATMENT. With specially trained paramedic teams, fibrinolytic therapy with either tPA or anistreplase has chopped off between 33 to 55 minutes of the "symptom-to-needle" time.[68,100] As shown by the MITI trial,[100] streamlining the patient's transit to hospital and, in particular, avoiding delays in the Emergency Room, can achieve as much as domiciliary institution of fibrinolysis. Hence there is currently emphasis on every step of the delay—the patient's recognition of symptoms, the arrival of paramedics, the transit time to hospital, and, above all, the lessening of the in hospital "door-to-needle" time. Nonetheless, it is difficult to escape the logic that if the first 70 minutes after the onset of symptoms represent the "golden time" (Fig. 9–7), that initiation of therapy at home must put more patients into the category of total prevention of the infarct.

RECOGNITION OF REPERFUSION. In the absence of early coronary angiography, two simple clinical criteria of reperfusion are rapid relief of chest pain and of ST-segment elevation.[116] Reperfusion arrhythmias, such as accelerated idioventricular rhythm or episodes of sudden sinus bradycardia are specific to reperfusion but not sufficiently common to be reliable. Other sophisticated techniques such as a rise in plasma myoglobin or troponin-T or creatine kinase isoenzymes may take too long to be of clinical use.

LYTIC FAILURE AND "RESCUE" ANGIOPLASTY. Some degree of resistance of thrombi to lysis can be expected in perhaps 10% to 15% of patients; the cause may include deep fissuring or rupture of the plaque with exposure of the platelet-rich thrombus which is very resistant to lysis. Rescue angioplasty is therefore becoming increasingly popular and in anterior infarcts benefits have been shown by one small trial.[107A] There is a very high mortality if it fails.[66]

REPERFUSION DAMAGE AND STUNNING. Benefits of reperfusion are diminished by the increased mortality on the first day, the **early hazard** of thrombolysis.[70] Reperfusion injury is the proposed cause. The agent closest to one having experimental and clinical support for this use is intravenous magnesium, given before thrombolysis, so that it can limit reperfusion calcium overload.[63]

REOCCLUSION. Reocclusion remains the "Achilles heel" of successful thrombolysis. It occurs in 5% to 20% of patients[10,31] with low rates in all arms of GUSTO. Early heparin lessens reocclusion according to the HART Study[82] which, however, only used an aspirin dose of 80 mg for comparative purposes. Possibly early full-dose aspirin might have been more effective.[109] Major contributory factors to restenosis include the presence of a residual luminal **stenosis,** and the persistence of residual thrombus (the latter is a powerful thrombogenic surface). Successful lysis re-exposes the site of the original thrombus, namely the plaque fissure. The potential for rethrombosis is easily understandable but not easily preventable.

*New approaches to preventing reocclusion* will probably involve the use of monoclonal antiplatelet glycoprotein IIb-IIIa antibodies;[127] monoclonal antibodies against the von Willebrand factor; inhibitors of the thromboxane and serotonin pathways; and prostacyclin derivatives. Hirudin and hirulog are very powerful antithrombins.

THROMBOLYSIS IN THE ELDERLY. Early reports described major side-effects in patients over the age of 75 years undergoing thrombolytic therapy, so that almost all trials have imposed an upper age limit. Even in thrombolytic-treated patients, the inhospital mortality rises from 2% in the young (less than 40 years) to 32% in the elderly (more than 80 years).[97] Nonetheless, the ISIS-2 trial documented a substantial mortality benefit in patients over the age of 70 years, confirmed for those over 75 in ISIS-4. The FTT meta-analysis[70] showed only a trend to mortality benefit in those over 75. Because of the greater risk of intracranial hemorrhage in this group, there are marginal arguments for preferring streptokinase over tPA. In elderly patients, it would be prudent to exclude hypertension with end-organ damage. Even transient hypertension with values exceeding 180 mmHg systolic or 120 mmHg diastolic could be contraindications. Those already taking aspirin (especially in high doses) are more likely to bleed.

THROMBOLYSIS IN WOMEN. The apparently worse prognosis of women after fibrinolysis can be accounted for by their worse baseline characteristics such as an increased incidence of hypertension, diabetes, and previous infarction.[131] Yet even allowing for all these factors, there is a higher risk of hemorrhagic stroke in women, largely limited to those treated by tPA.[118] Thus, if there is otherwise a rather balanced choice between tPA and streptokinase and the patient is female, there could be preference for streptokinase.

INTRACRANIAL HEMORRHAGE. This complication is clearly more frequent in tPA- than in streptokinase-treated patients.[118] Risk factors include age over 65 years, low body weight, hypertension, and female sex. In patients with three risk factors and treated by tPA, the probability of hemorrhage rises to between 3% and 4%.

ACTIVE INTERVENTION: ANGIOPLASTY OR SURGERY. The role of "primary" angioplasty without thrombolytic therapy in hospitals with suitable facilities is becoming established practice, particularly in patients with cardiogenic shock, early heart failure, or contraindications to thrombolysis. Facilities for cardiac surgery must be available in case angioplasty is contraindicated or fails. In the PAMI trial,[103] a 6 month follow-up showed improved short-term mortality and less reinfarction from the use of early primary angioplasty. A clear advantage is that there is no risk of intracerebral bleeding. A disadvantage is that the average treatment time ("door-to-balloon") is about 30 minutes longer with angioplasty than with fibrinolysis. The very high early patency rate (99%) may account for the much higher incidence of ventricular fibrillation, probably an example of a reperfusion arrhythmia. In another study, there was an excellent early patency rate of 91% in the angioplasty group.[133] In a third study from the Mayo Clinic,[75] a surprising advantage emerged for angioplasty versus tPA—namely it was cost-effective in that 3 days less were spent in hospital and there were fewer readmissions. But, in a subgroup, where "rescue" angioplasty had to be used, the cost was high. This study decisively showed that primary angioplasty is no better at reducing infarct size (sestamibi technique) than was tPA. Presumably the greater patency rate was offset by the longer delay in achieving reperfusion.

The "Achilles heel" of angioplasty (like that of fibrinolysis) is **restenosis**. There appears to be no benefit from aspirin, dipyridamole, warfarin or ACE inhibitors. Antiplatelet antibodies may help (p 258).

**Emergency angioplasty** after apparently succesful fibrinolytic therapy is not beneficial, but probably harmful and as such is contraindicated.

POSTFIBRINOLYTIC REMODELING. Following fibrinolysis, LV ejection fraction and echocardiographic indices of regional function improve for about 4 weeks and then start to deteriorate while the heart volume increases.[102] Such studies will bias physicians toward the use of postfibrinolytic ACE inhibitors, known to improve mortality in those with moderate LV impairment as in the SAVE study.[104] Because adverse remodeling is a consequence of a large infarct size, the most potent prophylaxis is by very early fibrinolytic therapy. The hypothetical benefit of late revascularization also needs to be considered (next section).

## Fibrinolytic Therapy: Recommendations

There is a growing consensus that the early administration (less than 6 hours after the onset of symptoms, ideally within 70 minutes, as in the MITI Trial[100]) of any of the standard fibrinolytic agents improves ventricular function and limits infarct size. The reduction in mortality is best when fibrinolysis is really early; even at 6 hours benefits are modest.[134] Nonetheless, later administration, even up to 12 hours, may still achieve some benefits. Thereafter, the "open artery hypothesis" predicts that mechanical revascularization may still improve remodeling. The difference in early mortality between tPA and streptokinase in favor of tPA is not large and the more crucial issue is to administer the lytic agent as soon as possible. Costwise, streptokinase retains its advantage.

*When does tPA justify the extra cost?* Not only does this agent cost more, but concurrent dose-adjusted heparin increases the demands on the doctors' time and laboratory costs. Fuster[73] suggests on the basis of subgroup analysis in the GUSTO trial[80] that streptokinase may be approppriate for those presenting more than 4 hours after the onset. The concept of risk stratification for hemorrhagic stroke helps. As patients age beyond 65 years, there is a progressive increase of risk.[118] Women are also more prone to intracranial hemorrhage,[131] with other risk factors being hypertension and a low body mass. Hence, it makes sense to prefer streptokinase in patients with two or more of these risk factors. For example, an elderly thin hypertensive woman is a relatively strong candidate for streptokinase. Conversely, younger patients (fewer collaterals and more rapid cell death) and those with large anterior infarcts will benefit more from rapid reperfusion with tPA. The earlier the patient is seen, the stronger the case for tPA. The greater early patency rate and improved mortality with tPA plus intravenous heparin when compared with streptokinase is likely to swing opinion in favor of this form of therapy, again subject to the problem of cost and the reservations concerning intracranial hemorrhage.[118] In unpublished data from GUSTO, long-term follow-up for 1 year shows that early patency achieves delayed benefits even in non-anterior infarcts, so that the arguments for early patency (however achieved) become powerful.[53A]

Regarding postfibrinolytic policy, this has not yet been clarified. The continued use of aspirin is routine. Beta-blockers, if not introduced earlier, are often given before the patient leaves hospital and continued indefinitely, although in ISIS-1[87] atenolol was only given for 1 month. In patients with residual LV dysfunction, ACE inhibitors are added. If rethrombosis occurs after streptokinase, tPA is the agent of choice to avoid allergic problems or resistance to streptokinase.

## Summary

Antithrombotic agents include platelet inhibitors, anticoagulants and fibrinolytics. *Aspirin* irreversibly inhibits the cyclo-oxygenase concerned in the synthesis of thromboxane $A_2$ with, in practice, a beneficial clinical effect over a wide dose range. Because side-effects, such as gastrointestinal hemorrhage are dose-related, the current trend is toward lower doses. Prophylactic aspirin is now indicated for all stages of symptomatic ischemic heart disease, including chronic effort angina, unstable angina, acute myocardial infarction (as early as possible), and postinfarct management. Other antiplatelet agents, such as sulfinpyrazone, dipyridamole, and ticlopidine are used less and less, although there are specific indications. For example, dipyridamole is still used to cover cardiac bypass operations and in combination for mechanical prosthetic valves in those having aspirin intolerance or requiring additional antithrombotic protection. Ticlopidine is preferred for stroke prevention in those intolerant of aspirin. In unstable angina, *intravenous heparin* is better than aspirin, but both are now started together. In the next few years, the emphasis is going to shift to much more *specific antithrombin agents* such as low molecular weight heparin, hirudin and hirulog. In uncomplicated AMI, warfarin may be omitted and only heparin used until the patient is mobile. When tPA is given, intravenous heparin is essential. With streptokinase, heparin is optional. Prolonged post-infarction anticoagulation is selected only for patients at definite risk of thromboembolism. Anticoagulation by *warfarin* should be considered for dilated cardiomyopathy and is essential for those with prosthetic mechanical heart valves. In atrial fibrillation, substantial evidence now shows the benefit of warfarin, failing which aspirin must be given, except in young patients with lone atrial fibrillation who need no specific therapy.

*Fibrinolytics* such as tissue plasminogen activator (tPA) or strepto-kinase are now the basis of therapy in the very early stages of AMI (within 6 to 12 hours of onset with ST-elevation or bundle branch block), and are combined with oral aspirin and in the case of tPA with dose-adjusted heparin. tPA has a mortality advantage over streptokinase but has a small but significant greater incidence of hemorrhagic stroke. Other risk factors for stroke are increasing age, female gender, low body mass, and hypertension on admission. In those with two or more risk factors for stroke, streptokinase seems preferable. In others, the tPA with a greater early patency and de-layed benefits (up to 1 year) or remodeling is preferable. Intravenous heparin is essential with tPA but optional with streptokinase. More important than the type of fibrinolytic used is the requirement to make the "symptom-to-needle" time as short as possible. Fibrinolysis is progressively less effective the longer the delay between the onset of symptoms and actual administration. After 12 hours the benefit on mortality is lost, yet the "open artery" hypothesis predicts benefits on remodeling and, therefore, less eventual CHF.

# References

*For references from Second Edition, see Gersh and Opie (1991)*

1.  Gersh BJ, Opie LH. Antithrombotic Agents: Platelet Inhibitors, Anticoagulants and Fibrinolytics. In: Opie LH (ed), Drugs for the Heart, Third Edition. WB Saunders Company, Philadelphia, 1991, pp 217–246.

*References from Third Edition*

2.  Antiplatelet Trialists' Collaboration. Br Med J 1988; 296:320–331.
3.  Balsano F, Rizzon P, Vroli F, et al. Circulation 1990; 82:17–26.
4.  Brand FN, Abbott RD, Kannel WB, et al. JAMA 1985; 254:3449–3453.
5.  CATS (Canadian-American Ticlopidine Study)—Gent M, Blakely JA, Easton JD, et al. Lancet 1989; 1:1215–1220.
6.  Clagett GP, Genton E, Salzman EW. Chest 1989; 95 (Suppl):128C–139S.
7.  Collen D. Ann Intern Med 1990; 112:529–538.
8.  Dunn M, Alexander J, de Silva R, Hildner F. Chest 1989; 96 (Suppl):118S–127S.
9.  ESPS (European Stroke Prevention Study) Group. Lancet 1987; 2:1351–1354.
10.  Fuster V, Stein B, Badimon L, et al. J Am Coll Cardiol 1988; 12 (Suppl A):78A–84A.
11.  Fuster V, Cohen M, Halperin J. N Engl J Med 1989; 321:183–185.
12.  Goldman S, Copeland J, Moritz T, et al. Circulation 1988; 77:1324–1332.
13.  Gurwitz JH, Goldberg RJ, Holder A, et al. Arch Intern Med 1988; 148:1733–1736.
14.  Hennekens CH, Buring JE, Sandercock P, et al. Circulation 1989; 80:749–756.
15.  Hogg KJ, Gemmill JD, Burns JMA, et al. Lancet 1990; 335:254–258.
16.  Hyers TM, Hull RD, Weg JG. Chest 1989; 95 (Suppl):37S–51S.
17.  Imanishi M, Kawamura M, Akabane S, et al. Hypertension 1989; 14:461–468.
18.  ISIS-2 (Second International Study of Infarct Survival) Collaborative Group). Lancet 1988; 2:350–360.
19.  Kopecky SL, Gersh BJ, McGoon MD, et al. N Engl J Med 1987; 317:669–674.
20.  Kopecky SL, Gersh BJ, McGoon MD, et al. Circulation 1989; 80 (Suppl II):II–409.
21.  Marder VJ, Sherry S. N Engl J Med 1988; 318:1512–1520.
22.  Neri Serneri GG, Gensini GF, Poggesi L, et al. Lancet 1990; 335:615–618.
23.  Neuhaus K-L, Feuerer W, Jeep-Tebbe S, et al. J Am Coll Cardiol 1989; 14:1566–1569.

24. Pacouret G, Charbonnier B for the IRS II Study. Circulation 1989; 80 (Suppl II):II–420.

25. Paganini-Hill A, Chao A, Ross RK, Henderson BE. Br Med J 1989; 299:1247–1250.

26. Penny WJ, Chesebro JH, Heras M, Fuster V. Curr Probl Cardiol 1988; 13:427–513.

27. Pfisterer M, Burkart F, Jockers G, et al. Lancet 1989; 2:1–7.

28. PRIMI Trial Study Group. Lancet 1989; 1:863–868.

29. Resnekov L, Chediak J, Hirsch J, Lewis HD. Chest 1989; 95:52S–72S.

30. Saour JN, Sieck JO, Mamo LAR, Gallus AS. N Engl J Med 1990; 322:428–432.

31. Sherry S. Am J Med 1987; 83:31–46.

32. Six AJ, Louwerenburg HW, Braams R, et al. Am J Cardiol 1990; 65:119–123.

33. Theroux P, Ouimet H, McCans J, et al. N Engl J Med 1988; 319:1105–1111.

34. TIMI Study Group. N Engl J Med 1989; 320:618–627.

35. Topol EJ, George BS, Kereiakes DJ, et al. Circulation 1989; 79:281–286.

36. Topol EJ. J Am Coll Cardiol 1990; 15:922–924.

37. UK-TIA Study Group. Br Med J 1988; 296; 316–320.

38. Van de Werf F, Arnold AER. Br Med J 1988; 297:1374–1379.

39. Wall TC, Phillips HR, Stack RS, et al. Am J Cardiol 1990; 65:124–131.

40. WARIS study—Smith P, Arnesen H, Holme I. N Engl J Med 1990; 323:147–152.

## New References

41. AIRE study—Acute Infarction Ramipril Efficacy (AIRE) Study Investigators. Effect of ramipril on mortality and morbidity of survivors of acute myocardial infarction with clinical evidence of heart failure. Lancet 1993; 342:821–828.

42. Anderson HV, Willerson JT. Thrombolysis in acute myocardial infarction. N Engl J Med 1993; 329:703–708.

43. Antiplatelet Trialists" Collaboration. Collaborative overview of randomised trials of antiplatelet therapy. I. Prevention of death, myocardial infarction, and stroke by prolonged antiplatelet therapy in various categories of patients. Br Med J 1994; 308:81–106.

44. APRICOT (Aspirin-Coumadin) Study—Meijer A, Verheught FWA, Werter CJPJ, et al. Aspirin versus Coumadin in the prevention of reocclusion and recurrent ischemia after successful thrombolysis: A prospective placebo-controlled angiographic study. Results of the APRICOT Study. Circulation 1993; 87:1524–1530.

45. Arnout JEF, Simoons M, de Bono D, et al. Correction between level of heparinization and patency of the infarct-related coronary artery after treatment of acute myocardial infarction with alteplase (rt-PA). J Am Coll Cardiol 1992; 20:513–519.

46. ASPECT Research Group—Anticoagulants in the Secondary Prevention of Events in Coronary Thrombosis (ASPECT) Research Group. Effect of long-term oral anticoagulant treatment on mortality and cardiovascular morbidity after myocardial infarction. Lancet 1994; 343:499–503.

47. ATACS trial—Cohen M, Adams PC, Parry G, et al, and the Antithrombotic Therapy in Acute Coronary Syndromes (ATACS) Research Group. Combination antithrombotic therapy in unstable rest angina and non-Q-wave infarction in nonprior aspirin users. Primary end points analysis from the ATACS Trial. Circulation 1994; 89:81–88.

48. Atrial Fibrillation Investigators. Risk factors for stroke and efficacy of antithrombotic therapy in atrial fibrillation: Analysis of pooled data from five randomized controlled trials. Ann Intern Med 1994; 154:1449–1457.

49. Becker RC, Corrao JM, Ball SP, Gore JM. A comparison of heparin strategies after thrombolytic therapy. Am Heart J 1993; 126:750–752.

50. Braunwald E. The open-artery theory is alive and well—again. N Engl J Med 1993; 329:1650–1652.

51. Buchalter MB. Are streptokinase antibodies clinically important? Br Heart J 1993; 70:101–102.

52. Cairns JA. Oral anticoagulants or aspirin after myocardial infarction? Lancet 1994; 343:497–498.

53. Cairns JA, Connolly SJ. Nonrheumatic atrial fibrillation. Risk of stroke and role of antithrombotic therapy. Circulation 1991; 84:469–481.

53A. Califf RM, van Der Werf F, Lee KL, Woodlief L for the GUSTO Investigators. One year follow-up from the GUSTO-I trial (abstr). Circulation 1994; 90 (part 2): I–324.

54. Cannegieter SC, Rosendaal FR, Briet E. Thromboembolic and bleeding complications in patients with mechanical heart valve prostheses. Circulation 1994; 89:635–641.

55. Caro JJ, Groome PA, Flegel KM. Atrial fibrillation and anticoagulation: From randomised trials to practice. Lancet 1993; 341:1381–1384.

55A. CARS study—Goodman SG, Langer A, Durica SS, et al. for the Coumadin Aspirin Reinfarction (CARS) Pilot Study Group. Safety and anticoagulation effect of a low-dose combination of warfarin and aspirin in clinically stable coronary artery disease. Am J Cardiol 1994; 74:657–661.

56. Clarke RJ, Mayo G, Price P, Fitzgerald GA. Suppression of thromboxane $A_2$ but not systemic prostacyclin by controlled-release aspirin. N Engl J Med 1991; 325:1137–1141.

57. Coughlin SR. Thrombin receptor function and cardiovascular disease. Trends Cardiovasc Med 1994; 4:77–83.

58. DAMAD Study Group. Effect of aspirin alone and aspirin plus dipyridamole in early diabetic retinopathy. A Multicenter randomized controlled clinical trial. Diabetes 1989; 38:491–498.

58A. Darius H, Sellig S, Belz GG, Darius BN. Aspirin 500 mg/d is superior to 100 and 40 mg/d for prevention of restenosis following PTCA. Circulation 1994; 90 (Part 2):I–651.

59. de Bono DP, Simoons ML, Tijssen J, et al. Effect of early intravenous heparin on coronary patency, infarct size, and bleeding complications after alteplase thrombolysis: Results of a randomized double blind European Cooperative Study Group trial. Br Heart J 1992; 67:122–128.

60. DiMarco JP. Further evidence in support of anticoagulant therapy before elective cardioversion of atrial fibrillation. J Am Coll Cardiol 1992; 19:856–857.

61. DUCCS-1 study—O'Connor CM, Meese R, Carney R, et al., for the DUCCS Group. A randomized trial of intravenous heparin in conjunction with anistreplase (anisoylated plasminogen streptokinase activator complex) in acute myocardial infarction: The Duke University Clinical Cardiology Study (DUCCS) 1. J Am Coll Cardiol 1994; 23:11–18.

62. Dutch TIA Trial Study Group. A comparison of two doses of aspirin (30 mg vs. 283 mg a day) in patients after a transient ischemic attack or minor ischemic stroke. N Engl J Med 1991; 325:1261–1266.

63. du Toit J, Opie LH. Modulation of severity of reperfusion stunning in the isolated rat heart by agents altering calcium flux at onset of reperfusion. Circ Res 1992; 70:960–967.

64. EAFT (European Atrial Fibrillation Trial Study Group. Secondary prevention in non-rheumatic atrial fibrillation after transient ischaemic attack or minor stroke. Lancet 1993; 342:1255–1262.

65. Eckman MH, Levine HJ, Pauker SG. Effect of laboratory variation in the prothrombin-time ratio on the results of oral anticoagulant therapy. N Engl J Med 1993; 329:696–702.

66. Ellis SG, van de Werf F, Ribeiro-da Silva E, Topol EJ. Present status of rescue coronary angioplasty: Current polarization of opinion and randomized trials. J Am Coll Cardiol 1992; 19:681–686.

67. EMERAS (Estudio Multicentrico Estreptoquinasa Republicas de America del Sur) Collaborative Group. Randomised trial of late thrombolysis in patients with suspected acute myocardial infarction. Lancet 1993; 342:767–772.

68. EMIP (The European Myocardial Infarction Project) Group. Prehospital thrombolytic therapy in patients with suspected acute myocardial infarction. N Engl J Med 1993; 329:383–389.

69. Feinberg WM, Albers GW, Barnett HJM, et al. Guidelines for the management of transient ischemic attacks. From the Ad Hoc Committee on Guidelines for the Management of Transient Ischemic Attacks of the Stroke Council of the American Heart Association. Circulation 1994; 89:2950–2965.

70. Fibrinolytic Therapy Trialists" (FTT) Collaborative Group. Indications for fibrinolytic therapy in suspected acute myocardial infarction: collaborative overview of early mortality and major morbidity results from all randomised trials of more than 1,000 patients. Lancet 1994; 343:311–322.

71. Fihn SD, McDonell M, Martin D, et al. for the Warfarin Optimized Outpatient Follow-up Study Group. Risk factors for complications of chronic anticoagulation. A multicenter study. Ann Intern Med 1993; 118:511–520.

72. Food and Drug Administration. Acetylsalicylic acid and the heart. JAMA 1993; 270:2669.

73. Fuster V. Coronary thrombolysis—a perspective for the practising physician. N Engl J Med 1993; 329:723–725.

74. Fuster V, Dyken ML, Vokonas PS, Hennekens C. Aspirin as a therapeutic agent in cardiovascular disease. Circulation 1993; 87:659–675.

75. Gibbons RJ, Holmes DR, Reeder GS, et al. Immediate angioplasty compared with the administration of a thrombolytic agent followed by conservative treatment for myocardial infarction. N Engl J Med 1993; 328:685–691.

76. Goldman S, Copeland J, Moritz T, et al. and the Department of Veterans Affairs Cooperative Study Group. Starting aspirin therapy after operation. Effects on early graft patency. Circulation 1991; 84:520–526.

77. Granger CB, Califf RM, Topol EJ. Thrombolytic therapy for acute myocardial infarction. Drugs 1992; 44:293–325.

78. GREAT (Grampian Region Early Anistreplase Trial) Group. Feasibility, safety, and efficacy of domiciliary thrombolysis by general practitioners: Grampian region early anistreplase trial. Br Med J 1992; 305:548–553.

79. Gruber S, Pal A, Kiss RG, et al. Generation of activated protein-C during thrombolysis. Lancet 1993; 342:1275–1276.

80. GUSTO (Global Utilization of Streptokinase and Tissue Plasminogen Activator for Occluded Coronary Arteries) Investigators. An international randomized trial comparing four thrombolytic strategies for acute myocardial infarction. N Engl J Med 1993; 329:673–682.

81. GUSTO Angiographic Investigators. The effects of tissue plasminogen activator, streptokinase, or both on coronary artery patency, ventricular function, and survival after acute myocardial infarction. N Engl J Med 1993; 329:1615–1622.

81A. GUSTO-IIa—The Global Use of Strategies to Open Occluded Coronary Arteries (GUSTO) IIa Investigators. Randomized trial of intravenous heparin versus recombinant hirudin for acute coronary syndromes. Circulation 1994; 90:1631–1637.

82. HART (Heparin-Aspirin Reperfusion Trial) Investigators—Hsia J, Hamilton WP, Kleiman N, et al. A comparison between heparin and low-dose aspirin as adjunctive therapy with tissue plasminogen activator for acute myocardial infarction. N Engl J Med 1990; 323:1433–1437.

83. Herlitz J, Hartford M, Aune S, Karlsson T. Occurrence of hypotension during streptokinase infusion in suspected acute myocardial infarction, and its relation to prognosis and metoprolol therapy. Am J Cardiol 1993; 71:1021–1024.

84. Hirayama A, Adachi T, Asada S, et al. Late reperfusion for acute myocardial infarction limits the dilatation of left ventricle without the reduction of infarct size. Circulation 1993; 88:2565–2574.

84A. HIT-III Study—Neuhaus K-L, van Essen R, Tebbe U, et al. Safety observations from the pilot phase of the randomized r-Hirudin for Improvement of Thrombolysis (HIT-III) study. A study of the Arbeitsgemeinschaft Leitender Kardiologischer Krankenhausarzte (ALKK). Circulation 1994; 90:1638–1642.

85. Hull RD, Raskob GE, Pineo GF, et al. Subcutaneous low-molecular-weight heparin compared with continuous intravenous heparin in the treatment of proximal-vein thrombosis. N Engl J Med 1992; 326:975–982.

86. Hunter JB, Lonsdale RJ, Wenham PW, Frostick SP. Heparin induced thrombosis: An important complication of heparin prophylaxis for thromboembolic disease in surgery. Br Med J 1993; 307:53–55.

87. ISIS-1 (First International Study of Infarct Survival) Collaborative Group. Randomized trial of intravenous atenolol among 16027 cases of suspected acute myocardial infarction: ISIS-I. Lancet 1986; 2:57–66.

88. ISIS-3 (Third International Study of Infarct Survival) Collaborative Group. ISIS-3: a randomised comparison of streptokinase vs. tissue plasminogen activator vs. anistreplase and of aspirin plus heparin vs. aspirin alone among 41,299 cases of suspected acute myocardial infarction. Lancet 1992; 339:753–770.

89. Israel DH, Sharma SK, Fuster V. Antithrombotic therapy in prosthetic heart valve replacement. Am Heart J 1994; 127:400–411.

90. Italian Study of Aspirin in Pregnancy. Low-dose aspirin in prevention and treatment of intrauterine growth retardation and pregnancy-induced hypertension. Lancet 1993; 341:396–400.

91. Karnash S, Granger S, Kline-Rogers E, et al., for the GUSTO Investigators. Menstruating women may be safely and effectively treated with thrombolytic therapy: Experience from the GUSTO trial (abstr). J Am Coll Cardiol 1994; 23:315A.

92. Kim CB, Braunwald E. Potential benefits of late reperfusion of infarcted myocardium. The open artery hypothesis. Circulation 1993; 88:2426–2436.

93. Kroll MH, Hellums JD, Guo Z, et al. Protein kinase C is activated in platelets subjected to pathological shear stress. J Biol Chem 1993; 268:3520–3524.

94. Lancet Editorial. Ticlopidine. Lancet 1991; 337:459–460.

95. LATE Study Group. Late Assessment of Thrombolytic Efficacy (LATE) study with alteplase 6–24 hours after onset of acute myocardial infarction. Lancet 1993; 342:759–766.

96. Linderer T, Schroder R, Arntz R, et al. Prehospital thrombolysis: Beneficial effects of very early treatment on infarct size and left ventricular function. J Am Coll Cardiol 1993; 22:1304–1310.

97. Maggione AP, Maseri A, Fresco C, et al. on behalf of the Investigators of the Gruppo Italiano per lo Studio della Sopravvivenza nell'Infarto Miocardico (GISSI-2). Age-related increase in mortality among patients with first myocardial infarctions treated with thrombolysis. N Engl J Med 1993; 329:1442–1448.

98. Manson JE, Stampfer MJ, Colditz GA, et al. A prospective study of aspirin use and primary prevention of cardiovascular disease in women. JAMA 1991; 266:521–527.

99. Meredith IT, Alison JF, Zhang F-M, et al. Captopril potentiates the effects of nitroglycerin in the coronary vascular bed. J Am Coll Cardiol 1993; 22:581–587.

100. MITI (The Myocardial Infarction Triage and Intervention) Trial—Weaver WD, Cerqueira M, Hallstrom AP, et al. for the Myocardial Infarction Triage and Intervention Trial). Prehospital-initiated vs. hospital-initiated thrombolytic therapy. JAMA 1993; 270:1211–1216.

101. Mueller HS, Cohen LS, Braunwald E, et al. Predictors of early morbidity and mortality after thrombolytic therapy in acute myocardial infarction: Analyses of patient subgroups in the thrombolysis in myocardial infarction (TIMI) trial, phase II. Circulation 1992; 85:1254–1264.

102. Nixdorff U, Erbel R, Pop T, et al. Long-term follow-up of global and regional left ventricular function by two-dimensional echocardiography after thrombolytic therapy in acute myocardial infarction. Int J Cardiol 1993; 41:31–47.

102A. O'Meara JJ, McNutt RA, Evans AT, et al. A decision analysis of streptokinase plus heparin as compared with heparin alone for deep-vein thrombosis. N Engl J Med 1994; 330:1864–1869.

103. PAMI (Primary Angioplasty in Myocardial Infarction) Study Group—Grines CL, Browne KF, Marco J, et al. A comparison of immediate angioplasty with thrombolytic therapy for acute myocardial infarction. N Engl J Med 1993. 328:673–679.

104. Pfeffer MA, Braunwald E, Moye LA, et al. Effect of captopril on mortality and morbidity in patients with left ventricular dysfunction after myocardial infarction. Results of the Survival and Ventricular Enlargement Trial. N Engl J Med 1992; 327:669–677.

105. PRACTICAL study—Foy SG, Crozier IG, Turner JG, et al. Comparison of enalapril versus captopril on left ventricular function and survival three months after acute myocardial infarction (the "PRACTICAL" Study). Am J Cardiol 1994; 73:1180–1186.

106. Pritchett ELC. Management of atrial fibrillation. N Engl J Med 1992; 326:1264–1271.

107. Purvis JA, McNeill AJ, Siddiqui RA, et al. Efficacy of 100 mg of double-bolus alteplase in achieving complete perfusion in the treatment of acute myocardial infarction. J Am Coll Cardiol 1994; 23:6–10.

107A. RESCUE Investigators. da Silva ER, Heyndrickx GR, Talley JD, et al. for the RESCUE Investigators. Long-term follow-up in the RESCUE Angioplasty Trial—does the benefit continue? Circulation 1994; 90 (Part 2):I–433.

108. Ridker PM, Manson JE, Gaziano M, et al. Low-dose aspirin therapy for chronic stable angina. A randomized, placebo-controlled trial. Ann Intern Med 1991; 114:835–839.

109. Ridker PM, Hebert PR, Fuster V, Hennekens CH. Are both aspirin and heparin justified as adjuncts to thrombolytic therapy for acute myocardial infarction? Lancet 1993; 341:1574–1577.

110. RISC Group. Risk of myocardial infarction and death during treatment with low-dose aspirin and intravenous heparin in men with unstable coronary artery disease. Lancet 1990; 336:827–830.

111. RISC Group. Wallentin LC and the Research Group on Instability in Coronary Artery Disease in Southeast Sweden. Aspirin (75 mg/day) after an episode of unstable coronary artery disease: Long-term effects on the risk for myocardial infarction, occurrence of severe angina and the need for revascularization. J Am Coll Cardiol 1991; 18:1587–1593.

112. SALT Collaborative Group. Swedish Aspirin Low-dose Trial (SALT) of 75 mg aspirin as secondary prophylaxis after cerebrovascular ischaemic events. Lancet 1991; 338:1345–1349.

113. Salzman EW. Low-molecular-weight heparin and other new antithrombotic drugs. N Engl J Med 1992; 326:1017–1019.

114. SAPAT (Swedish Angina Pectoris Aspirin Trial) Group—Juul-Moller S, Edvardsson N, Jahnmatz B, et al. Double-blind trial of aspirin in primary prevention of myocardial infarction in patients with stable chronic angina pectoris. Lancet 1992; 340:1421–1425.

115. Sasayama S. Effect of coronary collateral circulation on myocardial ischemia and ventricular dysfunction. Cardiovasc Drugs Ther 1994; 8:327–334.

116. Shah PK, Cercek B, Lew AS, Ganz W. Angiographic validation of bedside markers of reperfusion. J Am Coll Cardiol 1993; 21:55–61.

117. Silber H, Khan SS, Matloff JM, et al. The St Jude valve. Thrombolysis as the first line of therapy for cardiac valve thrombosis. Circulation 1993; 87:30–37.

118. Simoons ML, Maggioni AP, Knatterud G, et al. Individual risk assessment for intracranial haemorrhage during thrombolytic therapy. Lancet; 1993: 342:1523–1528.

119. Singer DE. Randomized trials of warfarin for atrial fibrillation. N Engl J Med 1992; 327:1451–1453.

120. Sugarman J, Powe NR, Guerci AD, Levine DM. Facts and fears regarding blood transfusions in decision making for thrombolytic therapy. Am Heart J 1993; 126:494–499.

121. Swedberg K, Held P, Kjekshus J, Rasmussen K, et al. on behalf of the CONSENSUS II Study Group. Effects of the early administration of enalapril on mortality in patients with acute myocardial infarction. Results of the Cooperative New Scandinavian Enalapril Survival Study II (CONSENSUS II). N Engl J Med 1992; 327:678–684.

122. TASS (Ticlopidine Aspirin Stroke Study) Group—Hass WK, Easton JD, Adams HP, et al. A randomized trial comparing ticlopidine hydrochloride with aspirin for the prevention of stroke in high-risk patients. N Engl J Med 1989; 321:501–507.

123. Theroux P, Waters D, Lam J, et al. Reactivation of unstable angina after the discontinuation of heparin. N Engl J Med 1992; 327:141–145.

124. Theroux P, Waters D, Qiu S, et al. Aspirin versus heparin to prevent myocardial infarction during the acute phase of unstable angina. Circulation 1993; 88 (part 1):2045–2048.

125. TIMI-IIIB Investigators. Effects of tissue plasminogen activator and a comparison of early invasive and conservative strategies in unstable angina and non-Q-wave myocardial infarction. Results of the TIMI-IIIB Trial. Circulation 1994; 89:1545–1556.

125A. TIMI-9A Trial—Antman EM for the TIMI-9A Investigators. Hirudin in acute myocardial infarction. Safety report from the Thrombolysis and thrombin Inhibition in Myocardial Infarction (TIMI) 9A trial. Circulation 1994; 90:1624–1630.

126. Topol EJ, Bonan R, Jewitt D, et al. Use of a direct antithrombin, hirulog, in place of heparin during coronary angioplasty. Circulation 1993; 87:1622–1629.

127. Topol EJ, Califf RM, Weisman HF, et al., on behalf of the EPIC Investigators.

Randomised trial of coronary intervention with antibody against platelet IIb/IIIa integrin for reduction of clinical restenosis: results at six months. Lancet 1994; 343:881–886.

128. Topol EJ, Fuster V, Harrington RA, et al. Recombinant hirudin for unstable angina pectoris. A multicenter, randomized angiographic trial. Circulation 1994; 89:1557–1566.

129. Turpie AFF, Gent M, Laupacis A, et al. A comparison of aspirin with placebo in patients treated with warfarin after heart-valve replacement. N Engl J Med 1993; 329:524–529.

130. Vaitkus PT, Barnbathan ES. Embolic potential, prevention and management of mural thrombus complicating anterior myocardial infarction: A meta-analysis. J Am Coll Cardiol 1993; 22:1004–1009.

131. White HD, Barbash GI, Modan M, et al. After correcting for worse baseline characteristics, women treated with thrombolytic therapy for acute myocardial infarction have the same mortality and morbidity as men except for a higher incidence of hemorrhagic stroke. Circulation 1993; 88 (part 1):2097–2103.

132. Willerson JT, Casscells W. Thrombin inhibitors in unstable angina: rebound or continuation of angina after argatroban withdrawal? J Am Coll Cardiol 1993; 21:1048–1051.

133. Zijlstra F, de Boer MJ, Hoorntje JCA, et al. A comparison of immediate coronary angioplasty with intravenous streptokinase in acute myocardial infarction. N Engl J Med 1993; 328:680–684.

## *Reviews*

134. Gersh BJ, Anderson JL. Thrombolysis and myocardial salvage. Results of clinical trials and the animal paradigm—paradoxic or predictable? Circulation 1993; 88:296–306.

135. Hirsh J, Fuster V. Guide to anticoagulant therapy. Part 1. Heparin. Circulation 1994; 89:1449–1468.

136. Hirsh J, Fuster V. Guide to anticoagulant therapy. Part 2. Oral anticoagulants. Circulation 1994; 89:1469–1480.

137. Patrono C. Aspirin as an antiplatelet drug. N Engl J Med 1994; 330:1287–1294.

# Notes

## Heparin Nomogram

Subtherapeutic APTT values were common in the TIMI-4 trial and lessened by the use of a heparin nomogram. The suggestion is as follows (Flacker, Arch Intern Med 1994; 154:1492–1496). If the APTT is 3 times control value, the infusion rate should be decreased by 50%; if the APTT is 2 to 3 times control values, the infusion rate should be decreased by 25%. If the APTT is 1.5 to 2 times control values there should be no change. If the APTT is less than 1.5 times control values, the infusion should be increased by 25% to a maximum rate of 2,500 units/hour. At the same time, overheparinization should be guarded against due to the risk of cerebral bleeding.

## High-dose Bolus Heparin

In the ongoing HEAP (Heparin in EArly Patency) study, intravenous front-loaded high-dose bolus heparin, 300 IU/kg, followed by a 48-hour infusion titrated to an APTT of 2 to 2.5 times baseline values, could induce full coronary reperfusion in patients with early AMI (Verheught et al., Circulation 1994; 90 Part 2:I–563). While awaiting further studies, "this simple, cheap and easily antagonizable treatment of AMI" could be used if conventional thrombolytic agents are not available.

# 10 Lipid-Lowering and Antiatherosclerotic Drugs

L.H. Opie ♦ W.H. Frishman

## Primary and Secondary Prevention

**Primary prevention** in those without evident coronary disease remains a desirable aim in those at high risk. In others, dietary but not drug prevention is the goal. Drugs for those at low risk may do more harm than good according to a large meta-analysis on over 57,000 patients.[30] The results of the national American campaign, emphasizing dietary modification, include a reduction in mean blood cholesterol levels and a fall in coronary heart disease mortality.[44] Although there were other lifestyle modifications, such as less smoking and more exercise, it is difficult to avoid the conclusion that dietary measures played an important role.

In those without overt coronary disease but at high risk, the combined impact of all risk factors including blood lipid profile, blood pressure levels, age, family history, possible diabetes and smoking habits, should be assessed before making a firm decision on drugs for lipid-lowering.[54] Large prospective trials are currently under way to test the further hypothesis that cholesterol reduction in those at high risk of coronary artery disease can also decrease total mortality.

For **secondary prevention**, cholesterol reduction by drugs or diet reduces heart attacks and overall mortality falls substantially in statin-treated postinfarct males.[62A] There is a small but consistent increase in noncoronary deaths among patients receiving the older cholesterol-lowering medications not found in the statin study.

Cholesterol reduction remains an essential component of a comprehensive secondary prevention program, where vigorous dietary measures are the first step in post-myocardial-infarction patients.[16] Current evidence is that in hyperlipidemic patients with coronary artery disease, cholesterol lowering leads to lessening of angiographic coronary stenosis[23] and clinical events.[66A] Cholesterol reduction by drugs, combined with vigorous lifestyle modification,[63] should theoretically be best.

The blood lipid profile is crucial in postinfarct management.

## Blood Lipid Profile

BLOOD CHOLESTEROL AND LIPOPROTEINS. The ideal blood cholesterol value may be about 180 to 200 mg/dL or 4.7 to 5.2 mmol/L.[53] The ideal **low-density lipoprotein** (LDL) level is less than 130 mg/dL and, in patients with coronary or other atherosclerotic disease, less than 100 mg/dL. LDL values above 130 mg/dL despite diet may warrant drug therapy in those with clinically coronary disease or more than two risk factors (Table 10–1). **High-density lipoproteins** (HDL) may aid in clearing cholesterol from the diseased arteries (Fig. 10–1). An HDL-cholesterol below 35 mg/dL (0.9 mmol/L)[1] is an added risk factor,[53] whereas a value above 60 mg/dL (1.6 mmol/L) is a negative (protective) risk factor. In the presence of a normal LDL value, a low HDL of itself does not warrant treatment. *Hence normalization of HDL is a desirable but not essential goal, secondary to the primary aim of reducing LDL-cholesterol (to below 100 mg/dL).*

BLOOD TRIGLYCERIDES. These are commonly high in patients with coronary artery disease, yet a specific causative role for hypertriglyceri-

## CHOLESTEROL ROUND – TRIPS

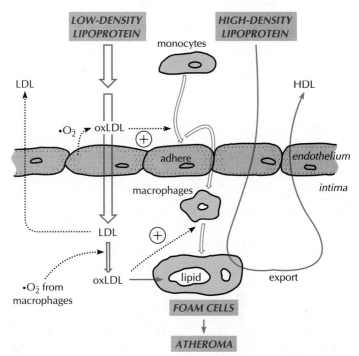

**FIGURE 10–1.** Proposed round-trip of cholesterol through the vascular endothelium and intima. LDL that is not oxidized (oxLDL) can potentially be re-exported. HDL acts hypothetically to help export lipid from the foam cells. $^{\bullet}O_2^-$, superoxide, representative of free radicals formed either in the endothelium or in foam cells. Vitamin E and other antioxidants are thought to prevent oxidation of LDL. For further details, see Kovanen[46] and Steinberg.[66] Fig. copyright L.H. Opie.

demia remains to be proven with the exception of some rare abnormalities. An elevated level (> 200 mg/dL) may be viewed with special concern when combined with high blood LDL or low HDL-cholesterol values (Table 10–1). Hypertriglyceridemia is often part of a **cluster of risk factors** including obesity, sedentary lifestyle, alcohol abuse, hypertension and diabetes mellitus.

OTHER LIPID FRACTIONS.   Whether elevations in the **lipoprotein(a)** fraction are predictive of coronary disease is open to question, at least in USA male physicians.[60] An elevation in **apolipoprotein B** may help to define a high-risk group of individuals even if they have not had previous symptoms,[70] yet the meaning of this fraction remains controversial. In patients with a family history of coronary disease, an increased apolipoprotein B (125 mg/dL or more) was an entry criterion in the FATS study.[37]

SECONDARY HYPERLIPIDEMIAS.   Diabetes mellitus, hypothyroidism, nephrotic syndrome, and alcoholism should be excluded and remedied if possible. Among drugs causing adverse lipid changes are diuretics, beta-blockers, progestogens and oral retinoids. The latter are supposedly able to retard age-related skin changes at the cost of increasing plasma cholesterol and triglycerides.

### Cholesterol in Special Population Groups

In the **elderly,** there is, in general, a less tight relationship between an elevated cholesterol and coronary disease. On the other hand, the absolute risk of clinical coronary disease in the elderly is much

TABLE **10–1**　**BLOOD CHOLESTEROL AND TRIGLYCERIDE VALUES IN MANAGEMENT OF CARDIAC PATIENTS**

| VALUES | MANAGEMENT |
|---|---|
| **Serum cholesterol levels** | |
| < 200 mg/dL (5.2 mmol/L) | *Ideal*; no changes |
| 200–240 mg/dL (5.2–6.2 mmol/L) | *Borderline*; fasting lipogram |
| > 240 mg/dL (6.2 mmol/L) | *High risk*; fasting lipogram |
| **Serum low-density cholesterol levels (most important)** | |
| < 100 mg/dL (2.6 mmol/L) | Aim in secondary prevention |
| < 130 mg/dL (3.4 mmol/L) | *Ideal* if no clinical CHD |
| 130–160 mg/dL (3.4–4.1 mmol/L) | *Borderline*; risk factor and lifestyle management; then drugs if CHD |
| > 160 mg/dL (4.1 mmol/L) | *High risk*; drugs if more than two risk factors* |
| > 190 mg/dL (4.9 mmol/L) | *Very high risk*; drugs even if less than two risk factors |
| **Triglyceride (fasting) levels** | |
| < 200 mg/dL (2.3 mmol/L) | *Normal* |
| 200–400 mg/dL (2.3–4.5 mmol/L) | *Borderline*; nondrug treatment (loss of weight, increased exercise, low alcohol intake, dietary therapy) |
| 400–1000 mg/dL (4.5–11.3 mmol/L) | *High*; lifestyle treatment; drugs if high LDL or low HDL-cholesterol. |
| > 1000 mg/dL (11.3 mmol/L) | *Urgent treatment needed*; risk of pancreatitis. |

*Overall risk factor for coronary heart disease (CHD) defined by NCEP[53] as family history of CHD, smoking, hypertension, diabetes mellitus, male gender over 45, women over 55 without estrogen replacement, and HDL-cholesterol < 35 mg/dL (0.9 mmol/L).

higher and therefore the blood cholesterol level remains an important consideration.[72] In elderly Swedish men, elevated blood triglyceride levels were much more predictive than cholesterol levels of the development of coronary heart disease.[68]

In **women,** a high blood cholesterol is not associated with increased all-cause or cardiovascular mortality.[43] A high LDL-cholesterol may be less predictive, whereas a low HDL-cholesterol or increased lipoprotein(a) may be stronger risk factors.[21A] In those with coronary disease, a high LDL-cholesterol remains a risk factor.

**Postmenopausal women,** not receiving estrogen replacement, have a cardiovascular risk equivalent to that of males.[53]

## Classification of Hyperlipidemias

The European Atherosclerosis Society[34] recommendations are extremely simple. Hypercholesterolemia is defined as a total cholesterol exceeding 200 mg/dL with a triglyceride value of below 200 mg/dL. Mixed hyperlipidemia consists of both fractions elevated above 200 mg/dL. Hypertriglyceridemia consists of triglyceride elevation above 200 mg/dL with a normal cholesterol. The latter condition when combined with a low HDL-cholesterol level is a risk factor for coronary disease. High triglyceride values of themselves are a risk for pancreatitis. This classification is easy to remember and

TABLE 10–2  DIETARY RECOMMENDATIONS OF AMERICAN HEART ASSOCIATION[1]

| DIETARY STEPS | FAT AS % OF CALORIES | DIETARY FAT COMPOSITION | DIETARY CHOLESTEROL INTAKE |
|---|---|---|---|
| 1 | 30 | Sat = mono* = polyunsat | < 300 mg |
| 2 | 25 | Sat = mono* = polyunsat | < 200 to 250 mg |
| 3 | 20 | Sat = mono* = polyunsat | 100 to 150 mg |

Sat = saturated fatty acids; mono = monounsaturated fatty acids; polyunsat = polyunsaturated fatty acids. *NCEP[53] recommends relatively more mono, up to 15%. For total calorie intake of 2,100 per day, 30% fat equals 70 grams.

readily blends with the recommendations of the National Cholesterol Education Program (Table 10–1).

### Dietary and Other Nondrug Therapy

Nondrug dietary therapy is basic to the management of all primary hyperlipidemias and frequently suffices as basic therapy when coupled with weight reduction, exercise, ideal (low) alcohol intake, and treatment of other risk factors such as smoking, hypertension or diabetes. Only 1 hour of brisk walking per week increased HDL-cholesterol in previously sedentary British women.[10] More vigorous training increases HDL-cholesterol in men with coronary heart disease.[3] High-intensity physical exercise is required to prevent progression or even to achieve regression of coronary heart disease.[41]

The **dietary recommendations of the American Heart Association**[25] are based on three phases, often applied consecutively (Table 10–2). In addition, sodium intake should be limited, as hypertension is often associated.

In practice, the dietary fatty acid recommendations can be simplified to a reduction of saturated fatty acids, largely of animal origin, and increasing other fatty acids from plants or fish oil. Exceptions: coconut oil and crustacean meat such as lobsters and prawns, are high in saturated fatty acids.

A **Mediterranean type diet** appears to confer postinfarct protection.[31] The monounsaturated oleic acid found in olive oil decreases LDL-cholesterol as much as the polyunsaturated linoleic acid[53] found in soybean oil or sunflower seed oil. Patients are told to eat more bread, more vegetables, more fish and less meat, "no day without fruit," and butter and cream are replaced by margarine. Increasing evidence suggests that long-chain **omega-3 fatty fish oils** may be protective, at least in the postinfarct period and when the benefit is largely independent of any change of blood lipid levels.[5] In the United Kingdom, tablets of **omega-3 marine triglycerides (Maxepa)** are licensed for reduction of plasma triglycerides in severe hypertriglyceridemia. Nonetheless, whatever the merits of the individual nonanimal fatty acid, total lipid intake must be restricted.

There should also be an increased intake of fruit, vegetables, probably specifically including carrots, nuts, seeds (especially sunflower seeds containing vitamin E), and cereal fibers. The ideal is a high-carbohydrate, high-fiber, cholesterol-lowering diet. (For role of dietary antioxidants, see last section).

## Drug-Related Hyperlipidemias

### Cardiac Drugs Causing Hyperlipidemias

Beta-blockers or diuretics may harmfully influence blood lipid profiles (Table 10–3), especially triglyceride values. Beta-blockers

TABLE 10–3    EFFECTS OF ANTIHYPERTENSIVE AGENTS ON BLOOD LIPID
PROFILES (PERCENTAGE INCREASE OR DECREASE)

| AGENT | TC | LDL | HDL | TG |
|---|---|---|---|---|
| **Diuretics** | | | | |
| Thiazides[1] | 14 | 10 | 2 | 14 |
| Low-dose TZ[2] | 0 | 0 | 0 | 0 |
| Indapamide[3] | 0 (+9) | 0 | 0 | 0 |
| Spironolactone[4] | 5 | ? | ? | 31 |
| **Beta-blockers** | | | | |
| Propranolol[1] | 0 | −3 | −11 | 16 |
| Atenolol[1] | 0 | −2 | −7 | 15 |
| Metoprolol[1] | 1 | −1 | −9 | 14 |
| Acebutolol[2] | −3 | −4* | −3 | 6 |
| Pindolol[1] | −1 | −3 | −2 | 7 |
| **Alpha-blockers** | | | | |
| (Grouped)[1] | −4 | −13 | 5 | −8 |
| Doxazosin[2] | −4* | −5* | 2 | −8 |
| **Alpha-beta-blocker** | | | | |
| Labetalol[1] | 2 | 2 | 1 | 8 |
| **Calcium antagonists** | | | | |
| (Grouped)[1] | 0 | 0 | 0 | 0 |
| Amlodipine[2] | −1 | −1 | 1 | −3 |
| **ACE inhibitors** | | | | |
| (Grouped)[1] | 0 | 0 | 0 | 0 |
| Enalapril[2] | −1 | −1 | 3 | −7 |
| **Central agents** | | | | |
| MD + TZ[3] | 0 | 0 | 0 | 0 |

TC = total cholesterol; LDL = low-density lipoprotein; HDL = high-density lipoprotein; TG = triglyceride; MD = methyldopa; TZ = thiazide.

1 = Frishman[72]

2 = TOHM Study;[67] chlorthalidone 15 mg/day; acebutolol 400 mg/day; doxazosin 2 mg/day; amlodipine 5 mg/day; enalapril 5 mg/day; data placebo-corrected.

3 = Opie[1]—Table 10–2.

4 = Plouin et al.[57]

* < 0.01 vs. placebo over 4 years.

tend specifically to reduce HDL-cholesterol. Diuretics, in addition, tend to increase total cholesterol. Beta-blockers with high intrinsic sympathomimetic activity (ISA) or high cardioselectivity may have less or no effect. Among the agents with the most consistent changes in triglycerides are chlorthalidone and propranolol as well as the combination propranolol-hydrochlorothiazide. However, total blood cholesterol levels are little changed: by only about 8% or less during diuretic therapy and even less with beta-blockade. Not all effects may be measured in the blood lipid constituents. Thus alpha-blockers move LDL particles to a larger less dense type of LDL, whereas beta-blockers tend to move particle size in the opposite direction.[19] The fact that both beta-blockers and diuretics also impair glucose metabolism is an added cause for concern when giving these agents to young patients.

BETA-BLOCKERS.  In angina, these agents may be replaced by calcium antagonists to avoid triglyceride elevation. Alternatively, agents with intrinsic sympathomimetic activity (ISA, p 16) such as pindolol or acebutolol may be used. During the therapy of hypertension, beta-blockers could be replaced by alpha-blockers, ACE inhibitors, calcium antagonists or centrally active agents. Nevertheless, in the TOMH study,[67] acebutolol given over 4 years to very mildly hypertensives reduced LDL significantly.

DIURETICS.  Doses should be kept low. Nonetheless, hydrochlorothiazide in a dose of only 12.5 mg may cause as much lipid disturbance as a dose of 100 mg although with many fewer other metabolic side-effects.[13] Chlorthalidone 15 mg daily over 4 years had no effect on blood lipids, after an early rise in total cholesterol at 1 year. Indapamide, not a classic thiazide diuretic, in an antihypertensive dose of 2.5 mg daily, appears to have little effect on lipids (Table 10–3).

ORAL CONTRACEPTIVES.  When these are given to patients with ischemic heart disease or those with risk factors such as smoking, possible atherogenic effects of high-estrogen doses merit attention. Not modifying the estrogen patterns and adding only progestins may induce least lipid changes.[39] In postmenopausal women, estrogen replacement reduces cardiovascular risk even when combined with progesterone (PEPI study, p 302).

### Cardiac Drugs not Causing Hyperlipidemias (Lipid-Neutral)

Cardiac drugs that have no harmful effects on blood lipids include the ACE inhibitors, the calcium antagonists, hydralazine and the centrally acting agents, such as reserpine, methyldopa, and clonidine.[1] The alpha-blockers, prazosin and doxazosin, appear favorably to influence the lipid profiles.[67]

## Drugs for Treatment of Hyperlipidemia

Lipid-lowering drugs may be required when dietary and risk-factor management fails, when cardiovascular drugs are not at fault, and when there are no predisposing diseases (hypothyroidism, poorly controlled diabetes mellitus, nephrotic syndrome; for hypertriglyceridemia, an excess alcohol intake or obesity). In general, lipid-lowering drugs frequently cause side-effects, usually subjective but sometimes serious. The statins, however, are well tolerated. Serial blood lipid profiles are required to confirm the benefits of therapy. Failure to improve within 6 weeks merits dose increase and, after 3 months, a drug change or combination therapy. Sometimes doses less than those usually recommended can be used in conjunction with dietary intervention or in drug combinations. The lipid-lowering drugs can be divided into the **major drugs,** namely the bile acid sequestrants, nicotinic acid and the statins, and the **minor drugs,** namely the fibrates and probucol.[53] These groups all act in different ways (Figs. 10–2 and 10–3) which are not yet fully understood; hence combination therapy may give additive results. An interesting recent concept is that lipid-lowering drugs may act in ways beyond regression of the atheromatous plaque, for example by improving endothelial function,[47] by stabilizing platelets, or by reduction of fibrinogen.[56,59]

## Bile Acid Sequestrants: The Resins

These drugs are especially valuable for patients with moderate LDL elevation and in younger men and premenopausal women who will be on therapy for a long time because of the good safety record.

**TABLE 10–4**   **Effects of Drugs (with Diet) on Blood Lipid Profiles in Patients with Coronary Heart Disease or Mild Hypercholesterolemia Studied for One Year or More**

| Drug | TC (% Change) | LDL (% Change) | HDL (% Change) | TG (% Change) | CHD | Angio | Mortality | Reference |
|---|---|---|---|---|---|---|---|---|
| Diet alone | −14 | −16 | 0 | −20 | ↓ | better* | same | 65 |
| Cholestyramine | −7 to −25 | −11 to −36 | 0 to +2 | 0 to +5 | ↓ | better | same | 11, 65 |
| Nicotinic acid | −12 | no data, ?↓ | no data, ?↑ | −29 | ↓ | no data | ↓ | 16 |
| Lovastatin | −17 to −29 | −24 to −40 | +7 to +10 | −10 to −19 | no data | better | ? less | 20A, 24, 36 |
| Pravastatin | −19 to −29 | −20 to −29 | +8 | −12 to −22 | ↓ | better | same | 56A, 59 |
| Simvastatin | −25 to −30 | −35 to −39 | +8 to +14 | −10 to −16 | ↓ | better | * | 21, 50A, 62A |
| Gemfibrozil | −8 to −10 | −8 to −10 | +9 to +14 | −35 to −40 | ↓ | no data | same | 19 |
| Bezafibrate | −17 | −16 | +23 | −16 | no data | no data | no data | 15 |
| Probucol | −15 | −14 | −17 | −2 | no data | no data | no data | 15 |
| Colestipol plus niacin | −22 | −34 to −38 | +35 to +41 | −17 | ↓ | better | ? same | 14, 23, 70 |
| Colestipol plus lovastatin | no data | −48 | +14 | no data | ↓ | better | ? same | 23, 70 |
| Exercise | no change | no change | +2 to +15 | −17 to −40 | no data | better | no data | 18, 41 |
| Multiple risk reduction | −16 | −24 | +12 | −17 | ↓ | better | same | 63 |

TC = total cholesterol; HDL = high-density lipoprotein cholesterol; LDL = low-density lipoprotein cholesterol; TG = triglycerides; CHD = coronary heart disease or cardiac events; Angio = angiographic demonstration of coronary disease. * Better = slows progress.

294

## LDL-RECEPTORS AND-CHOLESTEROL

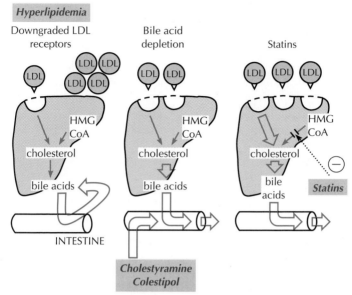

FIGURE 10-2.   Proposed mode of action of bile acid sequestrants and HMG CoA reductase inhibitors, together with their combination. Bile acid sequestrants such as cholestyramine increase the number of LDL-receptors so that more cholesterol is cleared from the circulation (middle panel). Statins increase receptors through a different mechanism. Note the advantage of combination therapy of two different types of agents. LDL = low-density lipoproteins. Fig. copyright L.H. Opie and modified from Reference 1.

### Cholestyramine (Questran) and Colestipol (Colestid)

These agents bind bile acids to interrupt the enterohepatic recirculation. Hence the hepatic LDL-receptor population increases in number so that the blood LDL is more rapidly removed and total cholesterol falls (Fig. 10–2); there may be a transitory compensatory rise in plasma triglycerides which is usually ignored. However, a second agent such as nicotinic acid or a fibrate may be required to adequately lower triglycerides.

DOSE.  Sequestrants are marketed as powders that must be mixed with liquid or sprinkled on food. Low initial doses are increased to cholestyramine 16 to 24 g daily (maximum 32 g) and colestipol 20 to 25 g daily, in 2 divided doses. Such high doses are seldom well tolerated, so that combination therapy (below) is often a viable alternative.

EFFECTS.  The major trial conducted was the Lipid Research Clinics Coronary Primary Prevention Trial,[11] in which cholestyramine modestly reduced coronary heart disease in hypercholesterolemic patients, yet there was no effect on overall mortality. The blood lipid profiles, however, did change in the desired direction. In the STARS study,[65] cholestyramine 8 g twice-daily with meals was combined with a cholesterol-lowering, high-fiber diet with increased omega-3 and omega-6 fatty acids. Diet alone achieved coronary angiographic regression and the effect was enhanced by cholestyramine.

SIDE-EFFECTS.  The major side-effects of these agents are gastrointestinal (GI): constipation, heartburn, and flatulence. With large doses, steatorrhea may occur (rare). Many patients need positive motivation from their physician to manage the GI side-effects of these agents. Some cannot manage more than a low dose which may nevertheless be useful when synergistically combined with other types of agents.[20]

HEPATIC EXPORT AND IMPORT OF LIPIDS

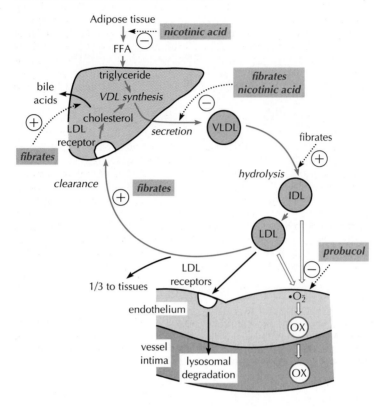

**FIGURE 10–3.** Proposed mechanism of action of fibrates, nicotinic acid and probucol. LDL = low-density lipoproteins; VLDL = very low-density lipoproteins; IDL = intermediate-density lipoproteins; FFA = free-fatty acids; OX = oxidized LDL. Fig. copyright L.H. Opie and modified from Reference 1.

New oral preparations of cholestyramine are often more acceptable though clearly more expensive.

**DRUG INTERACTIONS.** Watch for interference with the absorption of digoxin, warfarin, thyroxine and thiazides, which need to be taken 1 hour before or 4 hours after the sequestrant.[17] Impaired absorption of vitamin K may lead to bleeding and sensitization to warfarin.

**COMBINATION THERAPY.** In three studies,[23,26,45] colestipol has been combined with nicotinic acid and/or lovastatin to achieve angiographic regression of coronary disease.

## Inhibition of Lipolysis

### Nicotinic Acid (= Niacin)

This was the first hypolipidemic drug to reduce overall mortality.[6] It is the cheapest compound and can be bought over the counter. Nicotinic acid inhibits secretion of lipoproteins from the liver so that low-density lipoproteins are reduced including the triglyceride-rich component (VLDL). It consistently increases HDL-cholesterol. The basic effect of nicotinic acid may be decreased mobilization of free fatty acids from adipose tissue, so that there is less substrate for hepatic synthesis of lipoprotein lipid (Fig. 10–3). The lipid-lowering effects of nicotinic acid are not shared by nicotinamide and have nothing to do with the role of that substance as a vitamin.

DOSE.  The dose required for lipid-lowering is 1 to 2 g two to three times daily, achieved gradually with a low starting dose (100 mg twice daily with meals to avoid GI discomfort). The dose is increased until the target lipogram is reached or side-effects occur. In the latter case the dose is cut back and increased more slowly. Once 4 g daily is reached, another drug is usually added. The target dose could be lower (1.5 to 2 g daily) with still a marked effect on blood lipids and better tolerability and, furthermore, need be given only in two daily doses.[2] If taken with meals, flushing is lessened.

SIDE-EFFECTS.  On the debit side, this drug has numerous subjective side-effects, although these can be lessened by carefully building up the dose. Through ill-understood mechanisms, nicotinic acid causes prostaglandin-mediated symptoms such as flushing, dizziness and palpitations. Flushing lessens with time and if the drug is taken with meals. The NCEP[53] recommends that **aspirin** 325 mg should be taken 30 minutes before the morning dose of nicotinic acid, the latter taken with or just after breakfast. Impaired glucose tolerance and increased blood urate are reminiscent of thiazide side-effects with, however, an unknown basis. Hepatotoxicity may be linked to **long-acting preparations** (extended-release capsules or tablets), whereas flushing and pruritis are reduced.[32] Myopathy is rare.

CONTRAINDICATIONS.  Peptic ulcer, diabetes, pregnancy or a history of gout are contraindications to the drug.

COMBINATION THERAPY.  In three major studies, already cited, nicotinic acid was combined with colestipol (with or without lovastatin) to achieve a reduction in angiographic coronary disease. Note risk of myopathy with statin cotherapy.

## The Statins: HMG CoA Reductase Inhibitors

These agents are an exciting advance with relatively few side-effects and are now often the drugs of first choice. They are highly effective in reducing total and LDL-cholesterol, and long-term safety and efficacy is now established. The giant Simvastatin study (4S) showed a reduction in total mortality and in coronary events.[62A] Other studies show that these agents decrease angiographic coronary disease,[51] both slowing the progression of coronary disease and inhibiting the development of new lesions.[24,50A] The mechanism of action is shown in Fig. 10–2.

### Lovastatin (Mevacor)

This agent restrains progress of coronary and carotid atherosclerosis in hyperlipidemics, and may reduce cardiac clinical events.[20A,24,51]

DOSE AND EFFECTS.  In a dose of 5 to 40 mg once or twice daily, there is a dose response effect in reducing total cholesterol, LDL-cholesterol and triglycerides. HDL is increased.[51] In the EXCEL study[35] on over 8,000 patients for 48 weeks, the best lipid-lowering effect was seen with 40 mg twice daily, at the risk of slightly increased side-effects. In patients with moderate initial hypercholesterolemia (mean initial LDL-cholesterol 180 mg/dL), over 80% reduced LDL to below 160 mg/dL. All patients were receiving a Step 1 AHA diet (Table 10–2). Lovastatin decreases triglyceride levels modestly and increases HDL-cholesterol by 7% to 10% (Table 10–4). A single dose at night is nearly as effective as twice-daily dosage, perhaps because cholesterol synthesis occurs largely at night.

SIDE-EFFECTS.  These are few.[35] The incidence of liver damage increased from 0.1% to 1.5% in a dose-dependent manner. Myopathy, although rare, occurs especially during cotherapy with fibrates or nicotinic acid or with cyclosporine in transplant patients, and in the latter case up to one-third of the patients are at risk. **Myopathy** may be complicated by rhabdomyolysis and acute renal failure. Participation in severe physical exercise predisposes to myopathy. It is treated by drug discontinuation and fluid repletion. Ideally, patients should be monitored for liver enzymes[72] and creatine kinase. The previous fear of lens opacification, mentioned in the package insert, now falls away.[36] GI problems such as flatulence, diarrhea, constipation and nausea may lead to drug withdrawal. Pancreatitis is rare.

DRUG INTERACTIONS. There are no significant interactions with the common antihypertensive drugs including the beta-blockers and diuretics[58] nor with calcium antagonists or ACE inhibitors.[55] The adverse interaction with cyclosporine or fibrates or (possibly) nicotinic acid in relation to myopathy, however, needs to be considered.[53]

CAUTIONS AND CONTRAINDICATIONS. Hepatic damage is a greater risk with pre-existing hepatic pathology or in those at risk of hepatic injury. **Pregnancy** is a contraindication (category X). As cholesterol is an essential component of fetal development including steroid synthesis and membrane development, statins should not be given to women of child-bearing potential.

COMPARISONS AND COMBINATION THERAPY. In a comparative study, lovastatin 40 mg twice daily was more effective in changing blood lipid profiles than was cholestyramine 4 to 12 mg twice daily.[12] In a double-blind comparison with pravastatin, the two drugs were somewhat similar at equal doses,[49] while twice the dose of lovastatin was more effective than pravastatin. Nonetheless, the comparability of doses is fiercely debated.[61A] In a study with angiographic endpoints, lovastatin 20 mg twice daily combined with colestipol 10 g three times daily was approximately as effective as nicotinic acid 1 g four times daily and colestipol in the same dose.[23]

## Pravastatin (Pravachol, Lipostat)

The mechanism of action is identical to that of the other statins, so that all are clearly market competitors. Although not yet studied in as large a population as lovastatin or simvastatin, pravastatin has achieved the expected reduction of cardiovascular complications.[59,61A] In the PLAC studies, the rates of progression of coronary and carotid atheroma were reduced, as were clinical cardiac endpoints.[56A] By contrast, in a small angiographic trial in normolipidemic coronary patients, marked LDL-cholesterol reduction by pravastatin and nicotinic acid gave no clinical change over 2.5 years.[40A]

DOSE AND EFFECTS. There is a dose-dependent change in blood lipids over the range 10 to 40 mg given once a day with the evening meal.[49] At an average dose of 26.5 mg, given over 26 weeks, pravastatin reduced LDL by 26%, total cholesterol by 19%, triglycerides by 12%, and increased HDL by 8%.[59]

SIDE-EFFECTS. As in the case of lovastatin, liver damage and myopathy (see lovastatin) are rare but serious. Headache is increased (package insert).

CAUTIONS AND CONTRAINDICATIONS. These are similar to lovastatin.

DRUG INTERACTIONS. As for lovastatin.

COMPARATIVE STUDIES. Compared with gemfibrozil, pravastatin (40 mg once daily) reduced total and LDL-cholesterol more, whereas gemfibrozil (600 mg twice daily) more effectively reduced triglycerides and elevated HDL-cholesterol.[29]

## Simvastatin (Zocor)

This agent is similar to lovastatin and pravastatin, except that it is a prodrug which is enzymatically hydrolyzed to its active form. Experimentally, simvastatin but not pravastatin inhibits proliferation of isolated aortic myocytes.[28] The authors provide no explanation for this difference. It was the agent studied in the decisive Scandanavian 4S study.[62A]

EFFECTS. Its favorable effects on the lipid profiles are similar to those of the other statins. In the MAAS study, progression of coronary atheroma was slowed.[50A] For secondary prevention, a large prospective Scandinavian study (4S) on 4,444 patients with increased cholesterol levels, mostly males with past AMI, reduced LDL-cholesterol by 35% over 4 years,[62A] total mortality by 30%, cardiac death rate by 42%, and revascularization rates fell by 37%. There was no evidence of increased suicide or violent death. Differences between simvastatin and placebo arms started to emerge after 1 to 2 years of treatment, and most curves were still diverging at 4 years.

INDICATIONS. Similar to lovastatin.

DOSE. The initial dose is 5 to 10 mg once daily in the evening, with the lower dose recommended when the LDL is less than 190 mg/dL and the higher dose for higher LDL values. In the 4S study, the initial dose was 20 mg once daily just before the evening meal, increased to 40 mg if cholesterol lowering was inadequate after 6 weeks.[62A]

SIDE-EFFECTS. These include a rise in plasma creatine kinase (myopathy) and transaminase (hepatic damage). Repeated checks on blood transaminase levels advised. CNS toxicity (vascular lesions, optic nerve damage) has been found in dogs. In man, paresthesia has been associated with simvastatin in 22 cases in Australia with 4 cases of more serious neurologic damage.[69] A definite causal relationship still has to be established.

CAUTIONS AND CONTRAINDICATIONS. To minimize the risk of liver damage, avoid the drug in patients with liver damage shown or suspected (alcoholic history, past liver disease, high blood transaminase). The package insert advises that simvastatin should not be used or be temporarily suspended when there is risk of renal failure secondary to rhabdomyolysis and myopathy (severe acute infections, hypotension, major surgery, trauma, severe metabolic disorders). **Pregnancy** or risk thereof is a contraindication (category X; see lovastatin).

COMBINATION THERAPY. Combination with fibrates, nicotinic acid and cyclosporine should be avoided (increased risk of myopathy, also found with erythromycin). Combination with cholestyramine causes LDL-cholesterol to fall faster.

### Fluvastatin (Lescol)

This agent, relatively unknown and only recently approved in the USA, is claimed to have a number of advantages. First, the incidence of myopathy or rhabdomyolysis is apparently not increased, so that this statin in contrast to others can be coprescribed with nicotinic acid. Nonetheless, the package insert warns that diffuse myalgia, muscle tenderness or weakness, or an increase in plasma creatine kinase should lead to suspicion of myopathy. Second, this drug is relatively cheap. As for other statins, pregnancy or risk thereof remains a contraindication (category X), as does liver disease. The dose recommended by the manufacturers is 20 to 40 mg once daily in the evening. No outcome studies are available.

## The Fibrates: Activators of Plasma Lipoprotein Lipase

As a rule, none of the fibrates reduce blood cholesterol as much as do the statins or nicotinic acid. Therefore, they are not listed as major drugs by NCEP.[53] These agents may be preferable, however, when there are high blood triglycerides and are especially effective in Type III lipidemia. They are first-line therapy to reduce the risk of pancreatitis in patients with very high levels of plasma triglycerides. They all have risk of a myopathy-like syndrome especially in patients with renal impairment or during cotherapy with the statins. Although all belong to the same group, structural differences between the compounds seem important as judged by the very different results of large-scale trials on clofibrate (unfavorable) and gemfibrozil (favorable), stressing the requirement that each agent needs its own specific outcome trial.

### Gemfibrozil (Lopid)

This agent was used in the giant Helsinki Heart Study on 2,000 apparently healthy men with modest hypercholesterolemia, observed for 5 years.[9]

DOSE AND EFFECTS. In a dose of 600 mg twice daily there was a major increase in HDL (12%), a decrease in total cholesterol and LDL (8% to 10%) and a substantial reduction in triglycerides with an overall reduction in coronary events. Nonetheless, the total death rate was unchanged, due to a combination of nonsignificant increases in intracranial hemorrhage, accidents and violence.

SIDE-EFFECTS. Although there were somewhat more cataract operations and despite a theoretical risk of gallstone formation, no statistical significant changes were noted.

DRUG INTERACTIONS. Because it is highly protein-bound, it potentiates warfarin. When combined with lovastatin, there is a high risk of myopathy with myoglobinuria and further risk of acute renal failure.

CONTRAINDICATIONS. Cotherapy with any of the statins, or the presence of hepatic or severe renal dysfunction, and pre-existing gallbladder disease, because of the possible risk of increased gallstones.

### Bezafibrate (Bezalip, Under Evaluation by FDA)

This agent resembles gemfibrozil in its overall effects and side-effects and the alterations in blood lipid profile.[14] Whether its added effects on fibrinogen and platelets in patients with hypertriglyceridemia are of clinical relevance is not known. However, this property is not shared by gemfibrozil.[56] Because plasma glucose tends to fall with bezafibrate, this agent may be useful in diabetics or those with abnormal glucose metabolic patterns. As with other fibrates, warfarin potentiation is possible and cotherapy with lovastatin/simvastatin should be avoided. In addition, myositis, renal failure, alopecia and loss of libido may occur. The dose is 200 mg two to three times daily; however, once daily is nearly as good[14] and there is now a slow-release formulation available (**Bezalip-Mono,** 400 mg once daily). Some increase in plasma creatinine is very common and of unknown consequence. The major problem with this agent is that unlike gemfibrozil and simvastatin, there are as yet no long-term outcome trials.

### Fenofibrate (Lipantil)

This drug, used in Europe, is a prodrug converted to finofibric acid in the tissues. It may reduce the cholesterol more than the other fibrates.

## Increased Non-receptor Mediated Cholesterol Clearance

### Probucol (Lorelco, Lurselle)

This drug promotes the clearance of both HDL- and LDL-cholesterol from the circulation without any effect on triglycerides, possibly acting by increased excretion of cholesterol in the bile. Although the specific reduction of HDL-cholesterol is theoretically undesirable, the drug has a proven record for xanthoma regression.[72] An additional antioxidant effect is likely,[7] so that probucol can inhibit athero-oma independently of effects in the blood lipids. The dose is 500 mg twice daily with food. The side-effects, although potentially many, are usually not serious except for the threat of QT-prolonga-tion and torsades de pointes which, in turn, can be averted by avoiding the drug in patients with pre-existing QT-prolongation and by contraindicating the drug during cotherapy with antiarrhythmics likely to prolong the QT or with diuretics (Fig. 8–8). Hypokalemia should be excluded before therapy is started. Minor side-effects include vomiting, flatulence, abdominal pain and diarrhea; occasion-ally the latter can be really troublesome. Because probucol is highly lipophilic and persists in adipose tissue for up to 6 months, preg-nancy must not be embarked upon until the drug is withdrawn for that period. This is a clear disadvantage in women who are poten-tially child-bearing.

Despite these disadvantages, there is renewed interest in probucol in view of the mounting evidence that antioxidants can have benefi-cial effects on the basic atherosclerotic process independently of blood lipid changes. Yet in the PQRST study over 3 years, probucol added to cholestyramine failed to alter femoral atherosclerosis.[58A]

## Combination Therapy

The best combinations are those acting by different mechanisms, while avoiding statins combined with fibrates or nicotinic acid (risk of myopathy). In men with coronary disease at high risk for cardio-vascular events, two fixed-dose regimes were compared.[23,37] Colesti-pol 10 g three times daily was combined with either lovastatin 20 mg twice daily or nicotinic acid 1 g four times daily. Both regimes were equally effective, possibly that with nicotinic acid being mar-ginally better. However, symptoms were worse on the nicotinic acid regime. Both regimes were effective when compared with placebo or placebo plus colestipol. Angiographically measured coronary ste-nosis was lessened, especially in patients with modest elevations of LDL-cholesterol (130 to 160 mg/dL). Other important studies supporting the use of colestipol plus nicotinic acid are the CLAS study[26] and Kane et al.[45] Despite these claims for the benefit of triple therapy (diet plus bile acid sequestrant plus nicotinic acid or statin), it should not be forgotten that in the STARS study[65] strict diet plus cholestyramine was able to achieve coronary angiographic changes.

## Special Problems

PREGNANCY AND LIPID-LOWERING DRUGS.   As a group, lipid-lowering drugs are contraindicated during pregnancy because of the essential role of cholesterol in fetal development; *the bile acid sequestrants may be safest*. Women desiring to become pregnant should stop other lipid-lowering drugs especially probucol for about six months before conception. If a patient becomes pregnant when taking such drugs, therapy should be discontinued and the patient apprised of the potential hazard to the fetus (pravastatin package insert).

LIPID CLINIC REFERRALS.   Most lipid control in cardiac patients should be undertaken by cardiologists with the added help of a good dieti-cian. The primary aim is to reduce LDL-cholesterol to below 100 mg/dL. Advice from a Lipid Clinic should be obtained if there is severe hypercholesterolemia (including the familial homozygous variety) or severe hypertriglyceridemia, or if the lipid profile remains unfavorable despite vigorous diet, exercise, and two-drug treatment.

## Antiatherosclerotic Drugs

Quite apart from drugs which act to reduce blood cholesterol and to induce other favorable changes in the blood lipid profile, an entirely different approach is the use of drugs that are thought to prevent coronary atherosclerosis acting, for example, on the platelets or the vascular endothelium.[48] First, prophylactic **aspirin,** now in common use, is thought to protect by inhibiting the platelet participation in the atherosclerotic process. The hard evidence for this role of aspirin remains somewhat slender. Second, the **calcium antagonists** nifedipine and nicardipine have proved beneficial in preventing formation of new coronary lesions,[8] yet without evidence that cardiovascular events are reduced. A large study with isradipine (MIDAS)[52] showed small beneficial changes on carotid atheroma with, however, a possible increase in clinical events. Third, **beta-blockers** may prevent some types of atheroma in highly stressed primates, presumably acting by inhibition of FFA mobilization from adipose tissue and lessening platelet aggregation. The beta-blocker most likely to be studied for a possible effect in preventing atheroma is carvedilol, which has antioxidant properties. Fourth, the **ACE inhibitors** including captopril have a potent experimental antiatherosclerotic action, that may in part explain the effect of captopril in prevention of reinfarction in man.[62] Increased bradykinin, as a result of ACE inhibition, may protect the vascular endothelium.

## Natural Antiatherosclerotic Agents

ESTROGENS.  In postmenopausal women, users of estrogens have a 40% lower risk of mortality than those who never use estrogen.[42] The greater part of the reduction in mortality was because of fewer cardiovascular deaths. Simultaneously, an adverse effect of estrogen use was an increase in endometrial carcinoma. In another study, the incidence of gallstones increased.[22] The Postmenopausal Estrogen-Progesterone Intervention (PEPI) trial established that low-dose estrogen combined with progesterone reduced cardiovascular risk factors. In PEPI there was a favorable effect on the blood lipid profile including a decrease in LDL-cholesterol and an increase in HDL-cholesterol with, however, a concurrent increase in triglycerides. Other potential benefits of estrogens include an action on estrogen receptors in arteries, and a protective effect on the endothelium to promote coronary dilation—thus possibly explaining the benefit of estrogens in certain coronary syndromes in women.[27] In another study, estrogen-progesterone decreased lipoprotein(a).[21A] Therefore, estrogen-progesterone therapy is appropriate as part of preventative cardiological strategy except in those with pre-existing high blood triglyceride values. A further large trial is under way to assess whether such therapy, besides reducing risk factors, also lessens clinical coronary events.

Because, however, there are no data available from randomized control studies on the effects of estrogen addition, such therapy should presently only be undertaken in postmenopausal women at high risk of coronary disease or with prior infarction. Estrogen therapy is not effective in men.

DIETARY ANTIOXIDANTS.  The concept is that a high intake of dietary antioxidants, such as beta-carotene (pro-vitamin A) and vitamin E, protect against coronary artery disease hypothetically by helping to prevent oxidation of LDL-cholesterol. Two huge prospective studies in the USA support the protective role of dietary vitamin E.[61,64] Data for the protective role of carotene are clearest in smokers.[33,61] While awaiting the results of additional prospective studies, a reasonable recommendation is to increase dietary vitamin E (source: sunflower seeds) and where aggressive coronary risk reduction is required, to add oral vitamin E supplements. The case for increasing carotene (carrots, green leafy vegetables) is strongest in smokers.[50,61] Vitamin C remains controversial.

ALCOHOL.  There is a U-shaped relation between alcohol intake and coronary artery disease, with modest intake rates having a protective effect and higher rates an adverse effect, the latter probably by elevation of triglycerides and blood pressure. Modest quantities of alcohol may promote protection by (1) giving a more favorable blood lipid profile and, in particular, increasing HDL-cholesterol;[38] (2) red wine contains flavonoids which are protective antioxidants. For teetotallers, red grape juice could be equally antioxidant.

TEA.  In the Dutch Zutphen Elderly Study,[71] the major source of the apparently protective dietary flavonoid intake was tea and onions.

EXERCISE.  Besides the protective effects mediated by blood lipid profile changes, as already discussed, exercise may protect by increasing insulin sensitivity and lessening the risk of maturity onset diabetes.

## Summary

The basis for the usual therapy of hyperlipidemias, apart from the severe and hereditary types, is strict dietary modification. The ideal blood cholesterol level appears to be falling lower and lower, emphasizing the virtues of dietary advice for all cardiac patients. Similar principles apply to postinfarct management, where lipid-lowering (aim: LDL-cholesterol < 100 mg/dL) is an essential part of a comprehensive program of risk factor modification. Lipidemias secondary to drugs and diseases must be excluded. Among the cardiac drugs tending to cause hyperlipidemias are beta-blockers (especially propranolol) and thiazide diuretics. Careful attention to all other coronary risk factors is essential. The new HMG CoA reductase inhibitors (the statins) are increasingly impressive and widely used. The decisive 4S study has shown substantial total and cardiac mortality reduction when simvastatin was given over 4 years to postinfarct patients with modest hypercholesterolemia. Each of the existing agents can be used with success for specific indications when dietary management fails or is inappropriate. The new tendency is to start drug treatment with a statin. A forbidden combination is that of a statin with a fibrate because of the high risk of myopathy and renal failure; combination with nicotinic acid should also be avoided. In postmenopausal women, hormonal replacement therapy merits consideration in those without high blood triglyceride values. Increasing attention is being paid to the possible benefits of dietary antioxidants, such as carotene (especially in smokers), vitamin E, and flavonoids, the latter found in tea, red wine and red grape juice. The evidence for the protective role of dietary antioxidants is, however, chiefly epidemiological and rests on far less firm of a foundation than the benefits of aggressive dietary and drug lipid modification, which have proven value in reducing coronary artery disease.

## References

### For references from Second Edition, see Opie (1991)

1. Opie LH. Lipid-lowering and antiatherosclerotic drugs. In: Opie LH (ed), Drugs for the Heart, Third Edition. WB Saunders Company, Philadelphia, 1991, pp 247–261.

### References from Third Edition

2. Alderman JD, Pasternak RC, Sacks FM, et al. Am J Cardiol 1989; 64:725–729.
3. Arvan S, Rueda BG. J Am Coll Cardiol 1988; 12:662–668.
4. Blankenhorn DH, Nessim SA, Johnson RL, et al. JAMA 1987; 257:3233–3240.
5. Burr ML, Fehily AM, Gilbert JF, et al. Lancet 1989; 2:757–761.
6. Canner PL, Berge KG, Wenger NK, et al. J Am Coll Cardiol 1986; 8:1245–1255.
7. Carew TE. Am J Cardiol 1989; 64:18G–22G.
8. Fleckenstein A, Frey M, Zorn J, Fleckenstein-Grun G. In: Laragh JH, Brenner BM

(eds). Hypertension: Pathophysiology, Diagnosis and Management. Raven Press, New York, 1990, pp 471–509.

9. Frick MH, Elo O, Haapa K, et al. N Engl J Med 1987; 317:1237–1245.

10. Hardman AE, Hudson A, Jones PRM, Norgan NG. Br Med J 1989; 299:1204–1205.

11. Lipid Research Clinics Coronary Primary Prevention Trial Results. JAMA 1984; 251:351.

12. Lovastatin Study Group III. JAMA 1988; 260:359–366.

13. McKenney JM, Goodman RP, Wright JT, et al. Pharmacotherapy 1986; 6:179–184.

14. Monk JP, Todd PA. Drugs 1987; 33:539–576.

15. Mordasini R, Riesen W, Oster P, Riva G. Schweiz Med Woch 1982; 112:95–97.

16. Moss AJ, Benhorin J. N Engl J Med 1990; 322:743–753.

17. O'Connor P, Feely J, Shepherd J. Br Med J 1990; 300:667–672.

18. Reaven PD, McPhillips JB, Criqui MH, Barrett-Connor E. Circulation 1989; 80 (Suppl II):II–509.

19. Superko HR. Am J Cardiol 1989; 64:31G–38G.

20. Witztum JL. Circulation 1989; 80:1101–1114.

## New References

20A. ACAPS Research Group—Furberg CD, Adams HP, Applegate WB, et al., for the Asymptomatic Carotid Artery Progression Study (ACAPS) Research Group. Effect of lovastatin on early carotid atherosclerosis and cardiovascular events. Circulation 1994; 90:1679–1687.

21. Boccuzzi SJ, Keegan ME, Hirsch LJ, et al. Long term experience with simvastatin. Drug Invest 1993; 5:135–140.

21A. Bostom AG, Gagnon Dr, Cupples A, et al. A prospective investigation of elevated lipoprotein(a) detected by electrophoresis and cardiovascular disease in women. The Framingham Heart Study. Circulation 1994; 90:1688–1695.

22. Boston Collaborative Drug Surveillance Program. Surgically confirmed gallbladder disease, venous thromboembolism and breast tumors in relation to postmenopausal estrogen therapy. N Engl J Med 1974; 290:15–19.

23. Brown G, Albers JJ, Fisher LD, et al. Regression of coronary artery disease as a result of intensive lipid lowering therapy in men with high levels of apolipoprotein B. N Engl J Med 1990; 323:1289–1298.

24. CCAIT Study Group—The Canadian Coronary Atherosclerosis Intervention Trial. Waters D, Higginson L, Gladstone P, et al., for the CCAIT Study Group. Effects of monotherapy with an HMG-CoA reductase inhibitor on the progression of coronary atherosclerosis as assessed by serial quantitative arteriography. Circulation 1994; 89:959–968.

25. Chait A, Brunzell JD, Denke MA, et al. Rationale of the diet-heart statement of the American Heart Association. Report of the Nutrition Committee. Circulation 1993; 88:3008–3029.

26. CLAS (Cholesterol-Lowering Atherosclerosis Study)—Cashin-Hemphill L, Mack WJ, Pogoda JM, et al. Beneficial effects of colestipol-niacin on coronary atherosclerosis. JAMA 1990; 264:3013–3017.

27. Collins P, Rosano GMC, Jiang C, et al. Cardiovascular protection by estrogen—a calcium antagonist effect? Lancet 1993; 341:1264–1265.

28. Corsini A, Raiteri M, Soma M, et al. Simvastatin but not pravastatin inhibits the proliferation of rat aorta myocytes. Pharmacol Res 1991; 23:173–180.

29. Crepaldi G, Baggio G, Arca M, et al. Pravastatin versus gemfibrozil in the treatment of primary hypercholesterolemia. Arch Intern Med 1991; 151:146–152.

30. Davey Smith G, Song F, Sheldon TA. Cholesterol lowering and mortality: the importance of considering initial level of risk. Br Med J 1993; 306:1367–1373.

31. de Lorgeril M, Renaud S, Mamelle N, et al. Mediterranean alpha-linolenic acid-rich diet in secondary prevention of coronary heart disease. Lancet 1994; 343:1454–1459.

32. Etchason JA, Miller TD, Squires RW, et al. Niacin-induced hepatitis: A potential side-effect with low-dose time-release niacin. Mayo Clin Proc 1991; 66:23–28.

33. EURAMIC (European Community Multicenter Study on Antioxidants, Myocardial Infarction, and Breast Cancer) Study. Kardinaal AFM, Kok FJ, Ringstad J, et al. Antioxidants in adipose tissue and risk of myocardial infarction: the EURAMIC study. Lancet 1993; 342:1379–1384.

34. European Atherosclerosis Society. Prevention of coronary heart disease: scientific background and new clinical guidelines. Recommendations of the European Atherosclerosis Society prepared by the International Task Force for Prevention of Coronary Heart Disease. Nutr Metab Cardiovasc Dis 1993; 2:113–156.

35. EXCEL (Expanded Clinical Evaluation of Lovastatin) Study Results. Bradford RH, Shear CL, Athanassios DPH, et al. EXCEL (Expanded Clinical Evaluation of Lovastatin) Study Results. I. Efficacy in modifying plasma lipoproteins and adverse event profile in 8,245 patients with moderate hypercholesterolemia. Arch Intern Med 1991; 151:43–49.

36. EXCEL (Expanded Clinical Evaluation of Lovastatin) Study Results—Laties AM, Shear CL, Lippa EA, et al. Expanded clinical evaluation of lovastatin (EXCEL)

study results. II. Assessment of the human lens after 48 weeks of treatment with lovastatin. Am J Cardiol 1991; 67:447–453.

37. FATS study—Fendley Stewart B, Brown G, Zhao X-Q, et al. Benefits of lipid-lowering therapy in men with elevated apolipoprotein B are not confined to those with very high low-density lipoprotein cholesterol. J Am Coll Cardiol 1994; 23:899–906.

38. Gaziano JM, Buring JE, Breslow JL, et al. Moderate alcohol intake, increased levels of high-density lipoprotein and its subfractions, and decreased risk of myocardial infarction. N Engl J Med 1993; 329:1829–1834.

39. Godsland IF, Crook D, Simpson R, et al. The effects of different formulations of oral contraceptive agents on lipid and carbohydrate metabolism. N Engl J Med 1990; 323:1375–1381.

40. Grover SA. Modifying serum lipids to prevent coronary heart disease: do we have a consensus? Cardiovasc Drugs Ther 1993; 7:761–765.

40A. HARP Study—Sacks FM, Pasternak RC, Gibson CM, et al., for the Harvard Atherosclerosis Reversibility Project (HARP) Group. Effect on coronary athero-sclerosis of decrease in plasma cholesterol concentrations in normocholesterolae-mic patients. Lancet 1994; 344:1182–1186.

41. Hambrecht R, Niebauer J, Marburger C, et al. Various intensities of leisure time physical activity in patients with coronary artery disease: Effects on cardiorespira-tory fitness and progression of coronary atherosclerotic lesions. J Am Coll Cardiol 1993; 22:468–467.

42. Henderson BE, Paganini-Hill A, Ross RK. Decreased mortality in users of estrogen replacement therapy. Arch Intern Med 1991; 151:75–78

43. Hulley SB, Walsh JMB, Newman TB. Health policy on blood cholesterol. Time to change directions. Circulation 1992; 26:1026–1029.

44. Johnson CL, Rifkind RM, Sempos CT, et al. Declining serum total cholesterol levels among US adults. The National Health and Nutrition Examination Surveys. JAMA 1993; 269:3002–3008.

45. Kane JP, Malloy MJ, Ports TA, et al. Regression of coronary atherosclerosis during treatment of familial hypercholesterolemia with combined drug regimes. JAMA 1990; 264:3007–3012.

46. Kovanen PT. Atheroma formation: Defective control in the intimal round-trip of cholesterol. Eur Heart J 1990; 11 (Suppl E):238–246.

47. Leung W-H, Lau C-P, Wong C-K. Beneficial effect of cholesterol-lowering therapy on coronary endothelium-dependent relaxation in hypercholesterolaemic pa-tients. Lancet 1993; 341:1496–1500.

48. Liu JJ, Casley D, Wojta J, et al. Reduction of endothelin levels by the dihydropyri-dine calcium antagonist nisoldipine and a "natural factor" in cultured human endothelial cells. J Hypertens 1993; 11:977–982.

49. Lovastatin-Pravastatin Study Group. A multicenter comparative trial of lovas-tatin and pravastatin in the treatment of hypercholesterolemia. Am J Cardiol 1993; 71:810–815.

50. Margetts BM, Jackson AA. Interactions between people's diet and their smoking habits: the dietary and nutritional survey of British adults. Br Med J 1993; 307:1381–1384.

50A. MAAS study—Oliver MF, de Feyter PJ, Lubsen J, et al. Effect of simvastatin on coronary atheroma: the Multicentre Anti-Atheroma Study (MAAS). Lancet 1994; 344:633–638.

51. MARS study—The Monitored Atherosclerosis Regression Study. Blankenhorn DH, Azen SP, Kramsch DM, et al., and the MARS Research Group. Coronary angiographic changes with lovastatin therapy. Ann Intern Med 1993; 119:969–976.

52. MIDAS (Multicenter Isradipine/Diuretic Atherosclerosis Study) Research Group. Multicenter study with isradipine and diuretics against atherosclerosis. J Cardio-vasc Pharmacol 1990; 15 (Suppl 1):S23–S29.

53. NCEP (National Cholesterol Education Program—Second Report of the Expert Panel on Detection, Evaluation, and Treatment of High Blood Cholesterol in Adults (Adult Treatment Panel II). Circulation 1994; 89:1329–1445.

54. Oliver M. Doubts about preventing coronary heart disease. Multiple interventions in middle-aged men may do more harm than good. Br Med J 1992; 304:393–394.

55. Os I, Bratland B, Dahlof B, et al. Effect and tolerability of combining lovastatin with nifedipine or lisinopril. Am J Hypertens 1993; 6:688–692.

56. Pazzucconi F, Mannucci L, Mussoni L, et al. Bezafibrate lowers plasma lipids, fibrinogen and platelet aggregability in hypertriglyceridaemia. Eur J Clin Phar-macol 1992; 43:219–223.

56A. PLAC-II. Furberg CD, Byington RP, Crouse JR, Espeland MA. Pravastatin, lipids, and major coronary events. Am J Cardiol 1994; 73:1133–1134.

57. Plouin P-F, Battaglia C, Alhenc-Gelas F, Corvol P. Are angiotensin-converting enzyme inhibition and aldosterone antagonism equivalent in hypertensive pa-tients over fifty? Am J Hypertens 1991; 4:356–362.

58. Pool JL, Shear CL, Downton M, et al. Lovastatin and coadministered antihyper-tensive/cardiovascular drugs. Hypertension 1992; 19:242–248.

58A. PQRST Study—Walldius G, Erikson U, Olsson AG, et al. The effect of probucol on femoral atherosclerosis: The Probucol Quantitative Regression Swedish Trial (PQRST). Am J Cardiol 1994; 74:875–883.

59. Pravastatin Multinational Study Group for Cardiac Risk Patients. Effects of pravastatin in patients with serum total cholesterol levels from 5.2 to 7.8 mmol/liter (200 to 300 mg/dL) plus two additional atherosclerotic risk factors. Am J Cardiol 1993; 72:1031–1037.

60. Ridker PM, Hennekens CH, Stampfer MJ. A prospective study of lipoprotein(a) and the risk of myocardial infarction. JAMA 1993; 270:2195–2199.

61. Rimm EB, Stampfer MJ, Ascherio A, et al. Vitamin E consumption and the risk of coronary heart disease in men. N Engl J Med 1993; 328:1450–1456.

61A. Rosenson RS, Stein JH. Efficacy of low-density lipoprotein lowering with statins. Lancet 1994; 344:683.

62. SAVE study—Pfeffer MA, Braunwald E, Moye LA, et al. Effect of captopril on mortality and morbidity in patients with left ventricular dysfunction after myocardial infarction. Results of the Survival and Ventricular Enlargement Trial. N Engl J Med 1992; 327:669–677.

62A. Scandinavian Simvastatin Survival Study Group. Randomised trial of cholesterol lowering in 4,444 patients with coronary heart disease: the Scandinavian Simvastatin Survival Study (4S). Lancet 1994; 344:1383–1389.

63. SCRIP study—The Stanford Coronary Risk Intervention Project. Haskell WL, Alderman EL, Fair JM, et al. Effects of intensive multiple risk factor reduction on coronary atherosclerosis and clinical cardiac events in men and women with coronary artery disease. Circulation 1994; 89:975–990.

64. Stampfer MJ, Hennekens CH, Manson JE, et al. Vitamin E consumption and the risk of coronary disease in women. N Engl J Med 1993; 328:1444–1449.

65. STARS (St Thomas' Atherosclerosis Regression Study)—Watts GF, Lewis B, Brunt JNH, et al. Effects on coronary artery disease of lipid-lowering diet, or diet plus cholestyramine, in the St Thomas' Atherosclerosis Regression Study (STARS). Lancet 1992; 339:563–569.

66. Steinberg D. Antioxidants and atherosclerosis. A current assessment. Circulation 1991; 84:1420–1425.

66A. Superko HR, Krauss RM. Coronary artery disease regression. Convincing evidence for the benefit of aggressive lipoprotein management. Circulation 1994; 90:1056–1069.

67. TOMH Study—Neaton JD, Grimm RH, Prineas RJ, et al., for the Treatment of Mild Hypertension Study Research Group. Treatment of mild hypertension study. Final results. JAMA 1993; 270:713—724.

68. Welin L, Eriksson H, Larsson B, et al. Triglycerides, a major coronary risk factor in elderly men. A study of men born in 1913. Eur Heart J 1991; 12:700–704.

69. World Health Organization Report. Antihyperlipidaemic agents: Paraesthesia and neuropathy. WHO Drug Information 1993; 7:123.

70. Zhao X-Q, Brown G, Hillger L, et al. Effects of intensive lipid-lowering therapy on the coronary arteries of asymptomatic subjects with elevated apolipoprotein B. Circulation 1993; 88:2744–2753.

71. Zutphen Elderly Study—Hertog MG, Feskens EJM, Hollman PCH, et al. Dietary antioxidant flavonoids and risk of coronary heart disease. Lancet 1993; 342:1007–1011.

## Book

72. Frishman WH. Medical Management of Lipid Disorders. Focus on Prevention of Coronary Artery Disease. Futura Publishing Company Inc, Mount Kisco, NY, 1992.

# Notes

# 11 Which Drug for Which Condition?

B.J. Gersh  ♦  L.H. Opie

## Angina Pectoris

For **exertional angina pectoris,** initial treatment requires attention to any precipitating factors (hypertension, anemia, congestive heart failure (CHF), tachyarrhythmias, and valve disease). Sublingual nitroglycerin in combination with either a beta-blocker or calcium antagonist remains standard therapy, and the choice between these two types of agents may not be easy. Only in postinfarct patients is there hard evidence favoring the beta-blocker. Thereafter, the addition of long-acting nitrates is indicated. Nitrate tolerance is now an acknowledged problem. Eccentric dosage schedules are recommended for long-acting preparations (see Table 2–3). Alternatively, a new long-acting mononitrate may be given once a day in the morning; its duration of action is supposedly long enough to see the patient through the day yet providing a nitrate-free interval at night.

The *choice between a beta-blocker and a calcium antagonist* for first-line treatment of angina pectoris (combined with nitrates) is not always easy. Nevertheless, there are groups of patients for whom, on the whole, one of these agents might be preferable. First, in the presence of LV dysfunction, beta-blockers are presently preferred, because of their capacity to confer postinfarct protection even in the presence of features of heart failure, and because of their proposed use in cardiomyopathy including the ischemic variety. On the other hand, calcium antagonists are not well tested in the presence of LV dysfunction and diltiazem had adverse effects on mortality in patients with an LV ejection fraction below 40%. Whether a highly vascular-selective calcium antagonist such as felodipine is any better remains to be seen. Second, in patients thought to be at risk of developing unstable angina, the DHP calcium antagonists are contraindicated unless combined with a beta-blocker in view of the known adverse effects of nifedipine.[18] Third, in patients with angina associated with a relatively high heart rate (anxiety), beta-blockade is more logical, or if calcium antagonists are used they should be of the non-DHP variety (heart rate lowering agents). Conversely, when angina is associated with respiratory disease or insulin-requiring diabetes mellitus, beta-blockade is contraindicated and calcium antagonists are preferred. Even in non-insulin-dependent diabetes mellitus, the potential adverse effects of beta-blockade on lipid and glucose metabolism might be important, so that beta-blockers are relatively contraindicated.[110] In overt hyperlipidemia, beta-blockers as a group are relatively contraindicated, whereas calcium antagonists are lipid neutral. When coronary spasm is the established cause of the angina, as in Prinzmetal's variant angina, beta-blockers are ineffective and probably contraindicated.

Despite such guidelines, the choice between these two types of agents can often not readily be resolved. Of interest is that in the

TIBET study,[143] patients with mixed silent and symptomatic ischemia had an equal incidence of combined hard end-points when treated with either a beta-blocker (atenolol) or a calcium antagonist (long-acting nifedipine), whereas it was the combination that was more effective than either agent singly in reducing end-points.

The beta-blocker plus calcium antagonist combination seems safest in the case of dihydropyridines,[38] such as nifedipine, and is pharmacokinetically simplest with those beta-blockers, such as atenolol, that are not metabolized by the liver. The combination of verapamil or diltiazem with beta-blocker is also possible, although particular care should be taken in patients with left ventricular dysfunction or conduction defects.[22] "Triple therapy" with nitrates, calcium antagonists, and beta-blockers should not be automatically equated with maximal therapy because patients' reactions vary. In particular, excess hypotension should be avoided. When all else fails, bepridil (p 77) may benefit.

In true **Prinzmetal's angina,** relatively rare, beta-blockers are inferior to calcium antagonists and may aggravate the condition. In refractory cases of Prinzmetal's angina associated with coronary artery disease, bypass grafting combined with cardiac sympathetic denervation (plexectomy) appears superior to bypass alone.[1]

In **combined exertional and rest angina,** it has in the past been supposed without proof that calcium antagonists should be better than beta-blockers. Yet atenolol 100 mg daily gave better pain relief than either nifedipine 20 mg 3 times daily or isosorbide mononitrate 40 mg twice daily in a cross-over study.[33] Of particular note is that all three agents were equieffective for control of nocturnal angina and silent ST-changes.

In **unstable angina with threat of AMI,** the present emphasis is on antithrombotic therapy (heparin plus aspirin) combined with anti-ischemic therapy (beta-blockers and nitrates). Evidence for heparin is solid.[142] Therapy with aspirin should start immediately and all the other components introduced in the Emergency Room rather than later.[108] Aspirin plus heparin seems better than heparin alone[125] or aspirin alone.[52] Intravenous nitroglycerin is part of the standard therapy, although sometimes it is held in reserve for patients with recurrent pain despite oral nitrates.[52] There are no strong data indicating that beta-blockade is specifically beneficial. The often quoted HINT study[18] compared the beta-blocker metoprolol and placebo in unstable angina with inconclusive results, although the addition of nifedipine to prior beta-blocker therapy was clearly beneficial. With the ultrashort-acting beta-blocker esmolol, there are fewer episodes of anterior ischemia when compared with placebo.[3] Thus, the arguments for beta-blockade largely rest on first principles (reduced myocardial oxygen demand). Diltiazem, a calcium antagonist acting hemodynamically differently from nifedipine, may be used instead of a beta-blocker and is equieffective;[40] yet diltiazem has not been compared with placebo during the acute phase of unstable angina. In the absence of coronary spasm the case for nifedipine or any other DHP is very weak; two randomized trials in unstable angina, including the HINT study, have shown that nifedipine causes harm, presumably by excess hypotension or tachycardia, unless it is combined with a beta-blocker. Regardless of drug therapy, many patients require coronary revascularization (bypass or PTCA) within the first few months.[30] An early invasive strategy is no different in long-term outcome than a more conservative approach, though with fewer hospital admissions and drug requirements for those aggressively treated.[145] Thrombolytic therapy cannot be recommended and may be relatively contraindicated because only a minority of culprit lesions improve,[144] because the complication rate is increased (incidence of AMI; intracranial hemorrhage) and because "opening a closed artery and keeping an unstable artery open seem to require different tools."[151]

In **suspected non-Q-wave myocardial infarction,** there is, in general, a similar policy to that adopted for unstable angina.[145] In the early stages of onset of this condition, there would typically be ST-depression on the ECG, a situation not favorable for the effects of fibrinolytics.

CORONARY ARTERY BYPASS SURGERY FOR ANGINA PECTORIS. Multiple studies over the last 20 years have provided a clear message: In patients at high risk, revascularization prolongs survival in comparison with medical therapy alone.[13] High-risk patients are characterized by unstable angina, effort angina that is more than mild, left mainstem disease whether symptomatic or not, an age of 65 years or more, and LV dysfunction especially when the latter is combined with multivessel disease.[39] The *decision about surgery must be tailored to the individual* and needs to take into account all these complex factors and, in addition, the patient's lifestyle, occupation, other medical conditions, and tolerance for medical therapy.

PERCUTANEOUS TRANSLUMINAL CORONARY ANGIOPLASTY (PTCA). PTCA is extensively employed and works well, especially for severely symptomatic single vessel disease, when it relieves angina better than medical therapy without, however, any suggestion that it might improve survival.[46] **Restenosis** remains a significant problem and is the "Achilles heel" of angioplasty. Restenosis lessened the symptomatic benefit of PTCA in the ACME study.[46] The **antiplatelet antibody,** c7E3, directed against receptors IIa and IIIb, can be used to lessen restenosis in high risk-patients.[147] PTCA is more often followed by repeat angiography and repeat revascularization than is bypass grafting.[126] Nonetheless, in highly selected subsets of patients and in the short-term (1 to 3 years), there are no major differences in survival or freedom from myocardial infarction between PTCA and bypass grafting.[75,95A]

## "Silent" Myocardial Ischemia

"Silent" ECG ischemia, detected by ST-segment deviations on ambulatory monitoring, constitutes part of the total ischemic burden in coronary artery disease. Generally, such silent ischemia is associated with at least some painful component. Yet it is not known whether therapy should specifically be directed toward the silent component, whether silent ischemia needs to be shortened in duration or totally eliminated, or whether therapy may best be guided by clinically overt features such as chest pain. The ACIP study shows that revascularization is better than medical therapy over 1 year in suppressing ECG changes and decreasing hospitalization, while symptom-based therapy was as effective as a strategy based on the need to eliminate ECG ischemia.[45] The general rule seems to be that the same agents benefiting patients with overt angina also help for silent ischemia. The closest there are to outcome studies yet available compare the long-term effects on combined silent and symptomatic ischemia of (1) nifedipine with atenolol and with the combination, to show that the latter reduces cardiac death, myocardial infarction, and unstable angina when compared with each agent singly;[143] and (2) in patients with mild or no angina, atenolol reduces ambulatory ischemia as well as the aggravation of angina and the need for revascularization (ASSIST Study).[51]

## Early Phase Acute Myocardial Infarction

Principles of management are summarized in Table 11–1.

**Morphine** (2–5 mg slow IV every 5 to 30 minutes) combines a potent analgesic effect with hemodynamic actions that are particularly beneficial in reducing myocardial oxygen demand ($MVO_2$), namely a marked venodilator action reducing ventricular preload,

**TABLE 11–1    EARLY PHASE ACUTE MYOCARDIAL INFARCTION: PRINCIPLES OF MANAGEMENT**

1. Minimize pain-to-needle time, urgent hospitalization. Relieve pain by morphine.
2. Aspirin upon suspicion.
3. Thrombolysis as soon as possible. tPA plus dose-adjusted heparin *or* streptokinase without heparin.
4. Acute angioplasty in selected patients at specialized centers.
5. Continuing pain. Intravenous nitrates and/or beta-blockers. Consider angiography.
6. Consider indications for early beta-blockade, ACE inhibition.
7. Management of complications:
   - LVF (after Swan-Ganz catheterization)—ACE inhibitors, diuretics, nitrates.
   - Symptomatic ventricular arrhythmias: lidocaine; if refractory procainamide, bretylium, amiodarone.
   - Supraventricular arrhythmias (vagal procedures; intravenous adenosine or verapamil or diltiazem or esmolol).
   - Cardiogenic shock—acute angioplasty, intra-aortic balloon
   - bypass surgery.
   - RV infarction—fluids, inotropic support. Avoid nitrates.
   - Rupture of free wall, mitral valve, ventricular septum—cardiac surgery.
8. If patient non-insulin-dependent diabetic
   - Stop oral hypoglycemics
   - Replace by insulin (modified GIK regime).

a decreased heart rate, a mild arterial vasodilator action that may reduce afterload, and a decrease in sympathetic outflow.[92] In the presence of hypovolemia, morphine may cause profound hypotension. **Atropine** (0.5 mg intravenous aliquots to maximum of 2.0 mg) has a vagolytic effect that is useful for the management of bradyarrhythmias with atrioventricular (AV) block (particularly with inferior infarction), sinus or nodal bradycardia with hypotension, or bradycardia-related ventricular ectopy. Small doses and careful monitoring are essential since the elimination of vagal inhibition may unmask latent sympathetic overactivity, thereby producing sinus tachycardia and rarely even ventricular tachycardia (VT) or fibrillation (VF).[1] The role of prophylactic atropine for uncomplicated bradycardia is questionable.

**Sinus tachycardia** is a common manifestation of early phase sympathetic overactivity, which increases $MVO_2$ and predisposes to tachyarrhythmias. *The first step is to treat the underlying cause*—for example, pain, anxiety, hypovolemia or pump failure—and then to use a beta-blocker, which can be safe and effective provided that the patient is carefully observed.

**Acute hypertension** increases the load on the left ventricle yet improves perfusion of the ischemic zone. In experimental ischemia, the lower the heart rate the higher the blood pressure that can be tolerated.[1] Thus the benefits of blood pressure reduction in AMI are not clear unless there is LV failure (frequent in severe infarcts). Yet the blood pressure must be controlled in all patients in whom thrombolytic therapy is under consideration, to lessen the risk of bleeding. A smooth and careful reduction by intravenous nitroglycerin seems best; other tested drugs include intravenous atenolol or metoprolol (both often used in early AMI but not specifically tested for effects on blood pressure) or intravenous esmolol (p 26). The latter is especially suitable, because of its very short half-life, when there are possible contraindications including hemodynamic instability. The mean blood pressure should not fall below 80 mmHg.[19]

## Acute Reperfusion Therapy

THROMBOLYSIS. Removing the thrombotic obstruction to the blood supply remains the most effective mode of preserving the ischemic myocardium and reducing infarct size. Fibrinolytic therapy has come to dominate discussions on the management of early AMI (p 269). Very clearly the earlier the reperfusion takes place, the better. Likewise, the earlier the reperfusion, the stronger the theoretical arguments for the more rapidly acting tPA over streptokinase. Much of the delay is the "door-to-needle" time, i.e., from the time of entry into the Emergency Room to the administration of the thrombolytic agent. Aspirin needs to be given as early as possible. Three trials (MITI, EMIP, and GREAT, p 275) have shown the benefit of prehospital thrombolytic therapy, which, however, requires community organization to get the paramedical team there on time. Yet pivotal questions remain unanswered. Areas of persistent controversy include the efficacy of late reperfusion (more than 12 hours), which agent or combination of agents is best, and the possible role of adjuvant therapy such as beta-blockade to widen the therapeutic window.

Intravenous thrombolytic therapy has become standard for patients with evolving myocardial infarction, as shown by ST-segment elevation (ECG ischemia rather than necrosis) or fresh bundle branch block (Table 9–2). Numerous trials have documented a reduction in mortality compared with placebo. The greatest benefit is obtained with early administration, within 4 to 6 hours of the onset of symptoms. Within the first "golden" 70 minutes, benefits are spectacular (Fig. 9–7).

MECHANICAL REVASCULARIZATION. In selected centers, **primary coronary angioplasty** gives results at least as good as thrombolysis using tPA[87] and better than streptokinase.[71] Primary angioplasty is probably cheaper in the long run.[87] In other specialized centers, emergency bypass surgery is undertaken for AMI. Yet, for the vast majority of patients, logistics dictate that the most urgent requirement is for an intravenous thrombolytic agent.

REPERFUSION INJURY. Considerable experimental evidence points to a spectrum of reperfusion events, including ventricular arrhythmias, mechanical stunning, and microvascular injury.[27] Evidence for reperfusion-induced cell necrosis is less clear. Reperfusion injury occurs upon reperfusion, not later. The clinical counterpart may be the increased mortality with fibrinolytic therapy in the first 24 hours, the "early hazard."[80] Logically, intravenous magnesium with its anticalcium effect if given *before* the onset of thrombolysis should reduce reperfusion injury.[101] Post-thrombolytic magnesium had no proven benefit in the large ISIS-4 study (p 278).

REOCCLUSION. Successful thrombolysis is not an end in itself. The incidence of reocclusion was only 5% to 7% in the GUSTO trial (p 278). There are many contributory factors, including the severity of the underlying residual stenosis, the persistence of the initial thrombogenic substrate (plaque fissure), and activation of platelets and of the clotting cascade. Heparin started early helps to ensures higher patency rates in patients given tPA,[15] and should thereafter be maintained for about 5 days. In patients given streptokinase or anistreplase, heparin appears not to help. There are ongoing studies assessing the effects of hirudin and hirulog, as well as monoclonal antibodies to the platelet IIa/IIIb receptor (p 148). For example, hirudin plus streptokinase substantially improves the early patency rate,[100] while in the TIMI-5 trial[146] hirudin plus tPA was better at maintaining patency than heparin plus tPA.

Post-thrombolytic Angioplasty. Following thrombolytic therapy, routine emergency angioplasty is not helpful and may be harmful unless there is recurrent ischemia.[41] In the absence of thrombolytic therapy, **primary angioplasty** is now an established procedure, especially in cardiogenic shock.[93] In patients with failed thrombolytic therapy, **"rescue" angioplasty** is logical, especially in those with anterior infarcts.[122] The problem of how to assess reperfusion is currently under intense scrutiny. Changes in the 12-lead ECG or lessening of chest pain are useful indicators.[64,140] The reperfused myocardium also releases creatine kinase and muscle components, such as troponin and myoglobin.

### Prophylactic Early Beta-Blockade

Pooled data on trials of beta-blockers given early to about 29,000 patients suggest a 13% reduction in acute phase mortality.[141] It must be considered that almost all of these studies on early beta-blockade were gathered in the prethrombolytic era. With thrombolysis, intravenous atenolol was an integral part of the recent mega-trials, such as GUSTO and GISSI-3, and must be considered safe. Small-scale studies suggest that early beta-blockade may be combined with early reperfusion to reduce recurrent infarction and ischemia,[41] to reduce the risk of cerebral hemorrhage following tPA,[42] and to lessen chest pain[17] without, however, achieving solid long-term benefit. Logically, the earlier the reperfusion, the less the chest pain and the less the reflex adrenergic discharge. Hence, it is not imperative that beta-blockade be given with really early reperfusion unless there is concurrent hypertension or inappropriate tachycardia.[148] When reperfusion is later, say after 4 to 6 hours or more, or when thrombolytic therapy is contraindicated or not given, then the arguments for early beta-blockade remain strong. The best-tested drugs are metoprolol and atenolol, whereas the short-acting esmolol is preferred when the hemodynamic situation is potentially unstable.

It should not be forgotten that beta-blockade introduced after hemodynamic stabilization (late intervention, 25 studies, 24,000 patients) brings about a 23% reduction in late-phase mortality.[141]

### Therapy of Ventricular Arrhythmias in AMI

**Lidocaine** (lignocaine) has been widely used in the prophylaxis and therapy of early postinfarct arrhythmias. Whether prophylactic lidocaine therapy really benefits remains controversial. A meta-analysis of 14 trials shows that lidocaine reduces VF by about one-third, but may increase mortality by about the same percentage.[103] When hemodynamically serious VT fails to respond to lidocaine, procainamide or Class III agents (bretylium, intravenous amiodarone) are used. Pacing techniques (atrial or ventricular), stellate ganglion blockade or programmed ventricular stimulation may occasionally be lifesaving.

*Treatment of LV failure* is an essential adjunct to antiarrhythmic therapy. The possibility of drug-induced VT or of hypokalemia should always be borne in mind.

### Supraventricular Arrhythmias in AMI

Atrial fibrillation, flutter or paroxysmal supraventricular tachycardia are usually transient yet may be recurrent and troublesome. Precipitating factors requiring treatment include hypoxia, acidosis, heart failure with atrial distention, pericarditis, and sinus node ischemia. In the case of supraventricular tachycardia, initial therapy should be carotid sinus massage or other vagal maneuvers. In the absence of LV failure, intravenous diltiazem or verapamil or the ultrashort-acting beta-blocker esmolol are all effective in controlling the ventricular rate. Although intravenous diltiazem is licensed in the USA for acute conversion of supraventricular tachycardia, experience in AMI is limited and concurrent use of intravenous beta-blockade is a contraindication. In the presence of LV failure, intravenous adenosine (**Adenocard**) or the careful use of esmolol may be tried. Adenosine cannot be used for atrial fibrillation or flutter because of its ultrashort action. Cardioversion is limited to resistant cases with hemodynamic compromise. Recurrent atrial flutter may respond to atrial overdrive pacing.

## LV Failure with Pulmonary Congestion in AMI

Swan-Ganz catheterization to measure LV filling pressure and cardiac output allows a rational choice between various intravenous agents that reduce both preload and afterload or chiefly the preload. Nonetheless, the increasing use of bedside echocardiographic techniques to monitor LV function in AMI means that Swan-Ganz catheterization is being used less frequently. In the patient with AMI and pulmonary edema, excess diuresis with preload reduction and relative volume depletion must be avoided. Reduced ventricular compliance requires higher filling pressures to maintain cardiac output.

Where there are no intensive care facilities, intravenous unloading agents such as nitroprusside and nitrates are best avoided. In theory, sublingual agents that reduce the preload (short-acting nitrates) or the pre- and afterload (captopril) should be useful here.

The diuretic furosemide, although standard therapy and acting by rapid vasodilation as well as by diuresis, may sometimes paradoxically induce vasoconstriction.

Early use of ACE inhibitors in AMI is now becoming common. The AIRE study (p 115) has shown dramatic benefits for ramipril when clinical heart failure was diagnosed a few days after the onset of AMI. The GISSI-3 study[89] showed that lisinopril given prophylactically within 24 hours of the onset of symptoms of AMI was safe. The PRACTICAL study[117] started enalapril also within 24 hours in a very low initial dose (1.25 mg) and worked up to 5 mg three times daily; LV dilation and mortality decreased. Hence the early use of oral ACE inhibitors in clinical heart failure seems advisable. Combination with intravenous nitrates is not only permissible but positive, according to the GISSI-3 study.[89] In anterior infarcts, the case for very early oral ACE inhibition is good.[133A] It is imperative to avoid hypotension.

## "Forward Failure" in AMI

When cardiac output is low in the absence of an elevated wedge pressure or clinical and radiographic evidence of LV failure, it is crucial to exclude hypovolemia (possibly drug-induced), or right ventricular infarction. In the absence of these, the best strategy is to employ ACE inhibitors alone or in combination with a positively inotropic agent such as dopamine or dobutamine. Monitoring the hemodynamic response invasively is indispensible. Nitrates are usually contraindicated because their main effect is reduction of preload.

Inotropic support by digitalis in AMI remains controversial (p 152). The benefits of digoxin in AMI are probably small, so that its use is restricted to patients with frank LV failure not responding to furosemide, nitrates, or ACE inhibitors, or patients with atrial tachyarrhythmias in whom diltiazem or verapamil or esmolol fail or are contraindicated.

In **severely ill patients** with Killip Class III or IV, thrombolytic therapy is not of proven benefit and primary angioplasty must be considered to avoid cardiogenic shock (see next section).

## Cardiogenic Shock

**Acute angioplasty** may benefit in cardiogenic shock.[93] It is difficult to obtain prospective controlled data, so that a flexible approach is needed to achieve revascularization, whether by angioplasty, thrombolysis or bypass surgery.[93] Intra-aortic **balloon pumping** is used in most patients, who often also receive intravenous inotropes. Careful fluid management is essential. In thrombosis of the left main coronary artery, the ensuing severe cardiogenic shock is called the **left main shock syndrome.** Here the prognosis is so gloomy that heroics are redundant with only conservative therapy left.[118]

### Limitation of Infarct Size

Since myocardial infarction is ultimately the consequence of a serious imbalance between myocardial oxygen supply and demand, it is logical and prudent to employ measures aimed at redressing this imbalance. These measures include the treatment of arrhythmias, hypoxia, heart failure, hypertension, and tachycardia. Hypokalemia should be sought and treated. Despite much experimental evidence that numerous pharmacologic agents such as beta-blockers, nitrates, metabolic agents including glucose-insulin-potassium, or free radical scavengers will reduce infarct size, clinical evidence of benefit has been difficult to obtain.

**Intravenous nitroglycerin or nitroprusside** showed, in pooled data from 11 trials involving 2,000 patients, an average reduction of 35% in the odds of death, especially during the first week.[44,48] In contrast, oral or intravenous nitrates given within the first 24 hours in two mega-trials, ISIS-IV and GISSI-3 (p 41), had no effect. The timing of nitrate administration could be important. In the mega-trials, dosing was started as late as 24 hours after the onset of symptoms, whereas in one of the most careful of the smaller trials, best results were obtained in patients with ST-elevation and within 4 hours of the onset.[19] Therefore, the possible benefit of nitrates, given very early, remains. Also, nitrates may help relieve pain.

**Early beta-blockade** may confer part of its benefits by limitation of infarct size; there is reasonable evidence for a small benefit obtained in the prethrombolytic era.

**Calcium antagonists,** on the other hand, should not be given routinely in AMI,[16] especially not the dihydropyridines (DHPs), such as nifedipine. In non-Q-wave infarction, oral diltiazem was used with benefit but not tested in the acute phase.[14]

**Metabolic support** by glucose-insulin-potassium (GIK) appears to reduce in-hospital mortality in small trials in patients with Killip functional classes I-III.[1] When combined with reperfusion in a small study, there was again benefit from GIK.[36] Interest in GIK is reviving and several larger randomized trials are now in progress. At present, the strongest cases for GIK appear to be (1) when LV failure occurs after bypass surgery,[66] and (2) in a modified regime in diabetics with AMI.

## Long-Term Therapy After AMI

RISK FACTOR MANAGEMENT (Table 11–2). Long-term prognosis depends chiefly on the postinfarct LV function, the LV volume, the absence of ischemia, coronary anatomy, and electrical stability. Patency of the infarct-related artery[152] helps to prevent LV dilation, as does ACE inhibition.[117] Upon this background, control of risk factors remains essential. Cessation of smoking and rehabilitation exercise are of value. Aggressive lipid-lowering by statins is safe and effective (p 299). A Mediterranean type diet is the latest trend and appears to have scientific backing.[72] Reduction of blood pressure also helps.[26] All patients are given aspirin unless it is contraindicated. Recent studies draw attention to the possible prophylactic use of "nutriceuticals," such as vitamin E[86] and other antioxidants, including beta-carotene and flavonoids (p 302). Prospective trials proving protection are not yet available. Postmenopausal hormonal replacement therapy is reasonable in view of the PEPI study (p 302).[106]

TABLE 11–2 POSTINFARCT FOLLOW-UP: PRINCIPLES OF MANAGEMENT

1. **Risk factor modification**
   No smoking, full lipogram, control of hypertension, aerobic exercise, psychological support. Consider lipid-lowering drugs (statins).
2. **Assess extent of coronary disease**
   Residual ischemia? (symptoms, exercise test). Revascularize depending on extent and estimated viability of ischemic tissue.
3. **Assess LV function and size. Avoid LV dilation.**
   If LV dysfunction (low ejection fraction), ACE inhibitors.
4. **Prevention of reinfarction**
   Aspirin, if C/I another antiplatelet agent
   Beta-blockade if not C/I (respiratory disease, diabetes)
   Verapamil (or diltiazem) if beta-blockade C/I provided no LVF
   ACE inhibition (see above)
   Oral anticoagulation for selected patients
5. **Complications**
   Postinfarct angina: nitrates, consider revascularization
   Complex ventricular arrhythmias, symptomatic: consider amiodarone
   Overt LVF: diuretics, ACE inhibitors, nitrates, consider digoxin.
   Look for hibernating myocardium, consider revascularization.

PSYCHOSOCIAL FACTORS. Postinfarct patients who are single, isolated or stressed[62,128] or are depressed[84] may all be suffering from serious psychological depression. The latter is a relative contraindication to beta-blockade, especially propranolol (p 20). If tricyclic antidepressants have to be used, they may interfere with treatment of hypertension or cause tachycardia. Participation in a supervised exercise or rehabilitation program helps to contribute to an optimistic view of life.[48]

BETA-BLOCKADE. All the evidence is that postinfarct beta-blockade provides benefit,[48] reducing total late mortality by a mean of 23%.[141] Although the major benefit of beta-blockade is found in the first year or 18 months, there is documented benefit for up to 2 to 6 years, especially in those with an added indication such as angina or hypertension.[1,85] The present trend is to continue indefinitely, together with aspirin, and, whenever there is LV dysfunction, ACE inhibition. If, as some propose, the mechanism of benefit of beta-blockers is by heart rate reduction, then those with agonist activity should not be effective. Yet acebutolol was strikingly so in the APSI study.[49] More probably beta-blockers protect from the adverse effects of surges of catecholamines. Which subsets of patients are most likely to benefit? Paradoxically, those patients who appear to be at high risk also appear to benefit most. For example, beta-blockade may have its best effects in the presence of heart failure. Patients with a low ejection fraction (below 30%), pulmonary rales or congestion, or an S3 gallop, were all less likely to develop overt congestive heart failure when treated by beta-blockade.[99] ACE inhibitors were not used at that time; it is not clear whether diuretics were given in addition to beta-blockade. What is clear is that the SAVE study has shown that in patients with compromised postinfarct left ventricles, beta-blockers can beneficially be combined with ACE inhibitors, which is therefore the appropriate treatment. Obvious contraindications to beta-blockade remain severe bradycardia, hypotension, asthma, heart block greater than first degree, as well as insulin-dependent diabetes. Overt heart failure remains a contraindication to normal doses of beta-blockers; rather, very low initial doses, thereafter increasing, are now used in selected patients. In the presence of respiratory problems but in the absence of heart failure, verapamil is a viable alternative to beta-blockade (next section). In non-Q-wave infarction with **postinfarct angina,** diltiazem gives relief.[14]

CALCIUM ANTAGONISTS. As a group, these agents do not give postinfarct protection.[16] Yet there are good arguments for verapamil or diltiazem in the absence of LV failure,[82] or when beta-blockade is contraindicated by respiratory disease. In the large Danish postinfarct trial (DAVIT II) in which overt LV failure was prospectively excluded, verapamil 120 mg three times daily decreased reinfarction and cardiac mortality.[81]

PLATELET INHIBITOR AGENTS AND ANTICOAGULANTS. **Aspirin,** the simplest and safest agent, is now established therapy, starting with an oral dose as soon as possible after the onset of symptoms of AMI and continuing indefinitely thereafter. It prevents reinfarction, stroke, and vascular mortality as shown in numerous trials. The mega-trials have started with 160 to 325 mg, and the recent updated meta-analysis[47] suggests a maintenance dose of 75 to 325 mg daily. The lower doses should have fewer side-effects. Aspirin may also be selected for postinfarct follow-up of (1) those patients thought to be at risk of thromboembolism in whom oral anticoagulation is not advisable, and (2) those not likely to comply with the stringent requirements for prolonged oral anticoagulation therapy. When aspirin is contraindicated or not tolerated, then ticlopidine may be the next best.

**Anticoagulants** are usually given for 3 to 6 months postinfarct to patients with prior emboli, in those with LV thrombus (echocardiographically proven), or large anterior infarcts (threatened thrombus), or in those with established atrial fibrillation,[8,12] or in selected patients with overt congestive heart failure (p 265). In low-risk survivors of AMI not treated by aspirin, long-term anticoagulation protects from cerebrovascular events.[50] Under trial is a comparison of warfarin with aspirin or a low-dose combination.

DIGITALIS. The controversy whether digitalis contributes independently to cardiac death in the first year postinfarction has not been settled (p 152). Although several retrospective studies support the possibility that digoxin might contribute to postinfarct mortality,[97] there are no good prospective randomized data. Digoxin should neither be withheld from postinfarct patients with LV failure already treated by diuretics and ACE inhibitors, nor should it be given without careful evaluation of the risk-to-benefit ratio.

ACE INHIBITORS. Prevention of postinfarct LV enlargement is now a major aim.[134A] Apart from their use in postinfarct clinically evident heart failure, ACE inhibitors are now indicated in all patients with LV dysfunction and low ejection fractions to prevent eventual overt LVF, as shown for captopril in the SAVE study.[129] The benefit is not specific to captopril, because the SOLVD study[134] which used enalapril also showed benefit and 80% of the patients were postinfarct. Fascinating data from these trials suggest that these drugs reduce the rate of reinfarction, possibly acting via bradykinin (Table 5–2).

NITRATES. Although the routine use of nitrates in AMI is discredited by the recent mega-trials, it must not be forgotten that ACE inhibition by lisinopril combined with nitroglycerin for 6 weeks gave an impressive reduction in early mortality of 17% in GISSI-3 (Table 5–6).

ANTIARRHYTHMIC AGENTS. Complex ventricular ectopy and VT in the late-hospital phase of myocardial infarction are predictors of subsequent sudden death after discharge, independently of their frequent association with LV dysfunction.[1] Nonetheless, the hoped for benefit of antiarrhythmic therapy on postinfarct mortality is still elusive. Flecainide and other Class IC agents are clearly contraindicated.[5]

**TABLE 11-3** **ATRIAL FIBRILLATION (AF): PRINCIPLES OF MANAGEMENT**

**Acute onset**
- Correct precipitating factors (dehydration, alcohol, pyrexia, etc.).
- Use intravenous AV nodal inhibitors to control ventricular rate (diltiazem,[1] verapamil or beta-blocker; sometimes digoxin; not adenosine).
- If duration of AF < 48 hours, attempt chemical cardioversion[2] with procainamide infusion 15–20 mg/min up to 1,000 mg.
- Electrical cardioversion often required.

**Preparation for elective cardioversion**
- If AF < 3 months, left arrial size < 5 cm.
- Control ventricular rate (digoxin if CHF; otherwise can start with verapamil or diltiazem or beta-blockade). Exclude thyrotoxicosis.
- Oral anticoagulation for 3–4 weeks until after cardioversion. During this period, amiodarone often given as 800–1,600 mg/day for 1 week followed by 200–400 mg/day.
- Hospital admission.
- If patient not receiving amiodarone, start agents that might cardiovert: quinidine, disopyramide, sotalol. Quinidine or disopyramide require digoxin. Quinidine and amiodarone increase blood digoxin levels. Flecainide or propafenone are given only in the absence of structural heart disease, and usually with a beta-blocker or calcium-blocker to avoid a fast ventricular rate.
- Electrical cardioversion.

**Postcardioversion**
One of two policies.
- Aim to maintain sinus rhythm by chronic therapy. Use sotalol or low-dose amiodarone;[3] or in absence of structural heart disease, flecainide (approved in USA) or propafenone (not approved). Procainamide may be used for periods less than 6 months. Anticoagulation continued for 3–6 months, then stop if no recurrences.
- Alternate policy: Leave drug-free and if recurrence, control ventricular rate (digoxin if CHF, otherwise beta- or calcium-blockers). Oral anticoagulation essential.

1. Diltiazem preferred because of clearly defined dose guidelines in package insert, including rate for prolonged infusion.
2. Fenster et al., Am Heart J 1983; 106: 501.
3. Disch et al., Ann Intern Med 1994; 120: 449.

We thank Dr. Frank Marcus and Professor R. Scott Millar for advice.

Overall data with other Class I drugs are discouraging. Rather, beta-blockers and possibly amiodarone are the agents of choice.[141]

# Atrial Fibrillation

This, one of the most common of all arrhythmias, is often not easy to manage (Table 11-3). Two aspects currently emphasized are as follows. First, the use of antiarrhythmic drugs in patients with atrial fibrillation or after cardioversion has been increasingly questioned because the odds of dying from quinidine are increased three times over controls.[69] In general, the use of several other antiarrhythmic drugs may provoke a similar risk if not greater.[83] Hence, one current trend is toward early elective cardioversion whenever possible. A second trend is to acknowledge the risk of thromboembolism not only in recurrent atrial fibrillation, but also at the time of cardioversion. Because cardioversion is associated with a temporary atrial "stunning,"[79] there is probably a risk of thrombus formation even if the atrium is not enlarged. Thus, whenever possible, anticoagulation is required for cardioversion.

ACUTE ONSET ATRIAL FIBRILLATION. Precipitating factors must be treated (p 313). Urgent control of the ventricular rate is achieved by AV nodal inhibitors, such as (1) Class IV agents, verapamil or diltiazem, or (2) intravenous beta-blockade by esmolol, or (3) digoxin, or (4) combinations of these, of which the best documented is esmolol plus digoxin.[132] Other agents that can also be given intravenously include flecainide, propafenone, sotalol and amiodarone.[105] Elective cardioversion is then undertaken once the patient is anticoagulated.

**Urgent cardioversion** may be required if control of the ventricular rate cannot be achieved (consider WPW). In that case, standard practice has been not to anticoagulate for short-duration atrial fibrillation. In view of the newly described condition of atrial "stunning,"[79] logic would dictate that intravenous heparin should be used to cover the urgent cardioversion.

ELECTIVE CARDIOVERSION. Having achieved control of the ventricular rate, by AV nodal inhibitors, the patient is anticoagulated by warfarin while being maintained on drug therapy. Factors favoring drug conversion include a small left atrial size and atrial fibrillation less than 6 months in duration. The risk of embolization at the time of rhythm conversion is about 1% to 2%, so that prophylactic anticoagulation for 3 weeks is standard. Because hospitalization is required for cardioversion, it makes sense to admit the patient 2 days in advance and to attempt chemical cardioversion by one of the drugs inhibiting atrial refractoriness, such as procainamide, disopyramide, flecainide or propafenone. The latter two drugs may not be given in the presence of structural heart disease. If quinidine is given, then concurrent digoxin is essential to avoid a very fast ventricular rate that may result if the fibrillation is converted to flutter and there is enhanced conduction through the AV node resulting from the vagolytic action of quinidine. Post-cardioversion thromboembolism is not excluded by the absence of atrial thrombus on transesophageal echocardiogram.[56]

RECURRENT ATRIAL FIBRILLATION. After two attempts at cardioversion or when atrial fibrillation is known to be recurrent, the preferred drug therapy is probably by low-dose sotalol[95] or low-dose amiodarone.[90,109] At a mean dose of 277 mg, amiodarone maintained 76% of patients with refractory atrial fibrillation in sinus rhythm for over 2 years.[65] Only 3% of patients had pulmonary side-effects. Propafenone[121] or flecainide may also be used, despite their proarrhythmic effects, in selected patients without structural heart disease (both are licensed for this purpose in the USA, whereas sotalol and amiodarone are not).

Rather than aiming to maintain sinus rhythm by antiarrhythmic drugs, another major policy is to accept the existence of atrial fibrillation yet controlling the ventricular response by AV nodal inhibitors, and to provide oral anticoagulation. The logic for this line of therapy is that all the drugs that can be used to maintain sinus rhythm (quinidine, flecainide, propafenone, sotalol and amiodarone) have some potentially toxic side-effect. Hence, there is now a multicenter trial being organized to test whether maintenance of sinus rhythm or ventricular rate control is the better policy.

CHRONIC ATRIAL FIBRILLATION. Now all patients must receive warfarin or, if contraindicated, aspirin (p 267). Risk factor stratification helps to identify those patients who may be given aspirin, but in general the case for warfarin is strong (p 267). When using digoxin and when the ventricular rate seems not to respond, the first move is to check the patient's compliance and the digoxin blood level, to measure plasma potassium, and to reassess for thyrotoxicosis or other systemic or cardiac diseases. Thereafter the digoxin dose may be cautiously increased; however, optimal control of exercise heart rate usually needs a second AV nodal inhibitor such as verapamil, diltiazem, or beta-blockade.[1] In patients without LV failure, verapamil or diltiazem rather than digoxin would be the logical first choice, especially in the presence of angina or hypertension.

The **Maze operation** for atrial fibrillation is an important advance. Chronic atrial fibrillation, the most common of all sustained cardiac arrhythmias, increases morbidity and mortality, yet is often therapy-resistant. Hence, Cox et al.[70] decided to create an electrical maze. Numerous sutures in a labyrinthine pattern are made to stop potential macro-reentry circuits. Appropriate surgical incisions guide the impulse from the SA to the AV node with exiting blind alleys to allow normal atrial excitation. Initial results are encouraging, yet some patients require a permanent pacemaker.

## Other Supraventricular Arrhythmias

ATRIAL FLUTTER. Satisfactory control of the ventricular rate may be extremely difficult to achieve, but flutter is easily converted by a low-energy countershock. In the prevention of recurrent atrial flutter, sotalol or low-dose amiodarone may be tried. For resistant or recurrent cases, catheter ablation of the AV node with pacemaker implantation is increasingly used. After cardiac surgery, the use of temporary atrial pacing electrodes for rapid atrial pacing is particularly helpful in the management of postoperative paroxysmal atrial flutter.

CHAOTIC MULTIFOCAL ATRIAL TACHYCARDIA may respond to verapamil.[23] It is sometimes caused by theophylline toxicity. There appear to be no formal drug trials.

SUPRAVENTRICULAR TACHYCARDIA (Table 11–4). In the standard paroxysmal type (PSVT) with nodal re-entry, **vagotonic procedures** (Valsalva maneuver, facial immersion in cold water, or carotid sinus massage) may terminate the tachycardia. Always auscultate the carotid arteries before performing carotid sinus massage. If these measures fail, intravenous diltiazem, intravenous verapamil, intravenous esmolol, or intravenous adenosine are the choices (Chapter 8). Adenosine with its ultrashort duration of action is safest, especially if there is a diagnostic problem between PSVT with aberrant conduction and wide complex VT. If these steps fail, vagotonic maneuvers are worth repeating. *Thereafter the choice lies between intravenous digitalization*, or intravenous Class IC agents of which the best may be propafenone (intravenous use now approved in the USA), or cardioversion, and should be tempered by the clinical condition of the patient.

In **refractory paroxysmal supraventricular tachycardia,** innovative surgical approaches and **catheter ablation** have radically improved prognosis in refractory cases. Patients with supraventricular arrhythmias that are very rapid or refractory to standard drugs, or associated with a wide QRS complex on the standard electrocardiogram (implying either aberration, antegrade pre-excitation, or VT) warrant an invasive electrophysiologic study. In the majority of other patients, drug management is successful.

In the prevention of PSVT, the initiating ectopic beats may be inhibited by beta-blockade, verapamil, diltiazem, or by amiodarone. The latter is highly effective for supraventricular arrhythmias including paroxysmal atrial fibrillation and arrhythmias involving accessory pathways; potentially severe side-effects may be limited by a low dose (p 231). The Class IC drugs (propafenone or flecainide) are viable alternatives, but should not be used in the presence of structural heart disease in view of the CAST study,[5] as confirmed in the package inserts.

TABLE 11–4   PAROXYSMAL SUPRAVENTRICULAR TACHYCARDIA:
PRINCIPLES OF MANAGEMENT

**Entry point**
- Narrow QRS complex tachycardia; either AV nodal reentry or WPW. If *atrial flutter*, proceed straight to DC cardioversion.

**Emergency therapy: hemodynamically stable**
- Vagal maneuvers
- Intravenous AV nodal blockers (adenosine,[1] verapamil, diltiazem, esmolol; high success rate)
- Occasionally IV propafenone
- Synchronized DC cardioversion
- Burst pacing in selected cases, eg., post-bypass surgery

**Emergency therapy: hemodynamically unstable**
- Intravenous adenosine (not other AV nodal blockers)
- Must cardiovert if adenosine unsuccessful.

**Follow-up: PSVT with nodal reentry**
- Self-therapy by vagal procedures
- Prevention by long-acting AV-nodal blockers (verapamil, diltiazem, standard beta-blockers, digoxin)
- If repetitive attacks, perinodal ablation to inhibit re-entry through atrial slow pathways.[2] Some risk of AV nodal damage requiring permanent pacemaker

**Follow-up: WPW (delta wave during sinus rhythm)**
- Catheter ablation of bypass tract
- Sometimes surgery (young children; associated anomalies; multiple paths)
- Occasionally drug therapy: Class IC or Class III agents. Digoxin contraindicated, avoid other AV nodal blockers

**Follow-up: atrial flutter**
- Prevention by sotalol, amiodarone, or ablation of flutter circuits
- Rate control by AV nodal inhibitors (verapamil, diltiazem, beta-blocker, digoxin or combination)
- May consider AV nodal ablation and permanent pacemaker

**Catheter ablation**
- Being used earlier and earlier for follow-up of PSVT whether WPW present or not

1. Adenosine, ultrashort-acting preferred (see Reference 105); with esmolol, its action wears off relatively quickly allowing subsequent safer use of verapamil or diltiazem if needed.
2. Wu et al., J Am Coll Cardiol 1993; 21:1612.

We thank Professor R. Scott Millar for comments.

WOLFF-PARKINSON-WHITE SYNDROME   (Table 11–4). The acute treatment of choice is cardioversion if the patient is hemodynamically compromised. If presenting with narrow complex PSVT, the same intravenous therapy as for standard PVST may be followed (Table 11–4). For follow-up, because of the risk of **antegrade pre-excitation** via the bypass tract, then digoxin is *absolutely contraindicated* (because it shortens the refractory period of the tract). Verapamil, diltiazem, and beta-blockade may be dangerous by blocking the AV node and redirecting impulses down the bypass tract. Sotalol, with Class III properties, is an exception. In the prevention of paroxysmal supraventricular tachycardia including atrial fibrillation, surgical or catheter ablation of the accessory pathway is often highly successful and is now standard treatment. Otherwise, low-dose amiodarone is probably best (Fig. 8–4) followed by sotalol or propafenone.

## Bradyarrhythmias

Asymptomatic sinus bradycardia does not require therapy and may be normal, especially in athletes. For symptomatic **sinus bradycardia, sick sinus syndrome,** and **sinoatrial disease,** probanthine and chronic atropine are unsatisfactory in the long run so that pacing is usually required. First, however, the adverse effects of drugs such as beta-blockers, digitalis, verapamil, diltiazem, quinidine, procainamide, amiodarone, lidocaine, methyldopa, clonidine and lithium carbonate should be excluded.

In the **tachycardia/bradycardia syndrome,** intrinsic sinus node dysfunction is difficult to treat and once again may require pacemaking. Standard beta-blockers aggravate the bradycardic component of the syndrome, while pindolol with marked agonist activity (ISA) may be useful. Patients usually end up with a combination of a permanent pacemaker and antiarrhythmic agents.

For **AV block with syncope** or with excessively slow rates, atropine or isoproterenol or transthoracic pacing is used as an emergency measure, pending pacemaker implantation.

## Ventricular Arrhythmias and Proarrhythmic Problems

The criteria for instituting drug therapy are not clear-cut, although patients with sustained VT (Table 11–5), survivors of previous arrhythmia-related cardiac arrest, and those with severely symptomatic arrhythmias, all require treatment. *A full cardiologic assessment* is required. An essential adjunct to antiarrhythmic therapy lies in the management of underlying disease such as LVF, ischemia, anemia, thyrotoxicosis, or electrolyte imbalance. There is no evidence that therapy of asymptomatic ventricular arrhythmias, even in the presence of heart disease, prolongs life or prevents sudden death. Rather, the CAST study[5] warns that the proarrhythmic effects of some Class IC agents can actually increase mortality in patients with ischemic heart disease. The most effective way to prevent sudden death in patients with coronary disease is to eliminate ischemia and to improve LV function, often by coronary bypass surgery.[20]

The *choice of drug* for chronic use is ideally based on prior demonstration during acute and chronic Holter or electrophysiologic testing that the drug actually works and on its potential for toxicity in the individual under study. Class I agents including quinidine, disopyramide and mexilitine are still used. Propafenone is possibly the most effective and least harmful of the Class IC agents, although not as good as beta-blockade or amiodarone in the CASH study[63] in which the propafenone arm was discontinued. The antiarrhythmic effect of empiric beta-blockade monotherapy for VT is impressive and reportedly as good as electrophysiologic-guided drug choice.[135] Although the ESVEM study[76] has been much criticized, it did highlight that the Class III beta-blocker sotalol outperformed six Class I antiarrhythmics. Beta-blockers are among the few antiarrhythmic agents with positive long-term beneficial effects in postinfarct patients.[141] In those not responding to beta-blockade, or in whom beta-blockade is contraindicated, low-dose amiodarone is increasingly used, despite potentially serious side-effects. Like beta-blockade, amiodarone appears to give postinfarct protection although not all the studies have been completed.[141] In the CASCADE study,[61] empiric amiodarone was better than Class I agents in patients who were survivors of out-of-hospital ventricular fibrillation. Deciding between the agents

**TABLE 11–5 ACUTE SUSTAINED VENTRICULAR TACHYCARDIA OR SIMILAR TACHYCARDIA**

**Entry point: wide QRS complex tachycardia**

About 90% will be wide complex ventricular tachycardia; the others will include PSVT with aberration or WPW with anterograde conduction.

- DC cardioversion—procedure of choice, usually effective
- If DC cardioversion fails or if patient hemodynamically stable, IV lidocaine (safe but will only revert a minority)[1]
- IV procainamide (more effective but less safe)
- Or, where available, IV disopyramide (not in USA)
- Occasionally IV amiodarone (not in USA) or bretylium
- If torsades de pointes, IV magnesium sulfate
- If VT recurs soon after cardioversion, repeat the latter under cover of lidocaine or other IV drug
- (Only if PSVT presents as suspected VT, use IV adenosine for diagnosis but never verapamil nor diltiazem)

**Follow-up of acute attack**

- (If PSVT, see Table 11–4)
- If VT (majority), requires thorough cardiological evaluation. Need accurate diagnosis of rhythm, structural heart disease, and LV function.
- Empirical drug approach (sotalol, beta-blockers, sometimes amiodarone)
- or, Holter-guided choice
- or, electrophysiologic-guided choice
- Sometimes surgery (LV aneurysm)
- Catheter ablation if idiopathic refractory VT
- Implantable cardioverter/defibrillator if high risk of sudden death; or if other therapy ineffective

1. Griffiths et al., Lancet 1990, 336:670.
We thank Professor R. Scott Millar for comments.

currently available is somewhat of a personal choice and not entirely logical.

**Non-pharmacologic approaches** to the management of ventricular arrhythmias include sophisticated pacing modalities and surgery in conjunction with electrophysiologic mapping. Excellent results can be achieved in selected patients. The automatic **implantable cardioverter defibrillator (ICD)** is now an integral part of the management of patients with malignant ventricular arrhythmias. It is not yet certain whether an ICD gives a better outcome than a beta-blocker or amiodarone in survivors of sudden cardiac death[63] (see p 336).

# Congestive Heart Failure

GENERAL POLICY. Despite newer agents (particularly the ACE inhibitors), the long-term prognosis of CHF remains poor, unless a reversible cause, for instance valvular heart disease or hypertension, is present. The initial steps in a patient with heart failure are to investigate the cause and treat associated conditions including hypertension, thyrotoxicosis, and anemia. The past policy was to initiate treatment with diuretics, salt restriction, then digitalis before proceeding to conventional vasodilators. The current trend is to use ACE inhibitors from the start of symptoms (with diuretics), or even before, in asymptomatic LV dysfunction (without diuretics). The role of digitalis in patients with atrial fibrillation cannot be contested. In others, its hemodynamic benefits have now been re-established particularly in patients with more severe heart failure (p 147). Outcome studies on digitalis are still awaited. Combination "triple therapy" of diuretics, ACE inhibition, and digitalis is increasingly used as standard therapy for moderate to severe heart failure.

DIURETIC THERAPY. Doses and drugs should not be fixed. Diuretics may need to be reduced at the time of addition or increase of dose of the ACE inhibitor, or diuretic therapy may have to be stepped up in cases of refractory edema. Especially in severe right ventricular failure, the absorption of drugs given orally is impaired and a short course of intravenous furosemide can be very helpful. A pharmacokinetic adverse interaction of captopril and furosemide[123] needs to be considered. Therefore, ACE inhibitors other than captopril become the agents of choice when furosemide is used and a diuresis is critical. Alternatively, very low dose captopril is appropriate (p 124). The principle of sequential nephron blockade (Fig. 4–1) states that different types of diuretics can synergistically be added, such as a thiazide to a loop diuretic. An ACE inhibitor by its antialdosterone effect can act on the same site as spironolactone. Especially in patients with poor renal function, the combination of an ACE inhibitor and a potassium-retaining diuretic can precipitate hyperkalemia. **Posture** can influence diuretic efficacy.[2] To improve renal perfusion and to increase diuresis, the patient may have to return to bed for 1 to 2 hours of supine rest after taking a diuretic.

ACE INHIBITORS AND VASODILATORS. The most recent VA study (V-HeFT-II, p 115) with enalapril showed further benefit of ACE inhibition added to vasodilation by nitrates and hydralazine. The ACE inhibitor reduced sudden death, probably by an antiarrhythmic mechanism. The vasodilators were better at improving exercise capacity. In patients with pulmonary congestion, nitrates given at night can decisively improve sleep. As in angina, transdermal nitrates with 24-hour action cause tolerance.

BETA-BLOCKERS. Their use in congestive heart failure caused by cardiomyopathy remains highly controversial although steadily increasing. Some patients respond dramatically to cautious addition of low-dose metoprolol starting with 5 mg daily and working up to 150 mg daily over 6 weeks.[149] Others unexpectedly deteriorate. In 383 patients with dilated cardiomyopathy, metoprolol gave longterm symptomatic benefit without improving mortality.[149] Vasodilatory beta-blockers, well-tested in dilated cardiomyopathy, include carvedilol and bucindolol (p 14). Of these, carvedilol is closest to FDA approval, while a longer term trial with mortality as end-point will delay final assessment of bucindolol until about 1998.

VENTRICULAR ARRHYTHMIAS IN CHF. Amiodarone may be the drug of choice (p 241). Prophylactic antiarrhythmic therapy is contraindicated, especially since most antiarrhythmics inhibit the sinus node and there is a high incidence of bradyarrhythmic deaths in CHF.[24] Furthermore, the incidence of sudden death seems to be falling since the widespread introduction of ACE inhibitors.[114] There is no special place for the prophylactic use of amiodarone in patients with "high density" PVCs, as shown by the VA Co-operative study (p 241). Amiodarone does, however, improve CHF over 2 years in patients with NYHA Classes II and III.[85A,112] In **significantly symptomatic arrhythmias**, it is first essential to pinpoint precipitating factors such as hypokalemia, hypomagnesemia, or use of sympathomimetics, phosphodiesterase inhibitors or digoxin. The hemodynamic status of the myocardium must be made optimal because LV wall stress per se is arrhythmogenic. Antiarrhythmics are only given after documentation of benefit by electrophysiological studies or by ambulatory monitoring.[76] Logically, beta-blockers in initial low doses could be expected to improve LV function and the arrhythmias.

SEVERE INTRACTABLE CHF. Here invasive monitoring by Swan-Ganz catheterization may be necessary both to evaluate the hemodynamic status and, usually, to initiate tailored intravenous therapy as a bridge to oral agents. Theoretically, phosphodiesterase inhibitors, such as **amrinone** and **milrinone,** should be able to bypass the downgraded or uncoupled beta-receptors to evoke a better inotropic response than beta-receptor stimulants, such as dobutamine; yet a multicentered randomized study showed that **milrinone** (50 μg/kg bolus, followed by 0.5–0.625 μg/kg/min) gave similar effects to **dobutamine** with somewhat less initial chronotropic effect.[1] Further beta-receptor downgrading is a hazard in the case of dobutamine; there is loss of a sustained effect during one week of intravenous infusion.[1] **Dopamine** remains the agent of choice when it is thought that poor renal perfusion contributes to the clinical picture. Intermittent **intravenous nitroglycerin** tides some patients over,[74] and is the logical choice for ischemic cardiomyopathy. The dose of **ACE inhibitor** needs to be high to overcome intense renin-angiotensin activation, yet hypotension must be avoided.[116] Paradoxically, when a diuresis is required, lower ACE doses may improve renal perfusion and enhance diuresis.[138]

DIASTOLIC DYSFUNCTION.   Traditional concepts of heart failure emphasize the primary role of systolic ventricular dysfunction. In patients with a clinical diagnosis of heart failure, there is preserved LV systolic function in about 40%, thereby emphasizing the role of "diastolic dysfunction." The role of calcium antagonists and beta-blockers in this syndrome needs further evaluation; either therapy may work and can be combined with a mild diuretic if there is evidence of fluid retention. Fundamental therapy, however, is to aim for regression of massive LVH, the underlying cause of diastolic dysfunction. In hypertensive hearts, ACE inhibition is theoretically sound. In the elderly with increased myocardial stiffness, therapy is still indicated even though regression may not be achieved.

NEW AGENTS FOR CHF.   Of the various new agents, results with the vasodilator flosequinan, the inotrope vesnarinone, xamoterol (mixed beta-blocker plus partial agonist), nifedipine, and milrinone have all been disappointing when taking as end-point not short-term hemodynamic benefit but the long-term outcome. None of these are FDA-approved. Beta-blockade, initially in very low doses, seems a promising advance and is the subject of large American trials involving bucindolol and carvedilol. In Europe, metoprolol is best studied.

GENERAL MANAGEMENT.   Sodium restriction and, in severe cases, water limitation are important ancillary measures. It is often forgotten that in severe CHF there is delayed water diuresis. Weight loss and exercise rehabilitation, as well as psychological support, are all positive procedures.

CHF: SUMMARY.   In patients with mild CHF, initial therapy is a diuretic combined with an ACE inhibitor. In more severe CHF, digoxin is added. The triple combination of diuretics, ACE inhibitors and digoxin is now standard, followed by addition of vasodilators such as nitrates. An ACE inhibitor is often used as initial therapy in presymptomatic LV dysfunction. The lot of the individual patient with severe CHF can be improved by searching out underlying causes, by diuretic synergism, by adjustment of the dose of the ACE inhibitor and digoxin, by checking on serum potassium and magnesium, and by general management including salt restriction and exercise rehabilitation. Sometimes added beta-blockade started in very low doses and titrated upward may give decisive added benefit.

## Acute Pulmonary Edema

In acute pulmonary edema of cardiac origin, the initial management requires positioning the patient in an upright posture and oxygen administration. If the underlying cause is a tachyarrhythmia, restoration of sinus rhythm takes priority. **Morphine sulfate** is highly effective in relieving symptoms. Its mechanism of action is not precisely understood, but a venodilator action and a central sedative effect are likely.[1] **Intravenous furosemide,** which acts both as a diuretic and a vasodilator, is the other basic therapy. **Sublingual nitrates** are excellent for unloading of the left heart and relief of pulmonary congestion. If severe hypertension is the underlying cause, **intravenous nicardipine** or **intravenous sodium nitroprusside,** together with careful monitoring of pressures, may be required. Particular caution is necessary in the patient with a systolic blood pressure of less than 90 mmHg, if **vasodilators** are contemplated. In patients with pulmonary edema secondary to severe acute or chronic mitral or aortic regurgitation, intravenous nitroprusside is probably the agent of choice. **Oral ACE inhibitors** are started as soon as feasible, taking care to prevent hypotension. There is no reported experience with **intravenous enalaprilat,** a logical choice to achieve rapid ACE inhibition. Once acute pulmonary edema has been relieved and in the absence of AMI, **acute digitalization** is cautiously started (0.5 mg digoxin intravenously over 30 minutes, followed by oral digoxin to a total of 1.0 mg within 24 hours), and the patient continued on furosemide and ACE inhibitors. In AMI, xanthine compounds such as aminophylline or theophylline are also best avoided because of their proarrhythmic potential. Bronchospasm will usually respond to diuresis or load reduction. Otherwise, **aminophylline** may be given at 6 mg/kg intravenously over 30 minutes followed by 0.5 mg/kg/h with monitoring of plasma potassium, arrhythmias and respiration.

In refractory cases, resort to rotating tourniquets or intubation with mechanical ventilation. Pulmonary edema of cardiac origin must be differentiated from the adult respiratory distress syndrome, which requires specific therapy.

# Cardiomyopathy

## Hypertrophic Cardiomyopathy (IHSS)

Although many patients are asymptomatic, there is risk of sudden cardiac death, which mandates avoidance of competitive sports even in the absence of symptoms. Nonetheless, those who continue to play may not be entirely bent on suicide—a recent NIH series records 14 such patients alive and well.[107] The cornerstone of drug therapy in symptomatic patients is to avoid agents that increase cardiac contractility, such as digitalis, or those that reduce ventricular preload, such as nitrates or diuretics. The major new development is **dual chamber pacing,**[78] which gives benefit in patients resistant to verapamil or beta-blockade.

VERAPAMIL VS. PROPRANOLOL. Three basic drug therapies have been used: beta-blockade, calcium antagonists (especially verapamil), and disopyramide. Each has its advocates. **High-dose propranolol** is most widely used and frequently reduces symptoms. **Verapamil** is preferred in patients with asthma or other contraindications to beta-blockade and is usually well tolerated. Verapamil is logical therapy to relieve the diastolic relaxation problems found in hypertrophic cardiomyopathy.[1]

OBSTRUCTIVE CARDIOMYOPATHY. Verapamil plus myectomy was highly successful in a retrospective survey over 10 years.[131] It is not clear how many of these patients had clinical obstruction in which occasional dangerous or even lethal side-effects with verapamil have been reported. The afterload reducing effect of verapamil may be more vigorous than the negative inotropic effect, so that outflow tract obstruction is precipitated. Therefore, a cautious start with careful monitoring of verapamil effects is required. **Nifedipine** is contraindicated in patients with resting obstruction,[1] and this stricture applies to all DHPs with their greater vascular selectivity. **Disopyramide** (150 mg 4 times daily), but not propranolol or placebo, virtually abolished the subaortic pressure gradient in a small group of patients;[32] however, the use of propranolol is better established and has other documented benefits such as relief of symptoms.

ANTIARRHYTHMICS. When severe arrhythmias intervene or are feared, **amiodarone** is the antiarrhythmic of choice.[137] In patients with a family history of sudden death, syncope, or severe dyspnea, or in patients in whom malignant arrhythmias are suspected for other reasons, Holter monitoring for 48 to 72 hours is required to evaluate the need for, and the effects of antiarrhythmic therapy. **Disopyramide** should have antiarrhythmic as well as hemodynamic benefit. In those who have already experienced cardiac arrest, an automatic **implantable cardioverter defibrillator (ICD)** is the therapy of choice.

SURGERY. For refractory symptoms, **dual chamber pacing**[78] is usually undertaken before resorting to septal myectomy. The exact indications for operation are not widely agreed upon nor is the mechanism of benefit settled.[25] The role of mitral valve replacement is even more controversial.[21]

HYPERTENSIVE HYPERTROPHIC CARDIOMYOPATHY. In the elderly it responds to beta-blockers or verapamil.[1] Digitalis, diuretics and load reducers such as nifedipine or ACE inhibitors are all contraindicated.

## Dilated Cardiomyopathy

The standard therapy for CHF in this condition consists of diuretics, ACE inhibitors, and inotropic support. Beta-blockers (metoprolol and others, see p 14) are increasingly used starting with an ultra-low dose.[149] Metoprolol may be particularly useful in the presence of sinus tachycardia or ventricular arrhythmias.[96] Specific antiarrhythmic therapy is not as logical as previously thought because most antiarrhythmic drugs can depress LV function. For atrial fibrillation, anticoagulation is usual.[1] Immunosuppressive therapy by prednisone is not part of routine treatment, as shown in a multicenter study.[29] A large trial, not yet published, evaluated different immunosuppressives and showed no benefit. In severe disease, **dual chamber pacing** may help supposedly by avoiding the shortened time for ventricular filling.[58]

**Cardiac transplantation** is used for selected patients with cardiomyopathy failing to respond to comprehensive conservative therapy, including cautious beta-blockade. Select an experienced transplant center, expert in all phases of care, and do not wait until there is deterioration in the patient's general health. Conversely, the decision to transplant must not lightly be made until a full trial of modern anti-CHF therapy, probably including beta-blockade and optimal "tailored vasodilator treatment," has been undertaken.[136]

# Valvular Heart Disease

RHEUMATIC FEVER PROPHYLAXIS. Treatment should start as soon as a definitive diagnosis of streptococcal infection has been made; the treatment is either a single dose of benzathine penicillin—1,200,000 units for adults and half dose for children—or a full 10-day course of oral penicillin-V (125 to 250 mg three times daily). Thereafter, in selected patients in whom recurrences are feared, the penicillin injection is repeated monthly, or pencillin-V is given as 125 to 250 mg twice daily continuously.[37] The best route is by injection, which is used for 5 years followed by oral prophylaxis possibly for life.

GENERAL APPROACH TO VALVULAR HEART DISEASE. In most patients with symptomatic valvular regurgitation or stenosis, valve replacement or repair is indicated. As surgical techniques and the performance of prosthetic valves have improved, so have the surgical indications become less stringent. Now most patients with LV dysfunction are operated on even if asymptomatic. The indications for surgery for other patients with severe but asymptomatic valvular regurgitation are less clearly established. Concomitant therapy in patients with valvular heart disease may include diuretics, digitalis and, especially for certain nonstenotic lesions, vasodilators, including ACE inhibitors. Attention to arrhythmias, particularly atrial fibrillation, is essential and anticoagulants may be needed (p 266).

AORTIC STENOSIS. In valvular stenosis, the basic problem is obstructive and requires surgical relief. Sometimes excessive peripheral vasoconstriction requires relief by carefully titrated afterload reduction. For example, captopril initiated under hemodynamic monitoring improved a small group of nonoperable patients with severe aortic stenosis.[91] However, afterload reduction is generally contraindicated, because it increases the pressure gradient across the stenosed valve. In **aortic stenosis with angina,** preload reduction by nitrates must be cautious to avoid an excess fall in the filling pressure. Surgical therapy is required for those with angina, exertional syncope or symptoms of LV failure. Surgery can relieve the hypertrophy, to improve the coronary perfusion pressure, and often to correct accompanying coronary artery disease. Percutaneous aortic balloon valvuloplasty has been disappointing, but offers a reasonable alternative when surgery is contraindicated. In truly **asymptomatic aortic stenosis,** which is nonetheless hemodynamically significant, the key to the management is careful and regular supervision, with intervention as soon as symptoms appear.[115]

MITRAL STENOSIS. In **mitral stenosis with sinus rhythm,** beta-blockade by atenolol improves exercise capacity and is preferable to propranolol to lessen possible pulmonary symptoms. Prophylactic digitalization is still sometimes used supposedly to avoid a high ventricular rate during intermittent atrial fibrillation; this practice is not supported by the available data.[120] Balloon valvuloplasty is now established for relief of stenosis with selection of patients depending on the echocardiographic characteristics of the valve. **Paroxysmal atrial fibrillation** precipitating left-sided failure may require carefully titrated intravenous diltiazem, verapamil or esmolol, provided that the left ventricle itself is not depressed in function (associated mitral regurgitation). In **established atrial fibrillation,** digitalization is usually not enough to prevent an excessive ventricular rate during exercise, so that digoxin should be augmented by diltiazem, verapamil, or beta-blockade. Anticoagulation is essential for those with atrial fibrillation and merits consideration for those in sinus rhythm thought to be at high risk for atrial fibrillation (marked left atrial enlargement or frequent atrial extrasystoles).

MITRAL OR AORTIC VALVE REGURGITATION. Afterload reduction is much more effective in regurgitation than in stenosis. Either nifedipine[130] or enalapril[101A] benefits those with asymptomatic aortic regurgitation. In severe or symptomatic regurgitation, valve replacement is required. The current trend is to operate earlier both to prevent ventricular dilation and to "preserve the atrium," hence hopefully avoiding atrial fibrillation. Postinfarct mitral regurgitation, caused by chordal rupture or papillary muscle infarction, can precipitate sudden deterioration and has long-term risks, despite optimal therapy including ACE inhibitors.

# Infective Endocarditis

The management of **acute or subacute endocarditis** varies with the etiology and virulence of the infecting organism and the clinical manifestations of the episode. Consideration should be given to differences between prosthetic and native valve endocarditis in the prognosis, bacteriologic spectrum, and the response to therapy. Recently, an increase in endocarditis has occurred in drug addicts and in immunological compromised patients with more drug-resistant "exotic organisms."

Optimal therapy requires identification of the **causative organism,** which may delay initiation of therapy in subacute endocarditis for a short period. Definitive antibiotic therapy is based on susceptibility testing and requires the advice of an expert in infectious diseases. In culture-negative endocarditis therapy is empiric. The causative organism is still usually a streptococcus viridans, susceptible to penicillin-gentamicin. If a penicillin-resistant streptococcus is suspected, even if not proven, ampicillin-gentamicin is required. For penicillin allergy, **vancomycin** with or without **gentamicin** is used. Conditions predisposing the patient to infective endocarditis, such as poor dental hygiene or genito-urinary tract pathology, must be remedied.

INDICATIONS FOR SURGERY.   An increasing aggressive approach to early cardiac surgery has favorably influenced the outcome of infective endocarditis.[1] In patients with **native valve endocarditis,** the indications for surgery are heart failure resulting from valve dysfunction, uncontrolled infection, new conduction disturbances suggestive of ring abscess formation, fungal infection, relapse after initially successful therapy, and possibly recurrent emboli.[1] The approach to **prosthetic valve endocarditis,** particularly within three months of the initial operation, is also aggressive, with surgery for any signs of prosthetic valve dysfunction or any of the indications for surgery in native valves.[1] In the face of hemodynamic decompensation, surgery should not be delayed pending completion of antibiotic therapy.

ANTICOAGULANT THERAPY.   The decision to initiate or continue anticoagulant therapy in patients with infective endocarditis is often difficult. In those patients already on anticoagulants (eg., patients with mechanical prostheses or those in whom there are other indications for anticoagulation, such as thrombophlebitis) anticoagulant therapy should be continued or initiated. In the event of a cerebral thromboembolic complication, the risk of anticoagulant-induced hemorrhage must be balanced against the alternate risk of recurrent embolism.

ANTIBIOTIC PROPHYLAXIS.   Both American and European practice are based on **amoxycillin** prophylaxis (Tables 11–6 and 11–7). Chemoprophylaxis is indicated for patients with increased susceptibility to infective endocarditis, who must undergo dental procedures that may produce a bacteremia. In the case of GU or GI procedures, the organism is often an enterococcus. Standard prophylaxis is by the ampicillin-gentamicin-amoxycillin regime, or vancomycin (penicillin allergy) or oral amoxycillin alone (if risk is low). Cardiac indications for antibiotic prophylaxis are rheumatic or other acquired valvular heart disease, prosthetic heart valves or a prosthetic patch, hypertrophic obstructive cardiomyopathy, prior infective endocarditis, and congenital heart disease (excepting uncomplicated secundum atrial septal defects and repaired patent ductus arteriosus). In **mitral valve prolapse** with only a click, antibiotic prophylaxis is debatable; when there is a murmur, prophylaxis is definitely desirable.[6] Even in **high-risk patients** (prosthetic valves, a history of endocarditis, or surgical shunts or conduits), oral prophylaxis can be used although intravenous agents give maximal protection.[68]

## Cor Pulmonale

Therapy of right heart failure is similar to that of left heart failure, except that digitalis appears to be less effective because of a combination of hypoxemia, electrolyte disturbances, and enhanced adrener-

TABLE 11–6    AMERICAN RECOMMENDED ANTIBIOTIC REGIMENS FOR
DENTAL/RESPIRATORY TRACT PROCEDURES

| **Standard regimen** | |
| --- | --- |
| For **dental procedures** that cause gingival bleeding, and oral/respiratory tract surgery (can also use for high-risk patients[68]) | Amoxicillin 3.0 g 1 h before procedure, then 1.5g 6 h later. For patients unable to take oral medication, ampicillin 2.0g IV or IM 30 min before a procedure and 1 mU 6 h later |
| **Special regimens** | |
| Parenteral regimen for use when maximal protection desired; eg., for patients with prosthetic valves | Ampicillin 1.0–2.0 g IM or IV *plus* gentamicin 1.5 mg/kg IM or IV 1/2 h before procedure, followed by 1.5 g oral amoxicillin 6 h later |
| Oral regimen for amoxicillin or penicillin-allergic patients | Erythromycin stearate 1.0 g orally 2 h before, then 500 mg 6 h later |
| Parenteral regimen for ampicillin or penicillin-allergic patients | Clindamycin IV 300 mg* 30 min before procedure and 150 mg IV 6 h later |
| Parenteral regimen for high-risk patients | Vancomycin 1.0 g IV slowly over 1 h starting 1 h before. No repeat dose is necessary |

\* To avoid hypotension, give over 10 minutes (see Simmons et al.[133]).

From Committee on Rheumatic Fever.[68] "Later" = after the initial dose.

gic discharge. Thus when atrial fibrillation develops, cautious vera-pamil or diltiazem is preferred to reduce the ventricular rate. In general, all beta-blockers should be avoided because of the risk of bronchospasm. Bronchodilators should be beta$_2$-selective. For example, **albuterol** (**salbutamol**), has relatively little effect on the heart rate, while unloading the left heart by peripheral vasodilation.

## Pulmonary Hypertension

**Primary pulmonary hypertension** includes a variety of histologic appearances and probably pathogenic mechanisms, while excluding

TABLE 11–7    EUROPEAN RECOMMENDATIONS: ANTIBIOTIC PROPHYLAXIS
OF INFECTIVE ENDOCARDITIS FOR ADULTS DURING
DENTAL PROCEDURES

| NOT ALLERGIC TO PENICILLIN | | ALLERGIC TO PENICILLIN | |
| --- | --- | --- | --- |
| ORAL AMOXYCILLIN | IV OR IM AMOXYCILLIN | ORAL CLINDAMYCIN | IV TEICOPLANIN |
| 3 g 1 h before | 1 g just before 0.5 g 6 h later | 600 mg 1 h before | 400 mg IV plus gentamicin 120 mg IV **or** IV clindamycin 300 mg just before and 150 mg 6 h later |

Modified from Delaye et al.[7] and from Simmons et al.[133]

For cautions and instructions, see British National Formulary.[57]

pulmonary hypertension secondary to chronic pulmonary disease. Unless lung biopsy is performed, the pathogenesis cannot be established, and long-term anticoagulants are frequently used on the assumption that there is thromboembolism or thrombosis in situ.[124]

Calcium antagonists are increasingly being tried, one of the best documented being high-dose **nifedipine** (up to 240 mg daily).[34] Special care must be taken to watch for serious side-effects, such as hypotension or heart failure. This use is not FDA-approved. In one large study on 64 patients, 17 patients on high-dose nifedipine or diltiazem (720 mg daily) were alive after 5 years and the result was regarded as good.[124] Intravenous prostacyclin from a portable pump may provide a bridge to lung or heart-lung transplantation.

# Peripheral Vascular Disease

The basic problem is vascular atheroma, added to which are (1) variable degrees of arterial spasm and (2) variable severities of arterial thrombosis and platelet aggregation and embolization. Thus far, the medical therapy has been disappointing. The most effective attack on atheroma has been by surgery, where the big advance has been the use of catheter-based therapies including lasers and stents. The basis of present therapy is interventional whenever possible. Correction of coronary risk factors appears to play little role, except that cessation of smoking is essential in most types of active peripheral vascular disease. Exercise training benefits[10] and aspirin protects.[47] Chelation therapy does not work.[148A]

**Pentoxifylline** (**Trental**) decreases blood viscosity and maintains red cell flexibility of the erythrocytes as they are squeezed through the capillary bed. It is licensed for use in intermittent claudication[1] in the USA (600 to 1200 mg daily in three divided doses with meals; side-effect nausea).

In the future, therapy will logically be aimed at decreasing blood viscosity more effectively and lessening leucocyte activation.[102]

**Iloprost,** a prostacyclin analog, given by daily infusion for 4 to 28 days, healed ulcers and improved ischemic pain in patients with severe thromboangiitis obliterans (Burger's disease); aspirin was much less effective.[11] The serotonin antagonist, **ketanserin,** is of no benefit.[28]

**L-carnitine** (levocarnitine, **Carnitor;** not licensed for this indication)(2 g twice daily) improved the walking capacity of patients with intermittent claudication without hemodynamic effects, probably acting through a metabolic mechanism;[4] further confirmatory trials are required. L-propionylcarnitine seems more effective but must be given intravenously.[59]

CLAUDICATION PLUS HYPERTENSION.   Captopril maintains walking distance better than atenolol, labetalol, or pindolol.[127]

CLAUDICATION PLUS ANGINA.   Beta-blockers are still generally held to be contraindicated in the presence of active peripheral vascular disease, although a meta-analysis of 11 pooled trials showed no adverse effects on the walking distance in mild to moderate disease.[119] Calcium antagonists may, therefore, be preferred to beta-blockers, although there are no comparative studies. Experimentally, all ACE inhibitors and calcium antagonists inhibit the early stages of atheroma by complex mechanisms, yet cannot routinely be advised for this purpose.

*In summary,* the basis of medical therapy lies in cessation of smoking, exercise training, and aspirin. Interventional therapy is increasingly important. Pentoxifylline and, possibly, L-carnitine may be useful. Coronary artery disease is often associated, and requires therapy in its own right.

## Raynaud's Phenomenon

Once a secondary cause has been excluded (for example vasculitis, scleroderma, or lupus erythematosus), then **calcium channel antagonists** are logical. Nifedipine is best tested and one 10 mg capsule may be taken intermittently at the start of an attack.[35] Beta-blockers are traditionally contraindicated, although low-dose propranolol or metoprolol did not exaggerate primary Raynaud's phenomenon (see also absence of effect of beta-blockers in mild to moderate peripheral vascular disease[119]).

## Beri-Beri Heart Disease

This condition is characterized by high output CHF due to thiamine deficiency. Common in Africa and Asia, in Western countries it is underdiagnosed especially in alcoholics.[9] The basis of treatment is thiamine 100 mg parenterally followed by 50 to 100 mg daily with vitamin supplements, a balanced diet, and abstinence from alcohol. Even in Shoshin beri-beri with peripheral circulatory shock and severe metabolic acidosis, thiamine remains the mainstay of treatment because the acidosis responds poorly to treatment. Diuretics are needed when diuresis is delayed beyond 48 hours of thiamine therapy (Comment by courtesy of Dr D P Naidoo, University of Natal, South Africa).

## Heart Disease in Diabetics

The association between ischemic heart disease, hypertension, obesity, and diabetes mellitus has taken a new turn with the description of the unifying concept of **insulin resistance** (p 194). Thus, there is a metabolic syndrome that must be treated, requiring control of cholesterol and weight, as well as regulation of hypertension and diabetes. Because diabetes mellitus is a major risk factor for ischemic heart disease and often is an associated factor with hypertension, strict control of diabetes is required. It makes little sense that cardiologists carefully regulate blood pressure and angina, while being relatively lax on diabetic control. Tight control is essential to prevent complications.[73]

The preferential use of ACE inhibitors in **insulin-dependent diabetic nephropathy** is now established even in the absence of hypertension.[31,98,148B] Although many would argue that these agents are first choice in all **diabetic hypertensives,** nonetheless a variety of agents, including low-dose diuretics, are all acceptable.[110] Both the ACE inhibitors and calcium antagonists are free of adverse side-effects on glucose metabolism and on blood lipid profiles. These two agents can have additive beneficial effects on protein excretion in diabetic nephropathy.[54] Beta-blockers, previously thought not to impair glucose tolerance, are from this point of view the least desirable type of antihypertensive therapy.[110]

AMI IN DIABETICS. In insulin-requiring diabetics, careful regulation of blood sugar and potassium during a maintained insulin infusion is required. In non-insulin-requiring diabetics, continued use of oral antidiabetic agents might increase mortality because these agents are potassium channel closers with coronary constriction as a side-effect.[94] On recent evidence from Sweden, it is better to shift the therapy of the diabetes from an oral agent to insulin, during the early and follow-up phases of AMI;[104] one year mortality was reduced by 22%.

## Cardiovascular Drugs in Pregnancy

Most cardiovascular drugs are not well studied for safety in pregnancy. ACE inhibitors, warfarin, and the lipid-lowering statins are all clearly contraindicated (Table 11–8). For pregnancy hypertension,

**TABLE 11–8    CARDIOVASCULAR DRUGS IN PREGNANCY**

| DRUG CATEGORY | POTENTIAL ADVERSE EFFECT ON FETUS | SAFETY IN PREGNANCY CLASSIFICATION | TRIMESTER RISK (1, 2, 3) |
|---|---|---|---|
| Beta-blockers | Intrauterine growth retardation; neonatal hypoglycemia; bradycardia | C or D | 1, 3 |
| Nitrates | None; may benefit by delaying premature labour | C | None |
| Calcium antagonists | None; may delay labour; experimentally embryopathic | C | None |
| Diuretics Thiazides | May impair uterine blood flow; usually regarded as C/I yet meta-analysis suggests safety* | B or C | 3 |
| Furosemide | Experimentally embryopathic | C | (1) |
| Torsemide | None | B | None |
| Indapamide | None | B | None |
| ACE inhibitors | Embryopathic; may be lethal | D or X | (1), 2, 3 |
| Digoxin | None | C | None |
| Antihypertensives (see β-blockers, calcium antagonists, diuretics, ACEI) | | | |
| Methyldopa | Well tested in pregnancy | B | None |
| Antiarrhythmics | Generally no adverse effects | C | None |
| Amiodarone | Altered thyroid function | D | 2, 3 |
| Sotalol | None | B | None |
| Antithrombotics | | | |
| Warfarin | Embryopathic; crosses placenta with risk of fetal hemorrhage | X | 1, 3 |
| Heparin | None. Does not cross placental barrier. | C | None |
| Aspirin | High dose risk of premature close of patent ductus | none | 3 |
| Lipid-lowering agents | | | |
| Nicotinic acid | None | B | None |
| Gemfibrozil | None | C | None |
| Probucol | None | B | None |
| Statins + | Congenital anomalies | X | 1, 2, 3 |

For trimester risk, see British National Formulary.[57] (1) = risk in first trimester not established.

* Collins et al.[67]; + statins = lovastatin, simvastatin, pravastatin

C/I, contraindicated

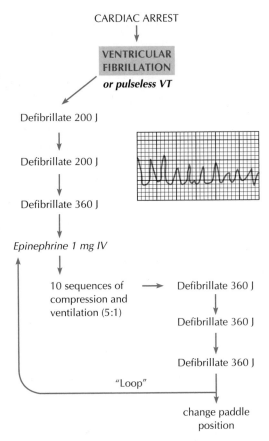

**FIGURE 11–1.** Algorithm for cardiopulmonary resuscitation (CPR) when there is ventricular fibrillation. Epinephrine, adrenaline. Modified from European Resuscitation Council Working Party.[77] Because there is no good evidence for high-dose epinephrine,[60] that has been omitted from the "loop." Modified from Reference 1.

methyldopa is best substantiated, while the diuretics are not as bad as often thought (Table 11–8).

## Cardiopulmonary Resuscitation

"Defibrillate as early and as often as possible."[150] The first essential is actually to shout for help, then to intubate, and to start compression/ventilation as soon as possible. If there is no intubation, clearing the airway is essential. Mouth-to-mouth breathing may be less effective than previously thought judging by animal data.[55] When there are three rescuers, one could manage ventilation, the second the chest compression, and the third could beneficially give interposed abdominal compression.[53] Active compression-decompression by a new device improves 24-hour survival.[147A]

New European[77] and American recommendations are basically similar. In the algorithm for **ventricular fibrillation** (Fig. 11–1), there are three rapid successive defibrillations followed by a "loop" of activity. Each loop includes three full dose (360J) defibrillatory shocks (Fig. 11–1). Each loop of activity is separated by ten sequences of 5:1 compression-ventilation sequences preceded by injection of vasoconstrictive doses of epinephrine (1 mg). Sodium bicarbonate is not recommended except in prolonged resuscitation when respiration is controlled. In the absence of adequate respiration, the $CO_2$ formed from the bicarbonate permeates into the cell to increase

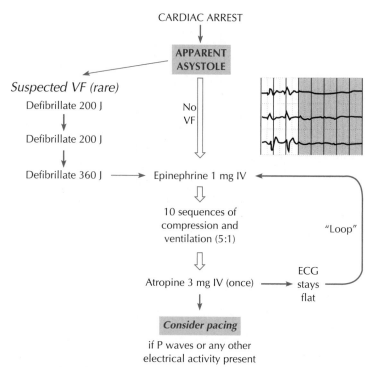

**FIGURE 11–2.** Algorithm for CPR in a patient with asystole. Epinephrine = adrenaline. Modified from Reference 1.

intracellular acidosis. No convincing data support the use of lidocaine or bretylium if early defibrillation fails.[111]

**Apparent asystole** (Fig. 11–2) has a dreadful prognosis.[111] Rarely, VF may masquerade as asystole,[111] so that the algorithm allows for three defibrillations. Otherwise epinephrine is followed by ten sequences of compression and ventilation, and then atropine (once only) and the loop repeated until P-waves or other electrical activity appears, when pacing may be considered.

In **electromechanical dissociation** (Fig. 11–3), the "loop" omits defibrillation and considers pressor agents and calcium. Epinephrine is again given early and in a randomized American study a high dose (0.2 mg/kg) was better than a standard dose.[60] Calcium chloride is thought to have specific value in the presence of hyperkalemia, hypocalcemia, or excess of calcium antagonists.

The ethics of when to stop the "loops" and when not to resuscitate are becoming increasingly complex.[111]

### Care of Cardiac Arrest Survivors

The patient will have been urgently hospitalized and cardiogenic shock is now the major risk. Prophylactic antiarrhythmic therapy by lidocaine or procainamide for 36 to 48 hours is common practice.[113] Some use intravenous amiodarone. Once stabilized, a full cardiac evaluation is required, including echocardiography and coronary angiography.

"The substrate for sustained monomorphic VT is seldom abolished by CABG,"[113] so that the indications for cardiac surgery must be decided in their own right. Nevertheless, it makes sense to consider an ischemic etiology in such patients, and aggressively to treat coronary heart disease and LV failure both medically and, where indicated, surgically. Empiric beta-blockade is the prime long-term antiarrhythmic treatment unless contraindicated, whereupon empiric amiodarone is the next choice. In the case of high-grade ventricular ectopics, Holter monitoring guides therapy as in the ESVEM study.[76]

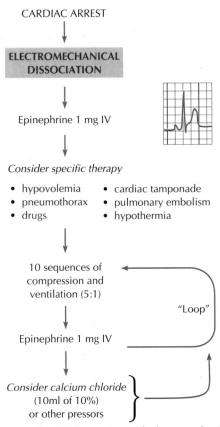

FIGURE 11–3. Algorithm for CPR in a patient with electromechanical dissociation. For use of high-dose epinephrine, see Brown et al.[60] Epinephrine = adrenaline. Modified from Reference 1.

Empiric beta-blockade might be just as good. The **implantable cardiac defibrillator (ICD)** is often regarded as the ultimate treatment and it undoubtedly reduces sudden cardiac death. It has "irrevocably altered the landscape for patients with malignant ventricular tachyarrhythmias,"[139] yet there are reservations. Sudden death may be avoided merely to be replaced by death from heart failure shortly thereafter ("not so sudden death"[139]). An important point is that the ICD should be selectively applied, specifically to patients at risk of sudden cardiac death yet otherwise having a reasonable expected overall cardiac prognosis. Thus far ICD is no better than amiodarone in the ongoing CASH study.[63]

# References

## For references from Second Edition, see Gersh and Opie (1991)

1. Gersh BJ, Opie LH. Which drugs for which condition? In: Opie LH (ed), Drugs for the Heart, Third Edition. WB Saunders Company, Philadelphia, 1991, pp 262–284.

## References from Third Edition

2. Abilgaard U, Aldershvile J, Ring-Larsen H, et al. Eur Heart J 1985; 6:1040–1046.
3. Boden WE, Ruble P, Mamby S and Multicenter Collaborating Investigators. Circulation 1989; 80:II–267.
4. Brevetti G, Chiariello M, Ferulano G, et al. Circulation 1988; 77:767–773.
5. CAST Investigators (Cardiac Arrhythmia Suppression Trial). N Engl J Med 1989; 321:406–412.

6. Danchin N, Voiriot P, Briancon S, et al. Lancet 1989; 1:743–745.
7. Delaye J, Etienne J, Feruglio GA, et al. Eur Heart J 1985; 6:826–828.
8. Douglas AS, Colwell L, Rose G. Br Heart J 1987; 57:413–415.
9. Editorial. Lancet 1982; 1:1287.
10. Ernst EEW, Matrai A. Circulation 1987; 76:1110–1114.
11. Fiessinger JN, Schafer M. Lancet 1990; 335:555–557.
12. Fuster V, Halperin JL. N Engl J Med 1989; 320:392–394.
13. Gersh BJ, Califf RM, Loop FD, et al. Circulation 1989; 79 (Suppl I):I-46–I-59.
14. Gibson RS, Boden WE, Theroux P, et al. N Engl J Med 1986; 315:423–429.
15. HART (Heparin-Aspirin Reperfusion Trial) Investigators—Hsia J, Hamilton WP, Kleiman N, et al. N Engl J Med 1990; 323:1433–1437.
16. Held PH, Yusuf S, Furberg CD. Br Med J 1989; 299:1187–1192.
17. Herlitz J, Hjalmarson A, Waagstein F. Br Heart J 1989; 61:9–13.
18. HINT Research Group (Holland Interuniversity Nifedipine/Metoprolol Trial). Br Heart J 1986; 56:400–413.
19. Jugdutt BI, Warnica JW. Circulation 1988; 78:906–919.
20. Kelly P, Ruskin JN, Vlahakes GJ, et al. J Am Coll Cardiol 1990; 15:267–273.
21. Krajcer Z, Leachman RD, Colley DA, et al. Circulation 1988; 78 (Suppl I):I-35–I-43.
22. Lessem JN, Singh BN. Cardiovasc Drugs Ther 1989; 3:355–373.
23. Levine JH, Michael JR, Guarnieri T. N Engl J Med 1985; 3123:21–25.
24. Luu M, Stevenson WG, Stevenson LW, et al. Circulation 1989; 80:1675–1680.
25. McIntosh CL, Maron BJ. Circulation 1988; 78:487–495.
26. Moss AJ, Rubison M, Oakes D, et al. Circulation 1989; 80 (Suppl II):II–268.
27. Opie LH. Circulation 1989; 80:1049–1062.
28. PACK Claudication Substudy Investigators. Circulation 1989; 80:1544–1548.
29. Parillo JE, Cunnion RE, Epstein SE. N Engl J Med 1989; 321:1061–1068.
30. Parisi AF, Khuri S, Depree RH, et al. Circulation 1989; 80:1176–1189.
31. Parving H-H, Hommel E, Nielsen MD, Giese J. Br Med J 1989; 299:533–536.
32. Pollick C. Am J Cardiol 1988; 62:1252–1255.
33. Quyyumi AA, Crake T, Wright CM, Mockus LJ, Fox KM. Br Heart J 1987; 57:505–511.
34. Rich S, Brundage BH. Circulation 1987; 76:135–141.
35. Roath S. Drugs 1989; 37:700–712.
36. Satler LF, Green CE, Kent KM, et al. Am Heart J 1987; 114:54–58.
37. Shulman ST, Amren DP, Bisno AL, et al. Circulation 1984; 70:1118A–1122A.
38. Strauss WE, Parisi AF. Ann Intern Med 1988; 109:570–581.
39. Taylor HA, Deumite J, Chaitman BR, et al. Circulation 1989; 79:1171–1179.
40. Theroux P, Taeymans Y, Morissette D, et al. J Am Coll Cardiol 1985; 5:717–722.
41. TIMI Study Group. N Engl J Med 1989; 320:618–627.
42. Topol EJ. J Am Coll Cardiol 1990; 15:922–924.
43. Waagstein F, Caidahl K, Wallentin I, et al. Circulation 1989; 80:551–563.
44. Yusuf S, McMahon S, Collins R, et al. Lancet 1988; 1:1088–1092.

## New References

45. ACIP study (Asymptomatic Cardiac Ischemia Pilot (ACIP) Study): 1 year follow-up. Rogers W, Bourassa MG, Andrews T, et al. Circulation 1994; 90 part 2:I–17 (abstr).
46. ACME Investigators—Parisi AF, Folland ED, Hartigan P on behalf of the Veterans Affairs ACME Investigators. A comparison of angioplasty with medical therapy in the treatment of single-vessel coronary artery disease. N Engl J Med 1992; 326:10–16.
47. Antiplatelet Trialists' Collaboration. Collaborative overview of randomised trials of antiplatelet therapy. I. Prevention of death, myocardial infarction, and stroke by prolonged antiplatelet therapy in various categories of patients. Br Med J 1994; 308:81–106.
48. Antman EM, Lau J, Kupelnick B, et al. A comparison of results of meta-analyses of randomized control trials and recommendations of clinical experts. Treatment for myocardial infarction. JAMA 1992; 268:240–248.
49. APSI study—Boissel J-P, Leizorovicz A, Picolet H, Peyrieux J-C for the APSI Investigators. Secondary prevention after high-risk acute myocardial infarction with low-dose acebutolol. Am J Cardiol 1990; 66:251–260.
50. ASPECT Research Group—Anticoagulants in the Secondary Prevention of Events in Coronary Thrombosis (ASPECT) Research Group. Effect of long-term oral anticoagulant treatment on mortality and cardiovascular morbidity after myocardial infarction. Lancet 1994; 343:499–503.
51. ASIST study (The Atenolol Silent Ischemia Study)—Pepine CJ, Cohn PF, Deedwania PC, et al. Effects of treatment on outcome in mildly symptomatic patients with ischemia during daily life. Circulation 1994; 90:762–768.
52. ATACS trial—Cohen M, Adams PC, Parry G, et al., and the Antithrombotic Therapy in Acute Coronary Syndromes Research Group. Combination antithrombotic therapy in unstable rest angina and non-Q-wave infarction in nonprior

aspirin users. Primary end points analysis from the ATACS Trial. Circulation 1994; 89:81–88.

53. Babbs CF, Sack JB, Kern KB. Interposed abdominal compression as an adjunct to cardiopulmonary resuscitation. Am Heart J 1994; 127:412–421.

54. Bakris GL, Barnhill BW, Sadler R. Treatment of arterial hypertension in diabetic humans: Importance of therapeutic selection. Kidney Int 1992; 41:912–919.

55. Berg RA, Kern KB, Sanders AB, et al. Bystander cardiopulmonary resuscitation. Is ventilation necessary? Circulation 1993; 88 (part I):1907–1915.

56. Black IW, Fatkin D, Sagar KB, et al. Exclusion of atrial thrombus by transesophageal echocardiography does not preclude embolism after cardioversion of atrial fibrillation. A Multicenter Study. Circulation 1994; 89:2509–2513.

57. BNF/British National Formulary (British Medical Association, London 1994; 27:207, 228, 524.

58. Brecker SJD, Xiao HB, Sparrow J, Gibson DG. Effects of dual-chamber pacing with short atrioventricular delay in dilated cardiomyopathy. Lancet 1992; 340:1308–1312.

59. Brevetti G, Perna S, Sabba C, et al. Superiority of L-propionylcarnitine vs L-carnitine in improving walking capacity in patients with peripheral vascular disease: An acute, intravenous, double-blind, cross-over study. Eur Heart J 1992; 13:251–255.

60. Brown CG, Martin DR, Pepe PE, et al. A comparison of standard-dose and high-dose epinephrine in cardiac arrest outside the hospital. N Engl J Med 1992; 327:1051–1055.

61. CASCADE study—The CASCADE Investigators. Randomized antiarrhythmic drug therapy in survivors of cardiac arrest (the CASCADE study). Am J Cardiol 1993; 72:280–287.

62. Case RB, Moss AJ, Case N, et al. Living alone after myocardial infarction. Impact on prognosis. JAMA 1992; 267:515–519.

63. CASH study—Siebels J, Cappato R, Ruppel R, et al., and the CASH Investigators. Preliminary results of the Cardiac Arrest Study Hamburg (CASH). Am J Cardiol 1993; 72:109F–113F.

64. Christian TF, Gibbons RJ, Hopfenspirger MR, Gersh BJ. Severity and response of chest pain during thrombolytic therapy for acute myocardial infarction: A useful indicator of myocardial salvage and infarct size. J Am Coll Cardiol 1993; 22:1311–1316.

65. Chun S, Sager P, Stevenson W, et al. Amiodarone is highly effective in maintaining NSR in refractory atrial fibrillation/flutter (abstr). J Am Coll Cardiol 1993; 21:203A.

66. Coleman GM, Gradinac S, Taegtmeyer H, et al. Efficacy of metabolic support with glucose-insulin-potassium for left ventricular pump failure after aortocoronary bypass surgery. Circulation 1989; 80 (Suppl I):I-91–I-96.

67. Collins R, Yusuf S, Peto R. Overview of randomised trials of diuretics in pregnancy. Br Med J 1985; 290:17–23.

68. Committee on Rheumatic Fever—Dajani AS, Bisno AL, Chung KJ, et al. Prevention of bacterial endocarditis. Recommendations by the American Heart Association. JAMA 1990; 264:2919–2922.

69. Coplen SE, Antman EM, Berlin JA, et al. Efficacy and safety of quinidine therapy for maintenance of sinus rhythm after cardioversion. A meta-analysis of randomized control trials. Circulation 1990; 82:1106–1116.

70. Cox JL, Boineau JP, Schuessier RB, et al. Successful surgical treatment of atrial fibrillation. Review and clinical update. JAMA 1991; 266:1976–1980.

71. de Boer MJ, Hoorntje JCA, Ottervanger JP, et al. Immediate coronary angioplasty versus intravenous streptokinase in acute myocardial infarction: Left ventricular ejection fraction, hospital mortality and reinfarction. J Am Coll Cardiol 1994; 23:1004–1008.

72. de Lorgeril M, Renaud S, Mamelle N, et al. Mediterranean alpha-linolenic acid-rich diet in secondary prevention of coronary heart disease. Lancet 1994; 343:1454–1459.

73. Diabetes Control and Complications Trial Research Group. The effect of intensive treatment of diabetes on the development and progression of long-term complications in insulin-dependent diabetes mellitus. N Engl J Med 1993; 329:977–986.

74. Dupuis J. Nitrates in congestive heart failure. Cardiovasc Drugs Ther 1994; 8:501–507.

75. ERACI Group—Rodriguez A, Boullon F, Perez-Balino N, et al., on behalf of the ERACI Group. Argentine randomized trial of percutaneous transluminal coronary angioplasty versus coronary artery bypass surgery in multivessel disease (ERACI): In-hospital results and 1-year follow-up. J Am Coll Cardiol 1993; 22:1060–1067.

76. ESVEM study—Mason JW, for the Electrophysiologic Study Versus Electrocardiographic Monitoring Investigators. A comparison of seven antiarrhythmic drugs in patients with ventricular tachyarrhythmias. N Engl J Med 1993; 329:452–458.

77. European Resuscitation Council Working Party. Adult advanced cardiac life support: The European Resuscitation Council guidelines 1992 (abridged). Br Med J 1993; 306:1589–1593.

78. Fananapazir L, Cannon RO, Tripodi D, Panza JA. Impact of dual-chamber permanent pacing in patients with obstructive hypertrophic cardiomyopathy with

symptoms refractory to verapamil and beta-adrenergic blocker therapy. Circulation 1992; 85:2149–2161.

79. Fatkin D, Kuchar DL, Thorburn CW, Feneley MP. Transesophageal echocardiography before and during direct current cardioversion of atrial fibrillation: Evidence for "atrial stunning" as a mechanism of thromboembolic complications. J Am Coll Cardiol 1994; 23:307–316.

80. Fibrinolytic Therapy Trialists" (FTT) Collaborative Group. Indications for fibrinolytic therapy in suspected acute myocardial infarction: Collaborative overview of early mortality and major morbidity results from all randomised trials of more than 1,000 patients. Lancet 1994; 343:311–322.

81. Fischer Hansen J and The Danish Study Group on Verapamil in Myocardial Infarction. Treatment with verapamil during and after an acute myocardial infarction: A review based on the Danish Verapamil Infarction Trials I and II. J Cardiovasc Pharmacol 1991; 18 (Suppl 6):S20–S25.

82. Fischer Hansen J. Postinfarct prophylaxis by calcium antagonists. In: Opie LH (ed). Myocardial Protection by Calcium Antagonists. Wiley-Liss, New York, 1994, pp 98–111.

83. Flaker GC, Blackshear JL, McBride R, et al. Cardiac mortality during antiarrhythmic drug therapy in the stroke prevention in atrial fibrillation (SPAF) study (abstr). J Am Coll Cardiol 1992; 19:227A.

84. Frasure-Smith N, Lesperance F, Talajic M. Depression following myocardial infarction. JAMA 1993; 270:1819–1825.

85. Frishman WH, Skolnick AE, Miller KP. Secondary prevention postinfarction: The role of beta-adrenergic blockers, calcium channel blockers, and aspirin. In: Gersh BJ, Rahimtoola S (eds). Acute Myocardial Infarction. Elsevier, New York, 1991, pp 469–492.

85A. GESICA study—Doval HC, Nul DR, Grancelli HO, et al., for Grupo de Estudio de la Sobrevida en la insuficiencia Cardiaca en Argentina (GESICA). Randomised trial of low-dose amiodarone in severe congestive heart failure. Lancet 1994; 344:493–498.

86. Gey KF, Puska P, Jordan P, Moser UK. Inverse correlation between plasma vitamin E and mortality from ischemic heart disease in cross-cultural epidemiology. Am J Clin Nutr 1991; 53:326S–334S.

87. Gibbons RJ, Holmes DR, Reeder GS, et al., for the Mayo Coronary Care Unit and Catheterization Laboratory Groups. Immediate angioplasty compared with the administration of a thrombolytic agent followed by conservative treatment for myocardial infarction. N Engl J Med 1993; 328:685–691.

88. Gibson RS, Young PM, Boden WE, et al., and the Diltiazem Reinfarction Study Group. Prognostic significance and beneficial effect of diltiazem on the incidence of early recurrent ischemia after non-Q-wave myocardial infarction: Results from the Multicenter Diltiazem Reinfarction Study. Am J Cardiol 1987; 60:203–209.

89. GISSI-3—Gruppo Italiano per lo Studio della Sopravvivenza nel' infarto Miocardico. GISSI-3: effects of lisinopril and transdermal glyceryl trinitrate singly and together on 6-week mortality and ventricular function after acute myocardial infarction. Lancet 1994; 343:1115–1122.

90. Gosselink ATM, Crijns HJGM, Van Gelder IC, et al. Low-dose amiodarone for maintenance of sinus rhythm after cardioversion of atrial fibrillation or flutter. JAMA 1992; 267:3289–3293.

91. Grace AA, Brooks NH, Schofield PM. Beneficial effects of angiotensin-converting enzyme inhibition in severe symptomatic aortic stenosis (abstr). Circulation 1991; 84 (Suppl II):II–146.

92. Gunnar RM, Bourdillon PDV, Dixon DW, et al. ACC/AHA guidelines for the early management of patients with acute myocardial infarction. A report of the American College of Cardiology/American Heart Association Task Force on assessment of diagnostic and therapeutic cardiovascular procedures (Subcommittee to develop guidelines for the early management of patients with acute myocardial infarction). Circulation 1990; 82:664–707.

93. Hibbard MD, Holmes DR, Bailey KR, et al. Percutaneous transluminal coronary angioplasty in patients with cardiogenic shock. J Am Coll Cardiol 1992; 19:639–646.

94. Hofmann D, Opie LH. Potassium channel blockade and acute myocardial infarction: Implications for management of the non-insulin requiring diabetic patient. Eur Heart J 1993; 14:1585–1589.

95. Juul-Moller S, Edvardsson N, Rehnqvist-Ahlberg N. Sotalol versus quinidine for the maintenance of sinus rhythm after direct current conversion of atrial fibrillation. Circulation 1990; 82:1932–1939.

95A. King SB, Lembo NJ, Weintraub WS, et al. A randomized trial comparing coronary angiography with coronary bypass surgery. N Engl J Med 1994; 331:1044–1050.

96. Koga Y, Toshima H, Tanaka M, Kajiyama K. Therapeutic management of dilated cardiomyopathy. Cardiovasc Drugs Ther 1995; 9:000–000.

97. Leor J, Goldbourt U, Behar S, et al, and the SPRINT Study Group. Digoxin and mortality in survivors of acute myocardial infarction: Observations in patients at low and intermediate risk. Cardiovasc Drugs Ther 1995; 9:000–000.

98. Lewis EJ, Hunsicker LG, Bain RP, Rohde RD for the Collaborative Study Group. The effect of angiotensin-converting enzyme inhibition on diabetic nephropathy. N Engl J Med 1993; 329:1456–1462.

99. Lichstein E, Hager WD, Gregory JJ, et al., for the Multicenter Diltiazem Post-

Infarction Research Group. Relation between beta-adrenergic blocker use, various correlates of left ventricular function and the chance of developing congestive heart failure. J Am Coll Cardiol 1990; 16:1327–1332.

100. Lidon R-M, Theroux P, Lesperance J, et al. A pilot, early angiographic patency study using a direct thrombin inhibitor as adjunctive therapy to streptokinase in acute myocardial infarction. Circulation 1994; 89:1567–1572.

101. LIMIT-2 Trial—Woods KL, Fletcher S. Long-term outcome after intravenous magnesium sulphate in suspected acute myocardial infarction: The second Leicester Intravenous Magnesium Intervention Trial (LIMIT-2). Lancet 1994; 343:816–819.

101A. Lin M, Chiang H-T, Lin S-L, et al. Casodilator therapy in chronic asymptomatic aortic regurgitation: enalapril versus hydralazine therapy. J Am Coll Cardiol 1994; 24:1046–1053.

102. Lowe GDO, Fowkes FGR, Dawes J, et al. Blood viscosity, fibrinogen, and activation of coagulation and keukocytes in peripheral arterial disease and the normal population in the Edinburgh artery study. Circulation 1993; 87:1915–1920.

103. MacMahon S, Collins R, Peto R, et al. Effects of prophylactic lidocaine in suspected acute myocardial infarction. An overview of results from the randomized, controlled trials. JAMA 1988; 260:1910–1916.

104. Malmberg K, Efendi S, Ryden L, for the multicenter study group. Feasibility of insulin-glucose infusion in diabetic patients with acute myocardial infarction. Diabetes Care 1994, in press.

105. Mannino MM, Mehta D, Gomes JA. Current treatment options for paroxysmal supraventricular tachycardia. Am Heart J 1994; 127:475–480.

106. Manolio TA, Furberg CD, Shemanski L, et al. Associations of postmenopausal estrogen use with cardiovascular disease and its risk factors in older women. Circulation 1993; 88 (part I):2163–2171.

107. Maron BJ, Klues HG. Surviving competitive athletics with hypertrophic cardiomyopathy. Am J Cardiol 1994; 73:1098–1104.

108. McCarthy M. Unstable angina guidelines in the USA. Lancet 1994; 343:788.

109. Middlekauff HR, Wiener I, Savon LA, Stevenson WG. Low-dose amiodarone for atrial fibrillation: Time for a prospective study? Ann Intern Med 1992; 116:1017–1020.

110. National High Blood Pressure Education Program Working Group. National high blood pressure education program working group report on hypertension in diabetes. Hypertension 1994; 23:145–158.

111. Niemann JT. Cardiopulmonary resuscitation. N Engl J Med 1992; 327:1075–1080.

112. Nul DR, Doval H, Grancelli H, et al. Amiodarone reduces mortality in severe heart failure (abstr). Circulation 1993; 88 (Suppl I):I–603.

113. O'Nunain S, Ruskin J. Cardiac arrest. Lancet 1993; 341:1641–1647.

114. Pahor M, Gambassi G, Carbonin P. Antiarrhythmic effects of ACE inhibitors: A matter of faith or reality? Cardiovasc Res 1994; 28:173–182.

115. Pellikka PA, Nishimura RA, Bailey KR, Tajik AJ. The natural history of adults with asymptomatic, hemodynamically significant aortic stenosis. J Am Coll Cardiol 1990; 15:1012–1017.

116. Pouleur H. High or low dose of angiotensin-converting enzyme inhibitor in patients with left ventricular dysfunction? Cardiovasc Drugs Ther 1993; 7:891–892.

117. PRACTICAL study—Foy SG, Crozier IG, Turner JG, et al. Comparison of enalapril versus captopril on left ventricular function and survival three months after acute myocardial infarction (the "PRACTICAL" Study). Am J Cardiol 1994; 73:1180–1186.

118. Quigley RL, Milano CA, Smith R, et al. Prognosis and management of anterolateral myocardial infarction in patients with severe left main disease and cardiogenic shock. The left main shock syndrome. Circulation 1993: 88 (part 2):65–70.

119. Radack K, Deck C. Beta-adrenergic blocker therapy does not worsen intermittent claudication in subjects with peripheral arterial disease. A meta-analysis of randomized controlled trials. Arch Intern Med 1991; 151:1769–1776.

120. Rawles JM, Metcalfe MJ, Jennings K. Time of occurrence, duration, and ventricular rate of paroxysmal atrial fibrillation: The effect of digoxin. Br Heart J 1990; 63:225–227.

121. Reimold SC, Cantillon CO, Friedman PL, Antman EM. Propafenone versus sotalol for suppression of recurrent symptomatic atrial fibrillation. Am J Cardiol 1993; 71:558–563.

122. RESCUE study—Ellis SG, da Silva ER, Heyndrickx GR, et al., for the RESCUE Investigators. Final results of the randomized RESCUE study evaluating PTCA after failed thrombolysis for patients with anterior infarction (abstr). Circulation 1993; 88:I–106.

123. Reyes AJ. Loop diuretics versus others in the treatment of congestive heart failure after myocardial infarction. Cardiovasc Drugs Ther 1993; 7:869–876.

124. Rich S, Kaufmann E, Levy PS. The effect of high doses of calcium channel blockers on survival in primary pulmonary hypertension. N Engl J Med 1992; 327:76–81.

125. RISC study—RISC Group. Risk of myocardial infarction and death during treatment with low dose aspirin and intravenous heparin in men with unstable coronary artery disease. Lancet 1990; 336:827–830.

126. RITA Trial Participants. Coronary angioplasty versus coronary artery bypass

surgery: The Randomised Intervention Treatment of Angina (RITA) trial. Lancet 1993; 341:573–580.

127. Roberts DH, Tsao Y, McLoughlin GA, Breckenridge A. Placebo-controlled comparison of captopril, atenolol, labetalol, and pindolol in hypertension complicated by intermittent claudication. Lancet 1987; 2:650–653.

128. Ruberman W, Weinblatt E, Goldberg JD, Chaudhary BS. Psychosocial influences on mortality after myocardial infarction. N Engl J Med 1984; 311:552–559.

128A. Santiago D, Warshofsky M, Mandri GL, et al. Left atrial appendage function and thrombus formation in atrial fibrillation-flutter: A transesophageal echocardiographic study. J Am Coll Cardiol 1994; 24:159–164.

129. SAVE study—Pfeffer MA, Braunwald E, Moye LA, et al. Effect of captopril on mortality and morbidity in patients with left ventricular dysfunction after myocardial infarction. Results of the Survival and Ventricular Enlargement Trial. N Engl J Med 1992; 327:669–677.

130. Scognamiglio R, Rahimtoola SH, Fasoli G, et al. Nifedipine in asymptomatic patients with severe aortic regurgitation and normal left ventricular function. N Engl J Med 1994; 331:689–694.

131. Seiler C, Hess OM, Schoenbeck M, et al. Long-term follow-up of medical versus surgical therapy for hypertrophic cardiomyopathy: A retrospective study. J Am Coll Cardiol 1991; 17:634–642.

132. Shettigar UR, Toole G, O'Came Appunn D. Combined use of esmolol and digoxin in the acute treatment of atrial fibrillation or flutter. Am Heart J 1993; 126:368–374.

133. Simmons NA, Ball AP, Cawson RA, et al. Antibiotic prophylaxis and infective endocarditis. Lancet 1992; 339:1292–1293.

133A. SMILE study—Borghi C, Ambrosioni E, Magnani B on behalf of SMILE Investigators. Effects of early ACE inhibition on long-term survival in patients with acute anterior myocardial infarction (abstr). Circulation 1994; 90 (Part 2):I–18.

134. SOLVD study—The SOLVD Investigators. Effect of enalapril on mortality and the development of heart failure in asymptomatic patients with reduced left ventricular fractions. N Engl J Med 1992; 327:685–691.

134A. St John Sutton M, Pfeffer MA, Moye LM, et al. Impact of LV shape and muscle/cavity ratio on survival and adverse events after acute myocardial infarction (abstr). Circulation 1994; 90 part 2:I–18.

135. Steinbeck G, Andresen D, Bach P, et al. A comparison of electrophysiologically guided antiarrhythmic drug therapy with beta-blocker therapy in patients with symptomatic, sustained ventricular tachyarrhythmias. N Engl J Med 1992; 327:987–992.

136. Stevenson LW, Sietsema K, Tillisch JH, et al. Exercise capacity for survivors of cardiac transplantation or sustained medical therapy for stable heart failure. Circulation 1990; 81:78–85.

137. Stewart JT, McKenna WJ. Management of arrhythmias in hypertrophic cardiomyopathy. Cardiovasc Drugs Ther 1994; 8:95–99.

138. Swanepoel CR. Which diuretic to use? Cardiovasc Drugs Ther 1994; 8:123–128.

139. Sweeney MO, Ruskin JN. Mortality benefits and the implantable cardioverter-defibrillator. Circulation 1994; 89:1851–1858.

140. TAMI 7 study—Krucoff MW, Croll MA, Pope JE, et al., for the TAMI 7 Study Group. Continuous 12-lead ST-segment recovery analysis in the TAMI 7 Study. Performance of a noninvasive method for real-time detection of failed myocardial reperfusion. Circulation 1993; 88:437–446.

141. Teo KK, Yusuf S, Furberg D. Effects of prophylactic antiarrhythmic drug therapy in acute myocardial infarction. An overview of results from randomized controlled trials. JAMA 1993; 270:1589–1595.

142. Theroux P, Waters D, Qiu S, et al. Aspirin versus heparin to prevent myocardial infarction during the acute phase of unstable angina. Circulation 1993; 88 [part 1]:2045–2048.

143. TIBET study—Dargie HJ, for the TIBET Study Group. Medical treatment of angina can favourably affect outcome (abstr). Eur Heart J 1993; 14 (Abstr Suppl):304.

144. TIMI-IIIA Investigators. Early effects of tissue-type plasminogen activator added to conventional therapy on the culprit coronary lesion in patients presenting with ischemic cardiac pain at rest. Results of the Thrombolysis In Myocardial Ischemia (TIMI IIIA) Trial. Circulation 1993; 87:38–52.

145. TIMI-IIIB Investigators. Effects of tissue plasminogen activator and a comparison of early invasive and conservative strategies in unstable angina and non-Q-wave myocardial infarction. Results of the TIMI-IIIB Trial. Circulation 1994; 89:1545–1556.

146. TIMI-5 Investigators—Cannon CP, McCabe CH, Henry TD, et al., for the TIMI-5 Investigators. A pilot trial of recombinant desulfatohirudin compared with heparin in conjunction with tissue-type plasminogen activator and aspirin for acute myocardial infarction: Results of the Thrombolysis In Myocardial Ischemia (TIMI) 5 Trial. J Am Coll Cardiol 1994; 23:993–1003.

147. Topol EJ, Califf RM, Weisman HF, et al. Randomised trial of coronary intervention with antibody against platelet IIb/IIIa integrin for reduction of clinical restenosis: Results at six months. Lancet 1994; 343:881–886.

147A. Tucker KJ, Galli F, Savitt MA, et al. Active compression-decompression resuscitation: effect on resuscitation success after in-hospital cardiac arrest. J Am Coll Cardiol 1994; 24:201–209.

148. Van de Werf F, Janssens L, Brzostek T, et al. Short-term effects of early intravenous treatment with a beta-adrenergic blocking agent or a specific bradycardiac agent in patients with acute myocardial infarction receiving thrombolytic therapy. J Am Coll Cardiol 1993; 22:407–416.

148A. Van Rij AM, Solomon C, Packer SGK, et al. Chelation therapy for intermittent claudication—double-blind randomized control trial. Circulation 1994; 90:1194–1199.

148B. Viberti G, Mogensen CE, Groop LC, Pauls JF, for the European Microalbuminuria Captopril Study Group. Effect of captopril on progression to clinical proteinuria in patients with insulin-dependent diabetes mellitus and microalbuminuria. JAMA 1994; 271:275–279.

149. Waagstein F, Bristow MR, Swedberg K, et al., for the Metoprolol in Dilated Cardiomyopathy (MDC) Trial Study Group. Beneficial effects of metoprolol in idiopathic dilated cardiomyopathy. Lancet 1993; 342:1441–1446.

150. Wardrope J, Morris F. European guidelines on resuscitation. Defibrillate as early and as often as possible. Br Med J 1993; 306:1555–1556.

151. Waters D, Lam JYT. Is thrombolytic therapy striking out in unstable angina? Circulation 1992; 86:1642–1644.

152. White HD, Cross DB, Elliott JM, et al. Long-term prognostic importance of patency of the infarct-related coronary artery after thrombolytic therapy for acute myocardial infarction. Circulation 1994; 89:61–67.

# Notes

# Notes

# Index

Note: Page numbers in *italics* refer to illustrations; page numbers followed by t refer to tables.